HIKE LIST

WITHIN BOSTON

1　The Freedom Trail
2　Charles River Loop
3　Back Bay Fens: Isabella's Loop
4　Muddy River Loop
5　Jamaica Pond Loop
6　Arnold Arboretum Tour

SEASIDE HIKES

7　Crane Beach: Dune Loop
8　Halibut Point: Quarry Loop
9　Plum Island: Hellcat Trail
10　Plum Island: Sandy Point Loop
11　Nasketucket Bay State Reservation Hike
12　World's End Tour

NORTH OF BOSTON

13　The Middlesex Fells Reservation West: Skyline Trail
14　Lynn Woods Hike
15　Agassiz Rock Hike
16　Manchester-Essex Woods: Cedar Hill–Pulpit Rock Hike
17　Ravenswood Park Hike
18　Dogtown Commons Hike
19　Great Meadow–Gerrish's Rock Hike
20　Maudslay State Park Hike
21　Ward Reservation Hike
22　Indian Ridge Loop
23　Skug River Loop
24　Goldsmith Woodlands Loop
25　Weir Hill Loop
26　Old Town Hill: Marsh and Farm Loop
27　Appleton Farms: Grass Rides Loop
28　Willowdale State Forest: Pine Swamp–Milldam Loop
29　Bald Hill Loop
30　Winnekenni Park: Lake, Forest, and Castle Hike
31　Beaver Brook Hike

SOUTH OF BOSTON

32　Blue Hills: Hemenway Hill Loop
33　Blue Hills: Skyline Trail
34　Wilson Mountain Hike
35　Noon Hill Loop (with Charles River extension)
36　Noanet Woodlands Hike
37　Borderland State Park: Pond and Quarry Hike
38　Whitney and Thayer Woods Hike (with Wompatuck State Park)
39　Destruction Brook Hike
40　Copicut Woods: Miller Brook Loop
41　Round Pond Hike
42　Slocum's River Hike

WEST OF BOSTON

43　Hammond Pond–Houghton Garden Hike
44　Hemlock Gorge Loop
45　Centennial Park Loop
46　Elm Bank Loop
47　Rocky Narrows Loop
48　Ogilvie Woods Hike
49　Cedar Hill to Sawink Farm Loop
50　In Thoreau's Footsteps
51　Foss Farm Hike
52　Great Brook Farm Loop
53　Callahan State Park Hike
54　Memorial Reservation Hike
55　Waters Farm Loop
56　Blackstone River and Canal Hike
57　Purgatory Chasm Hike
58　Mount Pisgah Hike
59　Mount Watatic–Nutting Hill Loop
60　Mount Wachusett Loop

MENASHA RIDGE PRESS
Birmingham, Alabama

60 HIKES WITHIN 60 MILES

BOSTON

INCLUDING
COASTAL AND INTERIOR REGIONS,
AND NEW HAMPSHIRE

HELEN WEATHERALL

60 Hikes within 60 Miles: Boston

Copyright © 2008 by Helen Weatherall
All rights reserved
Printed in the United States of America
Published by Menasha Ridge Press
Distributed by Publishers Group West
First edition, third printing 2012

Library of Congress Cataloging-in-Publication Data:
  Weatherall, Helen.
    60 hikes within 60 miles, Boston: including Essex, Middlesex, Suffolk,
  Norfolk, Plymouth, and Worcester counties / Helen Weatherall.—1st ed.
      p. cm.
    Includes index.
    ISBN-13: 978-0-89732-636-0
    ISBN-10: 0-89732-636-9
    1. Hiking—Massachusetts—Boston Region—Guidebooks. 2. Boston Region
  (Mass.)—Guidebooks. I. Title. II. Title: Sixty hikes with sixty miles, Boston.
  GV199.42.M42B67 2008
  796.5109744—dc22

                                            2007045529

Text and cover design by Steveco International and Scott McGrew
Cover photograph by Helen Weatherall
All other photographs by Helen Weatherall unless otherwise noted.
Author photograph by Flora Wadsworth
Cartography and elevation profiles by Lohnes+Wright, Scott McGrew, and
  Helen Weatherall

Menasha Ridge Press
P.O. Box 43673
Birmingham, AL 35243
www.menasharidge.com

To my mother, Sally Lunt Weatherall, as true a hero of the natural world, goodness, and truth as there will ever be.

TABLE OF CONTENTS

ACKNOWLEDGMENTS

THIS BOOK and a frighteningly great many of the most wonderful places in Massachusetts likely would not exist as open space if it wasn't for Charles Eliot, landscape architect and founder of the Trustees of Reservations. He did not work alone, but his accomplishments certainly demonstrate the vast difference one inspired individual can make to the betterment of the world. In getting to know each of these 60 hikes, I grew even more aware of the vulnerability of Massachusetts's natural places (including state parks!) and both humbled and heartened by the enormous amount of work myriad organizations are doing to preserve them. In the interest of fostering support, I would like to shine a halo of light on all those at the Essex County Greenbelt Association, the Sudbury Valley Trustees, the Dartmouth Natural Resource Trust, the Andover Village Improvement Society (AVIS), the Trust for Public Land, the Charles River Conservancy, the Appalachian Mountain Club, the Audubon Society, Friends of Lynn Woods, Friends of Middlesex Fells, Friends of Hemlock Gorge, Friends of Manchester-Essex Woods, the Waters family of Sutton, everyone behind the Bay Circuit Trail (Eliot's baby), the Wapack Trail, the Mid-State Trail, The Trustees of Reservations, and the gutsy, huge-hearted members of every last conservation commission in the state. Gratitude to friends and family who have maintained interest and support helped carry this book to fruition. Thanks to my tremendous brothers, Bobby and Alexander. Thanks, too, to my father, Robert Weatherall (who gave me his strong legs, curiosity, love of trees, and propensity for taking the long scenic route); thanks to my trusty and courageous hiking companion, Katy (my 14-pound terrier who always knows the right way), and with my deepest respect, appreciation, and love, thanks to my husband, Christopher.

—HELEN WEATHERALL

FOREWORD

Welcome to Menasha Ridge Press's *60 Hikes within 60 Miles*. Our strategy was simple: First, find a hiker who knows the area and loves to hike. Second, ask that person to spend a year researching the most popular and very best trails around. And third, have that person describe each trail in terms of difficulty, scenery, condition, elevation change, and all other categories of information that are important to hikers. "Pretend you've just completed a hike and met up with other hikers at the trailhead," we told each author. "Imagine their questions, and be clear in your answers."

You'll get more out of this book if you take a moment to read the Introduction explaining how to read the trail listings. The "Topographic Maps" section will help you understand how useful topos will be on a hike, and will also tell you where to get them. And though this is a "where-to," rather than a "how-to" guide, those of you who have hiked extensively will find the Introduction of particular value. As much for the opportunity to free the spirit as well as to free the body, let these hikes elevate you above the urban hurry.

All the best,
The Editors at Menasha Ridge Press

ABOUT THE AUTHOR

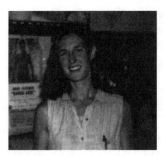 **HELEN WEATHERALL** is a writer, sculptor and environmentalist who prefers to spend her time outdoors. Having explored wildlands from Mt. Washington to Montana; the Amazon to Sri Lanka, and much in between, Helen recently settled in Ipswich, Massachusetts, where in the company of her husband, cat, and terrier, she is undertaking her first novel.

PREFACE

TODAY, WHEN THE NEW YORK MINUTE is thought slow from Boston to Beijing, and real people spend real cash for virtual homes for their pixel-rendered avatars, the time is right to lace on a reliable pair of walking shoes and head outdoors. The surest way to regain peace and clarity is to winnow down to a pair of legs and turn them loose on an open trail.

As a kid growing up near the town wharf where the Ipswich River turns salty, I had a favorite way to burn up an afternoon: rouse the dog and go out "marsh trotting." This pastime—invented by someone other than me—is hiking in one of its messiest and most delightful forms. Explained simply, to marsh trot is to hike from point A to point B, or Q, crossing salt marsh and jumping minnow-filled ditches to do so. Using boulders, tree stumps, and other landmarks to navigate, you're guaranteed by trip's end to be mud splattered, half soaked, and joyfully exhausted.

There are different reasons to hike: exercise, spend time with a friend, let the dog run, "get away from it all," reconnect with nature, explore—or lose oneself. There may be as many reasons as there are people who pick up this book. No reason is better than another.

The idea of choosing 60 hikes around Boston seemed easy at the start. *I know these parts* was my knee-jerk reaction. And then I started making a list. But as I began jotting down the *must-do* hikes, a question dogged me. Were they tired, too obvious? Too popular? Fortunately, family members and friends, whether solicited or not, gave their opinions and the vote was unanimous: include The Freedom Trail, Walden Pond, the Emerald Necklace, Crane Beach, Plum Island, Halibut Point, Old Town Hill, the Blue Hills, Dogtown Common, and World's End. No choice!

And so I set out to these favorites, to hike, map, and photograph them. And what I found was not the places I had explored when I was little, riding on my father's shoulders, and by my own loco-motion many times since, but new places. Looking into their history sometimes as far back as the last Ice Age, I discovered that there was much more to them than the composition of rocks, trees, and views I had previously thought them to be.

Besides hikes I know as old friends, this book includes marvelous hikes I dis-covered through research. One way to find lesser-known gems is to contact town conservation commissions and independent conservation groups. The hike In Tho-reau's Footsteps, which crosses town lines and includes three reservations, came about after a particularly inspiring conversation with Angela Seaborg, a conserva-tion planner for the town of Lincoln.

Each hike I took in writing this book brought me new revelations. Although I was well aware of the Middlesex Fells, I had never before set foot in them. Except on the evening that I spotted a coyote idling in the breakdown lane en route to the reserva-tion, the dark woods had always been but a blur seen through my windshield. One evening, a coyote biding its time in the breakdown lane waiting for a lull in the traffic caught my eye. I have wondered about the wily animal ever since.

What I discovered when I finally took myself to the Middlesex Fells was that they are not to be underestimated. I arrived at the reservation in late afternoon, and concerned that the hike would take longer than the number of daylight hours left me, I asked two others their opinion, I asked two others. One pleaded igno-rance, and the other assured me that I should have plenty of time if I kept up a good pace. So encouraged, I took to the trail. Three or so hours later, cricket chirps and dimming light forced the realization that the day was done though my hike was not. With no choice but to keep hiking I pressed on, relieved that the trail markers were reflective white. But when the glow of my cell phone wasn't enough to light the screen of my GPS unit and I couldn't find my dog, there was no choice left me but to accept that I was lost.

Informed by this episode, I packed a headlamp and fresh batteries for every hike I undertook thereafter. I came close to needing it on Mount Pisgah when the light began playing tricks. Later at Bald Hill when the daylight vanished as I navi-gated a pond swollen beyond the map's description, thanks to superheroes of the beaver world, exuberance replaced fear the instant I clicked on the light.

Today and tomorrow, Boston is a vibrant city with commerce, industry, art, the Red Sox, and occasional sirens. But for me since writing this book, Boston is also William Blackstone's peninsula, Shawmut, where the reverend and his white bull lived contentedly in the sparse company of the Massachusett people until John Winthrop and his tribe of black-cloaked Puritans scrambled up its rocky shore.

A place is a sum of its parts—its hills, ponds, woods, feathered and furry inhab-itants, and history, too. For this reason, in describing the hikes in this book, I have often included as much about the human and geologic history of the place as the trails' twists and turns. Just as the pleasure of spotting a bright red bird far up in a forest canopy is heightened by the knowledge that the bird is a South American–born scarlet tanager summering in the Blue Hills—so too is a hike to a beautiful vista made ever more thrilling by the knowledge that Miles Standish or the Wampanoag leader King Philip looked out from the peak three centuries ago.

Knowing more about a place gives added meaning to names on a map. When hiking over Wennepoykin Hill in the Middlesex Fells on a hot afternoon without knowing a thing about the hill's namesake, mundane physical details catch your notice; the crunch of granite gravel under your feet and the trickle of sweat on your brow. But once tipped off to the fact that Wennepoykin was a Massachusett who fought the English in King Philip's War, was captured, sent as a slave to Barbados, then returned to his homeland eight years later with the help of a Puritan minister, emotion and imagination will quickly revamp your perceptions.

No place is without history—but in Boston and its environs, place and history are all but synonymous. It may not matter that Herman Melville set sail on the whaling ship *Acushnet* from Fairhaven and later described what he experienced in *Moby-Dick,* that Judge Samuel Sewall of Salem Witch Trials fame got stranded on a sandbar off Plum Island in the 1600s and wrote of it in his journal—or that the Lynn Woods are a conserved remnant of woods where Hester Prynne intercepted Mr. Dimmesdale for a secret meeting in Nathaniel Hawthorne's novel *The Scarlet Letter.* But in each instance the place and the tale are forever meaningfully interwoven.

Like history, four seasons define New England. In Boston and surrounding areas, the seasons and accompanying weather are nothing if not assertive. For a Yankee like me "getting out into the weather" is reason itself to hike, not just in spring and summer when the air is warm and stirred gently by fresh breezes, but all year round.

HIKING RECOMMENDATIONS

LESS THAN 3 MILES

3 TO 6 MILES

3 TO 6 MILES *(continued)*

MORE THAN 6 MILES

HIKES GOOD FOR CHILDREN

HIKES ACCESSIBLE BY PUBLIC TRANSPORTATION

*Shuttle bus from commuter rail in summer

HIKES WITH WHEELCHAIR-ACCESSIBLE SECTIONS

HIKES WITH WHEELCHAIR-ACCESSIBLE SECTIONS
(continued)

RIVER HIKES

HIKES WITH SWIMMING

HIKES GOOD FOR BIRDING

MORE DEMANDING HIKES

DOG-FRIENDLY HIKES

All, with the following exceptions:

01 The Freedom Trail, although dogs are allowed on this hike through the historic heart of Boston, you and your dog are likely to be happier if you hike this one alone.

02 Charles River Loop, this urban hike is less than ideal for dogs.

07 Crane Beach: Dune Loop, dogs are welcome October 1 to March 31.

09 Plum Island: Hellcat Trail

10 Plum Island: Sandy Point Loop

51 Foss Farm, dogs are not allowed on the section of trail that crosses the Great Meadow National Wildlife Refuge

60 HIKES
WITHIN 60 MILES

BOSTON
INCLUDING
COASTAL AND INTERIOR REGIONS,
AND NEW HAMPSHIRE

INTRODUCTION

Welcome to *60 Hikes within 60 Miles: Boston*. If you're new to hiking or even if you're a seasoned trailsmith, take a few minutes to read the following introduction. It explains how this book is organized and how to use it.

HOW TO USE THIS GUIDEBOOK

THE OVERVIEW MAP AND OVERVIEW MAP KEY

Use the overview map on the inside front cover to assess the exact locations of each hike's primary trailhead. Each hike's number appears on the overview map, on the map key facing the overview map, and in the table of contents. As you flip through the book, a hike's full profile is easy to locate by watching for the hike number at the top of each page. The book is organized by region as indicated in the table of contents. A map legend that details the symbols found on trail maps appears on the inside back cover.

REGIONAL MAPS

The book is divided into regions, and prefacing each regional section is an overview map of that region. The regional provides more detail than the overview map, bringing you closer to the hike.

TRAIL MAPS

Each hike contains a detailed map that shows the trailhead, the route, significant features, facilities, and topographic landmarks such as creeks, overlooks, and peaks. The author gathered map data by carrying a Garmin eTrex Venture GPS unit while hiking. This data was downloaded into the Topo! digital mapping program and processed by expert cartographers to produce the highly accurate maps found in this book. Each trailhead's GPS coordinates are included with each profile (see page 2).

1

ELEVATION PROFILES

Corresponding directly to the trail map, each hike contains a detailed elevation profile. The elevation profile provides a quick look at the trail from the side, enabling you to visualize how the trail rises and falls. Key points along the way are labeled. Note the number of feet between each tick mark on the vertical axis (the height scale). To avoid making flat hikes look steep and steep hikes appear flat, height scales are used throughout the book to provide an accurate image of the hike's climbing difficulty.

GPS TRAILHEAD COORDINATES

To collect accurate map data, each trail was hiked with a handheld GPS unit (Garmin eTrex series). Data collected was then downloaded and plotted onto a digital USGS topo map. In addition to rendering a highly specific trail outline, this book also includes the GPS coordinates for each trailhead in two formats: latitude/longitude and Universal Transverse Mercator (UTM). Latitude/longitude coordinates tell you where you are by locating a point west (latitude) of the 0-degree meridian line that passes through Greenwich, England, and north or south of the 0-degree (longitude) line that belts the earth, aka the equator.

Topographic maps show latitude/longitude as well as UTM grid lines. Known as UTM coordinates, the numbers index a specific point using a grid method. The survey datum used to arrive at the coordinates in this book is WGS84 (versus NAD27 or WGS83). For readers who own a GPS unit, whether handheld or on board a vehicle, the latitude/longitude or UTM coordinates provided on the first page of each hike may be entered into the GPS unit. Just make sure your GPS unit is set to navigate using WGS84 datum. Now you can navigate directly to the trailhead.

Most trailheads, which begin in parking areas, can be reached by car, but some hikes still require a short walk to reach the trailhead from a parking area. In those cases, a handheld unit is necessary to continue the GPS navigation process. That said, however, readers can easily access all trailheads in this book by using the directions given, the overview map, and the trail map, which shows at least one major road leading into the area. But for those who enjoy using the latest GPS technology to navigate, the necessary data has been provided. A brief explanation of the UTM coordinates from Blue Hills: Skyline Trail (page 195) follows.

UTM Zone	19T
Easting	326699
Northing	4675115

The UTM zone number 19 refers to one of the 60 vertical zones of the Universal Transverse Mercator projection. Each zone is 6 degrees wide. The UTM zone letter T refers to one of the 20 horizontal zones that span from 80 degrees south to 84 degrees north. The easting number 326699 indicates in meters how far east or west a point is from the central meridian of the zone. Increasing easting coordinates on a topo map or on your GPS screen indicate that you are moving east; decreasing easting coordinates indicate you are moving west. The northing number 4675115 references in meters how far you are from the equator. Above and below the equator, increasing northing coordinates indicate you are traveling north; decreasing northing coordinates indicate you are traveling south. To learn more about how to enhance your outdoor experiences with GPS technology, refer to *GPS Outdoors: A Practical Guide for Outdoor Enthusiasts* (Menasha Ridge Press).

HIKE DESCRIPTIONS

Each hike contains seven key items: an "In Brief" description of the trail, a key at-a-glance box, directions to the trail, trailhead coordinates, a trail map, an elevation profile, and a trail description. Many also include a note on nearby activities. Combined, the maps and information provide a clear method to assess each trail from the comfort of your favorite reading chair.

IN BRIEF

A "taste of the trail." Think of this section as a snapshot focused on the historical landmarks, beautiful vistas, and other sights you may encounter on the hike.

KEY AT-A-GLANCE INFORMATION

The information in the key at-a-glance boxes gives you a quick idea of the statistics and specifics of each hike.

LENGTH The length of the trail from start to finish (total distance traveled). There may be options to shorten or extend the hikes, but the mileage corresponds to the described hike. Consult the hike description to help decide how to customize the hike for your ability or time constraints.

CONFIGURATION A description of what the trail might look like from overhead. Trails can be loops, out-and-backs (trails on which one enters and leaves along the same path), figure eights, or a combination of shapes.

DIFFICULTY The degree of effort an average hiker should expect on a given hike. For simplicity, the trails are rated as "easy," "moderate," or "difficult."

SCENERY A short summary of the attractions offered by the hike and what to expect in terms of plant life, wildlife, natural wonders, and historic features.

EXPOSURE A quick check of how much sun you can expect on your shoulders during the hike.

TRAFFIC Indicates how busy the trail might be on an average day. Trail traffic, of course, varies from day to day and season to season. Weekend days typically see the most visitors. Other trail users that may be encountered on the trail are also noted here.

TRAIL SURFACE Indicates whether the trail surface is paved, rocky, gravel, dirt, boardwalk, or a mixture of elements.

HIKING TIME The length of time it takes to hike the trail. A slow but steady hiker will average 2 to 3 miles an hour, depending on the terrain.

ACCESS A notation of any fees or permits that may be needed to access the trail or park at the trailhead. City and county parks typically do not require any permits or parking fees.

MAPS Here you'll find a list of maps that show the topography of the trail, including Green Trails Maps and USGS topo maps.

FACILITIES What to expect in terms of restrooms and water at the trailhead or nearby.

DIRECTIONS

Used in conjunction with the overview map, the driving directions will help you locate each trailhead. Once at the trailhead, park only in designated areas.

GPS TRAILHEAD COORDINATES

The trailhead coordinates can be used in addition to the driving directions if you enter the coordinates into your GPS unit before you set out. See page 2 for more information on GPS coordinates.

DESCRIPTION

The trail description is the heart of each hike. Here, the authors summarize the trail's essence and highlight any special traits the hike has to offer. The route is clearly outlined, including landmarks, side trips, and possible alternate routes along the way. Ultimately, the hike description will help you choose which hikes are best for you.

NEARBY ACTIVITIES

Look here for information on nearby activities or points of interest. This includes parks, museums, restaurants, or even a brew pub where you can get a well-deserved beer after a long hike. Note that not every hike has a listing.

WEATHER

Bostonians, or rather New Englanders as a whole, pay eager attention to forecasts while simultaneously regarding them with stubborn disdain. This is due both to something in their disposition and to the weather's high degree of variability, not just season to season but by minute by minute. A 20° drop or upward lurch in temperature is not unheard of either on a sultry summer evening or on a silvery afternoon in winter. Often the most reliable weather predictor is a stiff wind, for it likely signals a shift from humid to dry, hot to cool, or vice versa.

Average Temperature by Month

	Jan	Feb	Mar	Apr	May	Jun
High	36°	39°	46°	56°	67°	77°
Low	22°	24°	31°	41°	50°	59°
Mean	28°	29°	37°	47°	57°	67°

	Jul	Aug	Sep	Oct	Nov	Dec
High	82°	80°	73°	62°	52°	42°
Low	65°	64°	57°	46°	38°	28°
Mean	72°	71°	64°	54°	43°	32°

Boston's proximity to the sea and all that travels along the Gulf Stream from the Gulf of Mexico to Newfoundland and on across the Atlantic Ocean largely explains its weather's fickle temperament. In summer, the soggy winds of occasional Caribbean-born hurricanes add muscle and heft to the otherwise modest surf that smacks at the shore. These winds are known to drag in heat and humidity that settles on Boston's neighborhoods like a stifling blanket. Other storms like Canada-bred nor'easters deftly carve out the heat and replace perspiration with goose pimples. Bear in mind, too, that on any given day, the temperature at the shore is well below that of inland locations.

While there is no disagreement that a brilliant sunny day with the temperature between 65°F and 70°F is ideal for a hike in the hills, in today's GORE-TEX age, a pleasant hiking experience can be had in almost all conditions. Indeed, facing the elements when properly dressed is a distinctly satisfying pleasure. To ensure that you are in league with the weather when you set out on a hike, be sure to pack extra clothing. Having a Windbreaker or dry T-shirt to change into after a sweaty climb or cloudburst can make all the difference.

WATER

How much is enough? Well, one simple physiological fact should persuade you to err on the side of excess when deciding how much water to pack: a hiker working hard in 90°F heat needs approximately 10 quarts of fluid per day. That's 2.5 gallons—12 large water bottles or 16 small ones. In other words, pack one or two bottles even for short hikes.

Some hikers and backpackers hit the trail prepared to purify water found along the route. This method, while less dangerous than drinking it untreated, comes with risks. Purifiers with ceramic filters are the safest. Many hikers pack the slightly distasteful tetraglycine-hydroperiodide tablets to debug water (sold under the names Potable Aqua, Coughlan's, and others).

Probably the most common waterborne "bug" that hikers face is *giardia*, which may not hit until one to four weeks after ingestion. It will have you living in the bathroom, passing noxious rotten-egg gas, vomiting, and shivering with chills. Other parasites to worry about include *E. coli* and *cryptosporidium*, both of which are harder to kill than *giardia*.

For most people, the pleasures of hiking make carrying water a relatively minor price to pay to remain healthy. If you're tempted to drink "found water," do so only if you understand the risks involved. Better yet, hydrate prior to your hike, carry (and drink) 6 ounces of water for every mile you plan to hike, and hydrate after the hike.

CLOTHING

Nothing is certain about the weather in Boston and surrounding areas but its changeability. If it is a brilliant blue-sky morning when you prepare to head for the hiking trail, grab a sweater, or if you prefer, a warm, moisture-wicking, high-tech equivalent for later in the day when temperatures dip, especially in the deep shade of woods. Taking along a waterproof all-weather jacket made of GORE-TEX or the like is always an excellent idea. A mood- and possibly lifesaver, when weather conditions take a turn for the worse, a lightweight jacket also offers excellent protection against voracious bugs.

A cotton T-shirt is great to hike in on warm days when there's little change in temperature. But on longer, more challenging hikes, you are guaranteed to break a sweat no matter the season, and once damp, cotton loses utility and charm. Therefore if you are an incurable jeans and T-shirt type toss a back-up T in your knapsack, if only to have something to change into after hiking should you stop at an air-conditioned diner on your trip back home.

The person who packs a hat and mittens may get some teasing, but he or she may wind up the envy of all when icy winds blow down from Canada, catching your hiking party unprepared. The same can be said of wind and rain pants. Hypothermia can set in even when thermometers register temperatures above freezing.

Anyone who has gotten a blister or stubbed a toe knows the importance of appropriate footwear. The best shoes for hiking are boots with solid ankle support. The sneakers or sandals you wear every day may feel more comfortable, but their flimsy soles mean more work for your feet and ankles when hiking over rough terrain.

THE TEN ESSENTIALS

One of the first rules of hiking is to be prepared for anything. The simplest way to be prepared is to carry the Ten Essentials. In addition to carrying the items listed below, you need to know how to use them, especially navigation items. Always consider worst-case scenarios like getting lost, hiking back in the dark, broken gear (for example, a broken hip strap on your pack or a water filter getting plugged), twisting an ankle, or a brutal thunderstorm. The items listed below don't cost a lot of money, don't take up much room in a pack, and don't weigh much, but they might just save your life.

Compass: a high-quality compass

Extra clothes: rain protection, warm layers, gloves, warm hat

Extra food: have food in your pack when you've finished hiking

Fire: windproof matches or lighter and fire starter

First-aid kit: a good-quality kit including first-aid instructions

Knife: a multitool device with pliers is best

Light: flashlight or headlamp with extra bulbs and batteries

Map: preferably a topo map and a trail map with a route description

Sun protection: sunglasses, lip balm, sunblock, sun hat

Water: durable bottles, and water treatment like iodine or a filter

FIRST-AID KIT

A typical first-aid kit may contain more items than you might think necessary. These are just the basics. Prepackaged kits in waterproof bags (Atwater Carey and Adventure Medical make a variety of kits) are available. Even though there are quite a few items listed here, they pack down into a small space.

Ace bandages or Spenco joint wraps

Antibiotic ointment (Neosporin or the generic equivalent)

Aspirin or acetaminophen

Band-Aids

Benadryl or the generic equivalent diphenhydramine (in case of allergic reactions)

Butterfly-closure bandages

Epinephrine in a prefilled syringe (for people known to have severe allergic reactions to such things as bee stings)

Gauze (one roll)

Gauze compress pads (a half dozen 4 x 4-inch pads)

Hydrogen peroxide or iodine

Insect repellent

Matches or pocket lighter

Moleskin/Spenco "Second Skin"

Sunscreen

Whistle (it's more effective in signaling rescuers than your voice)

HIKING WITH CHILDREN

No one is too young for a hike in the outdoors. Be mindful, though. Flat, short, and shaded trails are best with an infant. Toddlers who have not quite mastered walking can still tag along, riding on an adult's back in a child carrier. Use common sense to judge a child's capacity to hike a particular trail, and always assume that the child will tire quickly and need to be carried.

When packing for the hike, remember the child's needs as well as your own. Make sure children are adequately clothed for the weather, have proper shoes, and are protected from the sun with sunscreen. Kids dehydrate quickly, so make sure you have plenty of fluid for everyone. To assist an adult with determining which trails are suitable for children, a list of hike recommendations for children is provided on pages xiv–xv.

GENERAL SAFETY

Feeling unease at the unfamiliar is a universal human response—which explains why crickets and birds are as jarring to city slickers counting sheep as street noises are to country folk longing for sleep. And though one of the pleasures of hiking is exploring the unknown, getting away from it all can have its stressful moments. The surest way to avoid danger and to ensure enjoyment on any hike, be it in an urban setting or remote mountain region, is to be prepared and to keep a level head at all times. The following are tips to improve your safety and enjoyment while hiking.

- **ALWAYS CARRY FOOD AND WATER, whether you are planning to go overnight or not.** Food will give you energy, help keep you warm, and sustain you in an emergency until help arrives. You never know if you will have a stream nearby when you become thirsty. Bring potable water or treat water before drinking it from a stream. Boil or filter all found water before drinking it.

- **STAY ON DESIGNATED TRAILS.** Most hikers get lost when they leave the path. Even on the most clearly marked trails, there is usually a point where you have to stop and consider which direction to head. If you become disoriented, don't panic. As soon as you think you may be off-track, stop, assess your current direction, and then retrace your steps back to the point where you went awry. Using map, compass, and this book, and keeping in mind what you have passed thus far, reorient yourself and trust your judgment on which way to continue. If you become absolutely unsure of how to continue, return to your vehicle the way you came in. Should you become completely lost and have no idea of how to return to the trailhead, remaining in place along the trail and waiting for help is most often the best option for adults and always the best option for children.

- **BE ESPECIALLY CAREFUL WHEN CROSSING STREAMS.** Whether you are fording the stream or crossing on a log, make every step count. If you have any doubt about maintaining your balance on a foot log, go ahead and ford the stream instead. When fording a stream, use a trekking pole or stout stick for balance and face upstream as you cross. If a stream seems too deep to ford, turn back. Whatever is on the other side is not worth risking your life.

- BE CAREFUL AT OVERLOOKS. While these areas may provide spectacular views, they are potentially hazardous. Stay back from the edge of outcrops and be absolutely sure of your footing; a misstep can mean a nasty and possibly fatal fall.

- STANDING DEAD TREES AND STORM-DAMAGED LIVING TREES POSE A REAL HAZARD to hikers and tent campers. These trees may have loose or broken limbs that could fall at any time. When choosing a spot to rest or a backcountry campsite, look up.

- KNOW THE SYMPTOMS OF HYPOTHERMIA. Shivering and forgetfulness are the two most common indicators of this insidious killer. Hypothermia can occur at any elevation, even in the summer, especially when the hiker is wearing lightweight cotton clothing. If symptoms arise, get the victim shelter, hot liquids, and dry clothes or a dry sleeping bag.

- BRING YOUR BRAIN. A cool, calculating mind is the single most important piece of equipment you'll ever need on the trail. Think before you act. Watch your step. Plan ahead. Avoiding accidents before they happen is the best recipe for a rewarding and relaxing hike.

- ASK QUESTIONS. Park employees are there to help. It's a lot easier to gain advice beforehand and avoid a mishap away from civilization when it's too late to amend an error. Use your head out there and treat the place as if it were your own backyard. After all, in the words of Chief Seattle, "This we know: the earth does not belong to man, man belongs to the earth. All things are connected like the blood that unites us all. Man did not weave the web of life, he is merely a strand in it. Whatever he does to the web, he does to himself . . ."

ANIMAL AND PLANT HAZARDS

TICKS

Ticks are often found on brush and tall grass waiting to hitch a ride on a warm-blooded passerby. Not so common in urban areas, they are, however, active and ubiquitous most everywhere else in all seasons except winter. Ticks come in several varieties of varying shapes and sizes, but the two species that raise the most concern are dog ticks and deer ticks, both of which latch onto humans as readily as they attach to any animal or bird. Although both these ticks are known to be carriers of disease, bear in mind that not every tick is infectious. Furthermore, to transmit a pathogen an infectious tick must be attached to the skin for several hours. By and large, the larger dog ticks are easy to detect since they tend to tickle as they creep under clothes. However, deer ticks, which can harbor Lyme disease, are often tiny and therefore nearly undetectable. There are a number of strategies for fending off tick attack. My personal favorites are to wear light clothing (to help make wandering ticks easier to spot), using natural insect repellent, and showering soon after hiking. If you do find a tick attached to a part of you (they prefer the softer places), stay calm and remove with tweezers. Fortunately or not, the first evidence of Lyme infection is an unmistakable mark that looks like a big red bulls-eye with the dot-sized tick at its epicenter. If you develop such a rash after hiking, visit a doctor immediately. Caught early, Lyme disease is easily treated with antibiotics.

SNAKES

Spend some time hiking in Boston and surroundings and you may be surprised by the variety of snakes you encounter. Most snakes sighted will be garter snakes, black racers, brown snakes, harmless water snakes, and perhaps the flashy, slender eastern ribbon snake. All but 2 of Massachusetts's 14 native snake species are harmless. The state's two venomous species, the timber

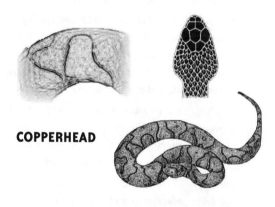

COPPERHEAD

rattlesnake and the copperhead, are not only shy and reclusive, but also woefully rare. Despite great efforts to protect them, both snakes are listed as "endangered" and therefore it is illegal to harass, kill, collect, or possess them. To calm your fears or add interest to your hiking experience, consider spending a few

minutes studying snakes before heading into the woods. If you do have the good fortune of spotting a snake while hiking, treat it with respect, give it a wide berth, and let it go its way.

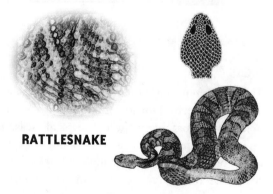

RATTLESNAKE

POISON IVY/POISON OAK/ POISON SUMAC

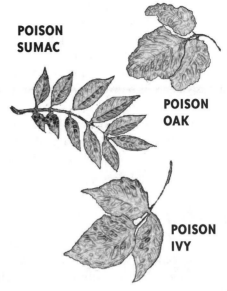

POISON SUMAC

POISON OAK

POISON IVY

Recognizing poison ivy, oak, and sumac and avoiding contact with them is the most effective way to prevent the painful itchy rashes associated with these plants. In the Northeast, poison ivy ranges from a thick, tree-hugging vine to a shaded groundcover, three leaflets to a leaf; poison oak occurs as either a vine or shrub, with three leaflets as well; and poison sumac flourishes in swampland, each leaf containing 7 to 13 leaflets. Urushiol, the oil in the sap of these plants, is responsible for the rash. Usually within 12 to 14 hours of exposure (but sometimes much later), raised lines and/or blisters will appear, accompanied by a terrible itch. Refrain from scratching, because bacteria under the fingernails can cause infection. Wash and dry the rash thoroughly, applying a calamine lotion to help dry out the rash. If itching or blistering is severe, seek medical attention. Remember that oil-contaminated clothes, pets, or hiking gear can easily cause an irritating rash on you or someone else, so wash not only any exposed parts of your body but also clothes, gear, and pets.

MOSQUITOES AND OTHER FLYING KILLJOYS

One of the advantages of hiking in fall, winter, or early spring is absence of biting insects. Boston is certainly well represented by winged tormentors. As a rule, conditions that suppress bugs include stiff breezes, dry air, and frost. Conversely, these six-legged killjoys love windless, humid air. When preparing for a hike, approach the bug issue as you would the weather: dress appropriately. Wearing a long-sleeved cotton shirt and loose cotton pants gives excellent protection from the swarms of mosquitoes that materialize around wetlands and elsewhere when the heat of the sun subsides in the later afternoon. Greenheads—a fierce variety of horsefly—unlike mosquitoes, gnats, deerflies, and no-se-ums, pose a threat only in areas near the salt marshes where they breed. Greenhead season on Crane Beach and Plum Island usually runs from mid-July through the first week of August.

Some swear by DEET, but years ago a hepatologist I met in the Peruvian Amazon persuaded me to stay clear of the powerful chemical. According to this scientist, DEET is a powerful solvent capable of dissolving nylon, and further-more is lethal to amphibians. Though the EPA deems DEET to be safe, the agency advises people who use the repellent to limit its use and to wash if off when its protections is no longer needed.

Before you reach for insect repellent, I recommend striking out on the trail just as you are if only to test for need. I enjoyed each one of the 60 hikes in this book without using any synthetic repellent at all. When on occasion I do apply bug repellent, I use a natural formula called Lewey's, bottled by Alison Lewey, a native Maliseet and Passamaquoddy from Maine. Having a refreshing scent of peppermint, thyme, lemongrass, and other herbs, Lewey's works wonderfully and is a true pleasure to wear.

TOPO MAPS

The maps in this book have been produced with great care and, used with the hiking directions, will direct you to the trail and help you stay on course. How-ever, you will find superior detail and valuable information in the United States Geological Survey's 7.5-minute series topographic maps. Topo maps are available online in many locations. A well-known free service is located at **www.terraserver .microsoft.com,** and another free service with fast click-and-drag browsing is located at **www.topofinder.com.** You can view and print topos of the entire United States from these Web sites and view aerial photographs of the same area at terraserver. Several online services such as **www.trails.com** charge annual fees for additional features such as shaded-relief, which makes the topography stand out more. If you expect to print out many topo maps each year, it might be worth paying for shaded-relief topo maps. The downside to USGS topos is that most of them are outdated, having been created 20 to 30 years ago. But they still provide excellent topographic detail.

Digital topographic map programs such as Delorme's TopoUSA enable you to review topo maps of the entire United States on your PC. Gathered while hik-ing with a GPS unit, GPS data can be downloaded onto the software, letting you plot your own hikes.

If you're new to hiking, you might be wondering, "What's a topographic map?" In short, a topo indicates not only linear distance but elevation as well, using contour lines. Contour lines spread across the map like dozens of intricate spiderwebs. Each line represents a particular elevation, and at the base of each topo, a contour's interval designation is given. If the contour interval is 20 feet, then the distance between each contour line is 20 feet. Follow five contour lines up on the same map, and the elevation has increased by 100 feet.

Let's assume that the 7.5-minute series topo reads "Contour Interval 40 feet," that the short trail we'll be hiking is 2 inches in length on the map, and that it crosses five contour lines from beginning to end. What do we know? Well, because the linear scale of this series is 2,000 feet to the inch (roughly 2 inches representing

1 mile), we know our trail is approximately four-fifths of a mile long (2 inches are 4,000 feet). But we also know we'll be climbing or descending 200 vertical feet (five contour lines are 40 feet each) over that distance. And the elevation designations written on occasional contour lines will tell us if we're heading up or down.

In addition to the outdoor shops listed in the Appendix, you'll find topos at major universities and some public libraries, where you might try photocopying the ones you need to avoid the cost of buying them. But if you want your own and can't find them locally, visit the United States Geological Survey Web site at **topomaps.usgs.gov.**

TRAIL ETIQUETTE

Whether you're on a city, county, state, or national park trail, always remember that great care and resources (from nature as well as from your tax dollars) have gone into creating these trails. Treat the trail, wildlife, and fellow hikers with respect.

- **Hike on open trails only. Respect trail and road closures (ask if not sure), avoid possible trespassing on private land, and obtain all permits and authorization as required. Also, leave gates as you found them or as marked.**

- **Leave only footprints. Be sensitive to the ground beneath you. This also means staying on the existing trail and not blazing any new trails. Be sure to pack out what you pack in. No one likes to see the trash someone else has left behind.**

- **Never spook animals. An unannounced approach, a sudden movement, or a loud noise startles most animals. Surprised animals can be dangerous to you, to others, and to themselves. Give them plenty of space.**

- **Plan ahead. Know your equipment, your ability, and the area in which you are hiking—and prepare accordingly. Be self-sufficient at all times; carry necessary supplies for changes in weather or other conditions. A well-executed trip is a satisfaction to you and to others.**

- **Be courteous to other hikers, bikers, equestrians, and others you encounter on the trails.**

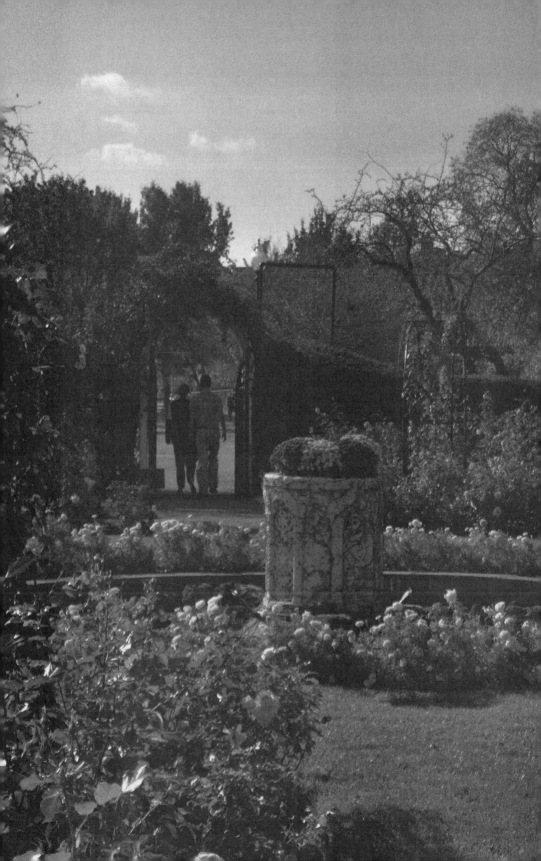

WITHIN BOSTON

01 THE FREEDOM TRAIL

KEY AT-A-GLANCE INFORMATION

LENGTH: 4.21 miles

CONFIGURATION: Point to point

DIFFICULTY: Easy

SCENERY: Boston's most historic streets; Boston Common, America's oldest public park; the Charles River; and views of Boston Harbor

EXPOSURE: Mix of sun and shade

TRAFFIC: Heavy

TRAIL SURFACE: Pavement

HIKING TIME: Allow at least 2 hours

SEASON: Most of the major sites on the Freedom Trail are open 7 days a week 9:30 a.m.–5 p.m. in the summer and 10 a.m.–4 p.m. in the off-season; however, times vary by site. The last tour of the USS Constitution is at 3:30 p.m. year-round. All sites are closed on Thanksgiving, Christmas, and New Years' Day.

ACCESS: Free

MAPS: See longer note at end of description.

FACILITIES: Restrooms can be found at the visitor centers on Boston Common and State Street and at Faneuil Hall, Quincy Market, the Charlestown Navy Yard, and Bunker Hill. In warm months, restrooms are available at the North End Visitor Center, located near the Old North Church.

WHEELCHAIR TRAVERSABLE: Yes

IN BRIEF

This hike, which is clearly marked with a painted red line or inlaid bricks—tours Boston in the footsteps of those who drove the American Revolution. Starting at the State House, the trail travels north, reaches Paul Revere's House, then crosses the Charles River to Charlestown, where it climbs to the Bunker Hill Monument and concludes at the USS *Constitution*—taking in a great many more historical sites along the way.

DESCRIPTION

Begin the hike on the steps of the "new" State House, located on Beacon Street just north of Boston Common. The Freedom Trail, marked with red paint or, in some places, brick, is easy to follow.

Before setting out, pause to look across the common. Before the ships of John Winthrop and company landed, these 44 acres belonged to William Blackstone (or Blaxton), the first white man to settle Shawmut. Eventually overwhelmed by shiploads of new arrivals, Blackstone retreated to Rhode Island, seeking peace and, ironically, freedom, from the Puritan's rigid code of law.

Long after being liberated from Blackstone's ownership, the ground on which the

---

The Freedom Trail

UTM Zone (WGS84) 19T

Easting: 330052

Northing: 4691567

Latitude: N 42° 21' 28"

Longitude: W 71° 03' 49"

Directions ——————————→

The best way to get to the start of the Freedom Trail is by public transit. If you're coming from outside the city, it's best to park near an outlying subway station and take the MBTA to Park Street. Both the Red and Green lines run directly to the Park Street Station, located on the Boston Common close to where the trail begins.

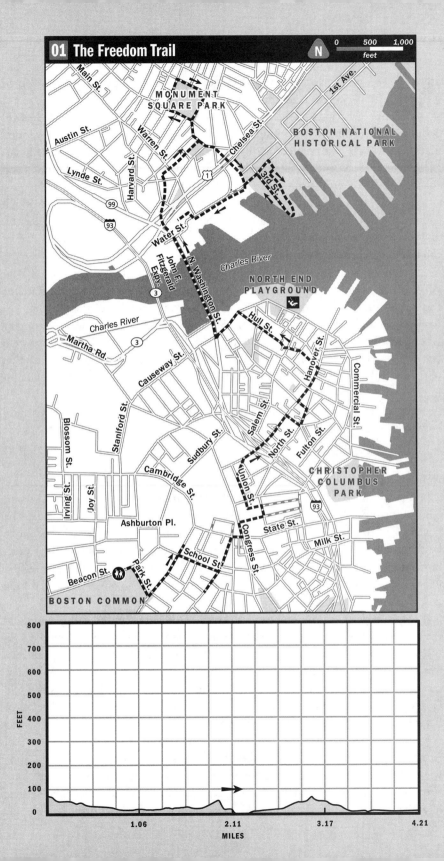

State House stands belonged to John Hancock, the commonwealth's first elected governor (1780–85), who used it to pasture his livestock.

Beacon Hill, located behind it, was the tallest of Boston's three once-prominent hills (linked by Tremont Street). Its name refers to the simple wooden alarm signal that was erected nearby in 1634. The hill once rose 60 feet higher. In the early 19th century, Hancock's heirs sold its top as fill for the millpond that lay at the base of its northern slope.

In 1787, newly back from studying architecture in Europe, Charles Bulfinch submitted plans for the new State House. Nine years later, on July 4, Paul Revere and acting governor Samuel Adams officiated at a highly ceremonial laying of the building's first cornerstone.

From the State House, the Freedom Trail heads south to the corner of Beacon and Tremont streets, where a granary once stood. Deemed inappropriate for the neighborhood after the gilded State House was completed, the granary was demolished and replaced with the Park Street Church. Thus, the humble granary where, among heaps of wheat and barley, the sails of the USS *Constitution* were cut and sewn was lost. But history continues, for in this evangelical Christian parish on July 4, 1829, William Lloyd Garrison gave a radical speech condemning slavery.

Although a place where the dead are interred, the Granary Burial Ground is where Boston's greatest historical figures come to life. Here tombstones for John Hancock, Peter Faneuil, Paul Revere, Samuel Adams, and the five victims of the Boston Massacre powerfully demonstrate that these indeed great men were mortal after all.

Continuing east to School Street, the trail arrives at King's Chapel, situated beside Boston's oldest cemetery. In 1688, finding no other available space, the governor of the Dominion of New England, Edmund Andros, seized this public land and built a wooden Anglican church beside the graves of prominent puritans, including Governor John Winthrop and Mary Chilton, said to be the first person to step ashore from the *Mayflower*. In 1689 the colonists, who had long despised Andros, deposed and arrested him.

After examining the fantastic carvings of skeletons brandishing swords at the Grim Reaper on many of the gravestones found in this burial ground, backtrack to School Street and proceed past Old City Hall (once the site of the Boston Latin School) to the Old Corner Bookstore, which faces Washington Street.

The white brick building with a double-pitch roof, still known as the Old Corner Bookstore, was once the address of Ticknor and Fields, the publisher of *Walden, The Scarlet Letter,* and *Hiawatha.*

Notably, only one other building ever occupied this spot—the home of Anne Hutchinson, who was banished from Massachusetts in 1638. Her crime was to hold Bible study classes explicitly for women at her house. In time, John Winthrop, the presiding judge of the General Court, condemned her actions in a civil trial in which he described her meetings as "a thing not tolerable nor

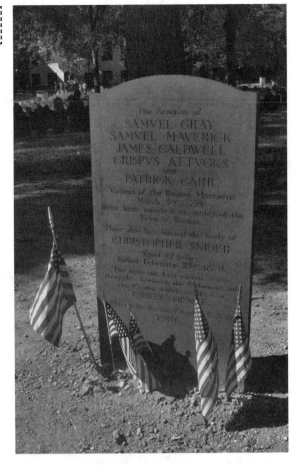

Gravestone for the victims of the Boston Massacre

comely in the sight of God, nor fitting for [her] sex."

Next, cross Washington Street and hike west several yards to the Old South Meeting House—one of the most important sites of the Revolution. Protesters gathered here following the Boston Massacre, and on December 16, 1773, 7,000 fiery citizens mobbed outside the building to condemn the Tea Act. Shortly thereafter, seizing on this collective passion, Samuel Adams organized the Boston Tea Party.

Before continuing on the Freedom Trail, walk a few steps up Milk Street (to the right of the Old South Church) to number 17. Benjamin Franklin was born in a modest house at this location on January 17, 1706.

From the Old Meeting House, hike north on Washington Street to the Old State House. Looking somewhat quaint now, with modern Boston built up around it, this brick building with a lion on one side and a unicorn on the other (both statues were replaced in 1882) was once Boston's most prominent edifice. Standing on the balcony here on July 18, 1776, Colonel Thomas Crafts read the Declaration of Independence to a triumphant crowd. Lighting bonfires in celebration, citizens burned reminders of the British rule, including the original lion and unicorn.

Proceeding farther north, the trail leads to a marketplace built in 1742 as a gift to Boston by Peter Faneuil. Of Huguenot descent, Faneuil inherited a great fortune from an uncle; with one stipulation—Faneuil had to remain a bachelor or forfeit the money. To appease those resistant to the market, Faneuil elected to include a public meeting hall. In 1763 James Otis dedicated the room to the "Cause of Liberty." Centuries later, the hall is still an important meeting place; this is where in 1960 John F. Kennedy made his last campaign speech.

Continuing on the same trajectory, the trail passes along the Blackstone Block on Union Street. The names of the little cobblestone passageways—Marsh Lane, Creek Square, Salt Lane, to name some—bespeak the locale's age and original character. The Union Oyster House, at the end of the block, is both hard to miss and hard to pass up. Louis-Philippe, the eventual king of France, lived here in the 1790s when in exile—reportedly giving French lessons to while away the time!

Turning the corner on Hanover Street, the Freedom Trail passes through a marketplace now called simply "Haymarket." Filled with vendors selling everything from flounder to artichoke and havarti (Fridays and Saturdays), the market has been alive and well since Boston's founding.

Beyond Blackstone Street, Hanover Street crosses the site of Boston's "Big Dig," now the Rose Kennedy Greenway. Follow the Freedom Trail (marked red) as it jogs left to Salem Street then back to Hanover, to reach the "Isle of North Boston" or "the North End," as it is called today.

In the early days, its residents relied on two drawbridges to cross Mill Creek, which flowed between the isle and the mainland. Having a colorful history in its own right, the neighborhood shifted from being quiet and upright to being dangerously raucous as Boston's port prospered and grew after the Revolution. Settled by Irish immigrants, Eastern European Jews, and, in most recent decades, Italians, the neighborhood is ever evolving.

From Hanover Street, the trail turns right onto Richmond Street—"The Black Hole"—as it was called in the 1830s when people came here to gamble and indulge in carnal pleasures.

Reaching North Street (which follows the original shoreline), the trail bears left to pass two noteworthy houses, the Pierce-Hichborn House and the House of Paul Revere. Built in 1680, 50 years after Boston's founding, Paul Revere's house stands where the childhood home of Cotton Mather stood before a fire consumed it and 44 other residences in 1676.

Follow the trail left at Prince Street to pass Mariner's House and, shortly after, turn right to rejoin Hanover Street. Ahead, at the Bulfinch-designed St. Stephen's Church (where Rose Kennedy was baptized), the trail bears left to continue west through the Paul Revere Mall to the Old North Church (officially, Christ Church in Boston). This church merits a book of its own—its claim to fame is its contribution to the launching of the Revolution, for it was from the steeple of the Old North Church that Paul Revere's comrades Robert Newman and Captain Pulling sent a signal to Charlestown to warn of British aggression.

Continuing toward Charlestown, the Freedom Trail climbs uphill to another burial ground—this one named for the man who sold it to the Puritans—the shoemaker William Copp. Aside from Increase and Cotton Mather, few of the people buried here are well-known. However, the cemetery boasts many interesting epitaphs, ranging from quite peculiar to poignant. One reads, "Stop here my friend & cast an Eye, As you are now, so was I, As I am now, so you must be, Prepare for Death and follow Me."

After leaving the cemetery, follow the trail down Hull Street, go left on Commercial Street, then cross the Charlestown Bridge (first opened in 1786). From Chelsea Street in Charlestown, the trail makes a loop. Those concerned with getting to the USS *Constitution* in time for a tour (the last one is at 3:30 p.m.) should hike to the right. Otherwise, cross the street to City Square.

When a group of Puritans left Salem seeking ever greener pastures, they settled here on "Mishawum." On this central spot, then called "Market Square," they erected "The Great House," which served as the seat of government and the home of Governor Winthrop—but only temporarily—since the area lacked potable water. Lured by the springs of Shawmut, Winthrop and company soon crossed the river for good.

From the square, follow the trail along Main Street to Winthrop Street, which leads north to Monument Square at the top of "Breeds Hill," where the (misnamed) pivotal Battle of Bunker Hill occurred on June 17, 1775.

The Bunker Hill Monument is the last official site on the Freedom Trail, but round out the tour with a visit to the USS *Constitution*. To get there, follow the red line back to Winthrop Square then on to the Charlestown Navy Yard.

After taking in marvelous "Old Ironsides"—as she was nicknamed for the impenetrability of her hull hewn of live oak—either backtrack to Boston or get a lift via the MBTA bus line, T, or the water shuttle, which leaves from Pier 4 in the Navy Yard at quarter to and quarter past the hour until 6:15 p.m.

Note: To fully enjoy this hike, it is best to either start early and allow plenty of time for its many historical diversions or plan to complete it over the course of two days.

Maps: Boston's official visitor information center on Boston Common sells a foldout Freedom Trail map for $2. The Park Service, which has two visitor centers, one at 15 State Street across from the Old State House and another at the Charlestown Navy Yard next to the USS *Constitution,* offers its own excellent foldout Freedom Trail map free of charge.

NEARBY ATTRACTIONS

The New England Aquarium (Central Wharf, [617] 973-5200), the Institute of Contemporary Art (100 Northern Avenue, [617] 478-3100), China Town, the Kennedy Library (Columbia Point, [866] JFK-1960), the Science Museum (Science Park, [617] 723-2500), and the Children's Museum (300 Congress Street, [617] 426-6500) are all located near the Freedom Trail. For those who love wonderful food or sipping espresso while watching soccer among fans cheering in Italian, an extended visit to the North End is a must. One historical site not included on the Freedom Trail is The Boston Tea Party Ship and Museum, anchored at the Congress Street Bridge.

02 CHARLES RIVER LOOP

KEY AT-A-GLANCE INFORMATION

LENGTH: 7.78 miles
CONFIGURATION: Loop
DIFFICULTY: Easy to moderate
SCENERY: The lovely Charles River, and life and leisure along its banks, with historic Boston on the south bank and Cambridge to the north
EXPOSURE: A mix of sun and shade
TRAFFIC: Light to heavy depending on the day and time of day
TRAIL SURFACE: Pavement with stretches of grass or packed earth
HIKING TIME: 2.5–3 hours
SEASON: Year-round sunrise–sunset
ACCESS: Free
MAPS: Available online at: www.mass.gov/drc/parks/metroboston/maps/ch_east.gif
FACILITIES: Public restrooms, snacks, soft drinks, sandwiches, hotdogs, pretzels, and coffee are available for purchase at the Esplanade Café, open 10 a.m.–6 p.m.
SPECIAL COMMENTS: See longer comment at end of description.
WHEELCHAIR TRAVERSABLE: Yes
DRIVING DISTANCE FROM BOSTON COMMON: Driving to the river is not recommended. However, if you do drive look for parking at Boston Common where there are plenty of meters and a parking garage.

IN BRIEF

To get to know Boston, the best place to start is the Charles River basin. Once a sprawling tidal river with winding estuaries and thousands of acres of salt marsh, the Charles today is wholly reinvented. In an exploration of the lower Charles, this hike takes you on a tour of Boston's lagoon and tree-lined Esplanade, and then crosses to Cambridge where it follows the Embankment to Harvard University. Looping back to Boston's shore via a scenic footbridge, the hike returns to the start at Longfellow Bridge.

DESCRIPTION

After taking ownership of the land mass shaped like a balled hand attached to a delicate wrist, two generations of Puritan settlers were too consumed with pleasing God and spurning the crown of England to bother with reconfiguring the earth beneath their feet. Victory in the Revolution, however, shifted minds from fear and loathing to health concerns and the pursuit of wealth.

Separated by a channel, Charlestown and Boston are close neighbors and yet far removed by land. Since Winthrop's landing in 1630, travel between the two had always been arduous and time consuming. The public

Charles River Loop

UTM Zone (WGS84) 19T

Easting: 329467

Northing: 4691909

Latitude: N 42° 21' 39"

Longitude: W 71° 04' 15"

Directions

The Charles River is best reached by foot, bicycle, or public transportation. Using the "T", take the Silver, Green, or Orange line to the Red line and get off at the Charles Street station. On exiting the station, cross to Charles Street via the crosswalk, then bear right to cross Embankment Road to the pedestrian bridge.

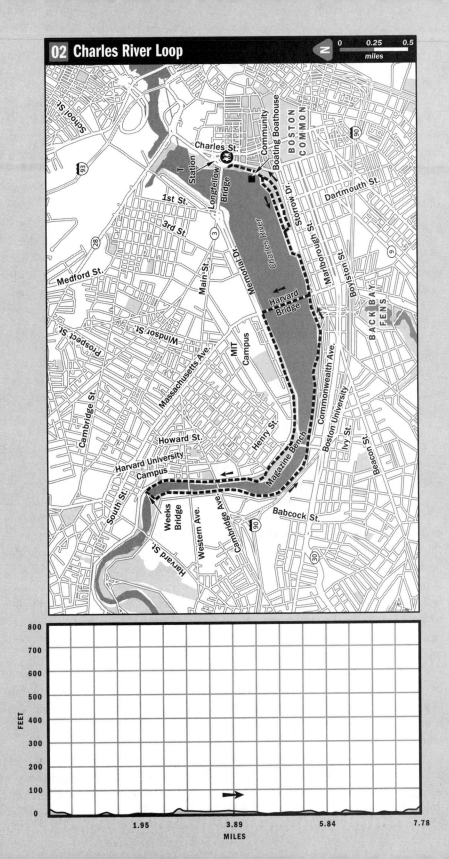

pined for a bridge, but for a century no one had the gumption to build one.

Finally in 1786, John Hancock petitioned the General Court of Massachusetts for permission to build a toll bridge to link the towns. Though the court had snubbed other, perhaps less resolute proposals, Hancock got his way on the condition that he compensate Harvard College for fares lost to the institution's preexisting ferry service.

A year later, on the anniversary of the Battle of Bunker Hill, Hancock opened his drawbridge.

"The Charles River Bridge" (engineered by Lemuel Cox) was a success of astounding magnitude, so much so that everyone began fancying a bridge of their own. But Hancock, who a year later had reclaimed the governor's seat, protected his interests by using his authority to dictate where any new bridge could be built. By this cunning, the next bridge proposed, that of Francis Dana, was restricted to a site beside the city's Pest House; and like Hancock, Dana was required to compensate Harvard.

Dana's bridge—said to be even more impressive than Cox's—opened in 1793, and it, too, turned a pretty profit.

With so much money being made from two bridges, and so much river left to cross, another proposal soon materialized. This time from Andrew Craigie, a showy man with wealth and reputation to match Hancock.

By 1808 Craigie owned 300 acres of East Cambridge and had the trustees of Harvard firmly on his side. Thus empowered, Craigie built his bridge despite protests from Dana and Hancock (then united in a partnership) and, to ensure steady traffic, he also built the requisite access roads.

In the years that followed, bridge fever showed no signs of abating. Rather it raged hotter until the court had had enough. In 1846, to end future dreams of easy money from traffic crossing the Charles, the court granted Isaac Livermore—the largest shareholder of the Hancock Corporation—the right to build a bridge between the Dana and Craigie bridges. This right, however, was granted with the stipulation that upon reaping $150,000 in profits, Livermore would be required to first buy the Dana and Craigie bridges then turn over all four bridges—his own included—to the commonwealth.

This roadblock placed on the avenue to wealth may have been a disappointment, but one the coming railroad boom soon erased. Amid the loud and messy dealings for bridge-building rights, tracks were being laid for railroad lines connecting Boston with Providence, Worcester, and Lowell. As soon as the steam engines were fired up, all eyes and betting odds were steered from boats and bridges to mighty locomotives. Pristine in Blackstone's time, before the Puritans landed, the river began to take on a different life as industry gained traction.

Near Brighton's salt marsh where salt hay was still being harvested in 1872, an enormous slaughterhouse ran a brisk business. In Cambridgeport, on the marshy shore opposite, a slew of soap makers dug in, and all along the Charles's 80-mile length, mills and tanneries spilled their waste into the water flowing by.

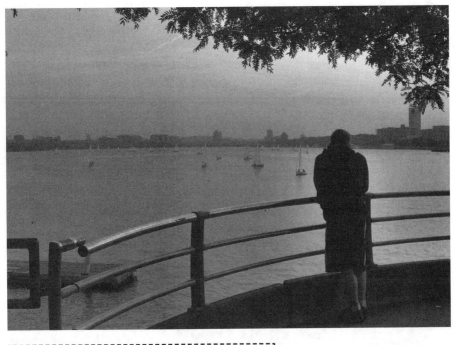

A peaceful moment looking westward on the Charles River

As the 20th century approached, the Charles was a fetid approximation of its former self and, not least of all, a threat to human health. Finally, despite vehement opposition by some—mostly blueblood residents of Beacon Street—advocates for damming the river won out.

By luck, the movement to establish a Greater Boston park system coincided with the reinvention of the Charles. Acting independently but toward the same end, Cambridge, then Boston, took possession of the river's banks and converted them to open space for public enjoyment.

Cross the traffic-clogged tide pool at the foot of the Charles Street MBTA subway station to Charles Street, then stride over quiet Embankment Road to access the south bank of the Charles River via the pedestrian footbridge dead ahead. As you are lifted above the exhaust of rushing cars into air softened with organic scents, the city abruptly gives up the chase.

Instead of asphalt, traffic signs, and parking meters, you will see the rippling waters of the Charles and, to the immediate right, the elegant carbon-smudged silhouette of the Longfellow Bridge, renamed in 1927 to honor the poet Henry Wadsworth Longfellow, who professed his love for the river in a poem titled "To the River Charles."

At the foot of the pedestrian bridge, hike left on the paved walkway in the shade of willows and Norway maples past the Sailing Center to a cove protected by a breakwater. Immediately after the cove, the path arrives at the Hatch Shell,

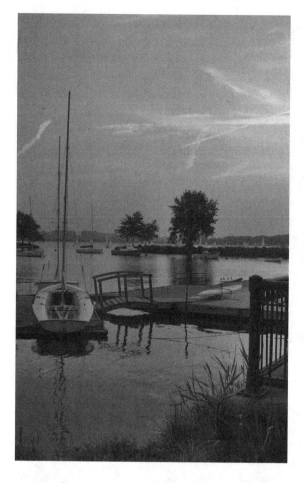

made famous by Arthur Fiedler and the "Boston Pops" orchestra. Bear right here to cross a granite footbridge outfitted with snarling lions.

Never mind as Lycra-bound joggers and skateboarders in jeans blur by, but slow your pace to take in other sites, including a Dragon boat biding its time at a mooring in the cove between races. Unmistakably oriental in line and color, these boats draw the eye like an ocelot among house cats. Look to the lagoon to the left and you will likely spot an authentic gondola being guided by a man in stripes and a straw hat looking thoroughly Venetian.

Arching around two more lagoons—the first sunken like a Roman bath and decorated with a fountain, the next less formal and surrounded by bankings and fawning willows—the path crosses another picturesque footbridge and arrives at a junction. To keep clear of bicyclists and others on wheels, stay with the path beside the water.

A thick grove of trees shade a playground gracefully integrated into the park and recently updated with the latest in swings and slides. Looking diagonally west across the water, you can see the dome of Massachusetts Institute of Technology (MIT) resting on the horizon looking like the bald head of a scientist pondering string theory.

Mount the stairs of the Harvard Bridge directly ahead and, once at the top, bear right to cross the river to Cambridge. Among the smorgasbord of standard sights, two in particular draw the eye: the Citgo sign lighting the sky above Kenmore Square (once the tip of Judge Samuel Sewell's farm on the bay now filled and home to Fenway Park), and, directly underfoot, a measurement notated as "Smoots."

The distance between each Smoot is exactly 5' 7"—the length, or height, of Oliver Smoot, MIT class of 1962. In 1958 MIT's Lambda Chi Alpha fraternity conceived a prank, or "hack" to determine the distance from the MIT dorms in Boston to the MIT campus for the benefit of brothers making the trek on cold, foggy nights. To serve as a measuring unit, Lambda Chi Alpha's pledge master chose Smoot, who was a handy height and carried a name that "sounded scientific." So they lay Smoot down end-to-end again and again from Boston to Cambridge and found the distance to be 364.4 Smoots + 1 ear. And so it was that Oliver Smoots found his calling, for he went on to become president of the International Organization for Standardization (ISO) and chairman of the American National Standards Institute (ANSI).

On the Charles's northern bank, bear left to hike west toward Harvard University, either on the paved bicycle route or on the winding footpath closer to the water. Across traffic whooshing by on Memorial Drive sits the MIT campus.

This mile-long academic stretch to the Boston University Bridge is quiet and focused, with few distractions but teams of rowers skimming up river and down like giant water bugs.

In 1858 one boatload of Harvard rowers (including the future president of Harvard Charles W. Eliot) thought to set themselves apart from other boats on a race day by tying red silk scarves around their heads. Not only did they soundly trounce the competition in a 3-mile race that day, but they out-rowed the field in a 6-mile race two weeks later. From then on, crimson was their lucky color, and by 1910 it was adopted by the university.

After passing the Boston University (BU) boathouse on the left, the ziggu-ratlike Hyatt, and the once but now no longer bustling home of Polaroid on the right, stay close to the river to navigate the BU Bridge.

Ahead is a five-acre piece of land that was known in colonial times—when it was a hillock surrounded by salt marsh—as Captain's Island. Toward the turn of the century, the spit of land was converted to Magazine Beach, complete with sand and a bathhouse built out of granite blocks salvaged from a powder magazine that once stood on the site. Immediately popular, the beach attracted swimmers right up to 1951, when unchecked pollution led the city to turf over the sand and build a public swimming pool.

Once past the soccer field and fitness station, bear left on a paved drive to enter the park and reunite with the riverbank, following the path as it curves back to meet Memorial Drive.

Bending northward, the path crosses Cambridgeport. Before the first bridge to Cambridge was built, this tract of land was a marshy tidal zone with Pelham's Island at its epicenter. Once made accessible, the marsh was drained and filled, and in 1805 the port was officially opened.

Approaching Harvard, the path along the embankment crosses streets at two more bridges, River Street and Western Avenue. Piebald-trunked London plain (or sycamore) trees planted in 1900 by the landscape architect Charles

Eliot lend grace and shade to Memorial Drive from here on up the river.

One day back in 1974, a Cambridge woman named Isabella Halsted, who, with others, had fended off a development plan that would have condemned the plain trees, struck on the idea of a riverfront "park" that would see Memorial Drive closed to cars. Halsted handily garnered popular support then sealed victory by attending a charity auction and placing the winning bid for a lunch date with Senator Edward Kennedy. One year later, and to this day, the road is closed on Sundays.

Shortly after Western Avenue, where the river winds west opposite Harvard's handsome red-brick campus, the path leads to the lovely John W. Weeks footbridge. Built in 1926 for the benefit of students at Harvard Business School, it is the only footbridge across the Charles. Having reached the hike's halfway point, bear left to make the river crossing.

On arriving at the Charles's south side, on the edge of a Boston neighborhood named for the 19th-century painter Washington Allston, turn left to loop back east. For approximately 1.2 miles, the path is quite narrow and exposed to the rush of traffic on Storrow Drive, but in a dramatic return to peace, the path swings away from the riverbank at the BU Bridge. Here, a boardwalk runs under a railroad trestle, taking the path through the realm of nursery-tale ogres before reemerging at the BU boathouse.

Here the path splits. Stay to the left to hike beside the river. Over the past few decades, efforts by the Charles River Watershed Association and other groups have restored the health of the Charles to such an extent that the newly formed 20-member Charles River Swimming Club held their first 1-mile race on the Charles on July 21, 2007.

As you walk and contemplate a swim, keep an eye out for fish feeding at the water's edge, cottontail rabbits in the undercover, and stealthy night herons winging by in the dimming light of late day.

On arriving back at the Harvard Bridge crossed earlier, continue east and bear left at the first footbridge to retrace your steps to the chain of lagoons. Then to vary the return route, turn off at the next footbridge to switch to the south side of the Esplanade and make your way to the Italianate lagoon adorned with an exuberant fountain. On a summer evening with the moon rising in the warm light of the setting sun there is no place more transcendently beautiful.

Beyond this poetic pool is another lagoon of equal charm and intrigue. Slow to a stroll to watch and listen as gondoliers propel their curvaceous crafts across a silken sheet of water to Old World tunes played on accordion.

The Hatch Shell lies directly ahead, and farther south, the docks and boathouse of Boston Community Boating. Follow the path past these familiar sites meandering on whim to reach the pedestrian bridge that leads back to Charles Street.

Note: Memorial Drive north of the Western Avenue Bridge in Cambridge is off limits to cars from 11 a.m.–7 p.m. every Sunday from late April to early November.

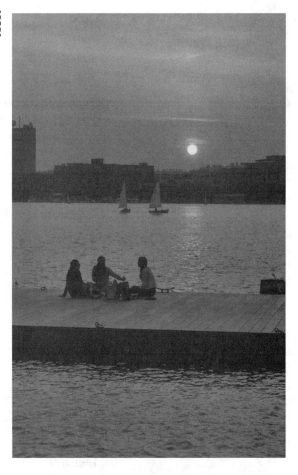

Picnicking on the Charles at sunset

NEARBY ATTRACTIONS

In addition to the count-less points of interest and diversions to be found in Boston, Cambridge, and Charlestown, the Charles River itself offers several notable attractions espe-cially for those itching to get out on the water. Arrange canoe and kayak rentals with Charles River Canoe and Kayak (open Thursday through Sunday, [617] 965-5110), riverboat sightseeing tours with the Charles Riverboat Com-pany (100 Cambridgeside Place, Suite 320, Cam-bridge, [617] 621-3001), and romantic gondola cruises courtesy of Gon-dola di Venezia (Tuesday through Friday, 7 a.m. to 11 a.m., and Wednesday through Sunday, 2 p.m. to midnight). For information or to purchase tickets visit **www.BostonGondolas .com** or call (800) 979-3370). Those with a romantic bent who prefer to stay on dry land might like to attend a night of tango dancing on the Weeks Bridge. Evenings of Tango by Moonlight, sponsored by the Tango Society of Boston, are held every full moon (give or take) in summer from 7:30 to 11 p.m. or there-abouts. In addition to watching accomplished dancers, those who drop by can partake of impromptu 15-minute minilessons. Visit **www.bostontango.com** for a schedule and additional information.

03   BACK BAY FENS: Isabella's Loop

KEY AT-A-GLANCE INFORMATION

LENGTH: 1.8 miles
CONFIGURATION: Loop
DIFFICULTY: Easy
SCENERY: A rose garden, the Fenway Victory Gardens (many are very elaborate), and the neighborhood surrounding the historic Fenway Baseball Park
EXPOSURE: Mixed sun and shade
TRAFFIC: Moderate to heavy
TRAIL SURFACE: Clay, turf, and pavement
HIKING TIME: 1–1.5 hours
SEASON: Year-round, 7:30 a.m.–dusk
MAPS: Available through the Emerald Necklace Conservancy, www.emeraldnecklace.org, (617) 232-5374
FACILITIES: This hike combines nicely with a visit to the Isabella Stewart Gardner Museum, which has restrooms and a café.
SPECIAL COMMENTS: This hike can easily be extended. In fact, the driving notion behind Frederick Law Olmsted's Emerald Necklace was that Bostonians should be able to move among neighborhoods via healthy green space.
DRIVING DISTANCE FROM BOSTON COMMON: 2.5 miles

IN BRIEF

Following a route that the renowned art collector Isabella Stewart Gardner herself may have taken, this hike sets out from Gardner's mansion (now the Isabella Stewart Gardner museum) for a tour of the Back Bay Fens.

DESCRIPTION

In 1623, when the Anglican clergyman William Blackstone laid down his small collection of worldly goods—186 books in a variety of languages and, it is supposed, a bag of apple cores—on the awkward peninsula called Shawmut by the Sagamore, the loudest sound to mar the quiet was the racket of gulls excited by the ebbing tide, or the anxious beating of the reverend's heart. Newly arrived from Liverpool, England, on a boat captained by a son of Fernando Gorges, Blackstone was not in a party of Puritans; he was alone. Over the next eight years, he built a house, planted an orchard, and generally thrived on the 800 acres he claimed for himself.

In 1626, while Blackstone was planting an orchard on his hill, Roger Conant and a group of others dissatisfied with Cape Ann settled Salem. Four years later, armed with a charter from King Charles I that granted his party all that lay between 3 miles south of the

---

Back Bay Fens:
Isabella's Loop
UTM Zone (WGS84) 19T
Easting: 327085
Northing: 4689551
Latitude: N 42° 20' 20"
Longitude: W 71° 05' 56"

Directions ⟶

The hike begins at the Isabella Stewart Gardner Museum, at 280 The Fenway. There is both on-street metered parking and paid parking at the Museum of Fine Arts garage and in the parking lot on Museum Road, two blocks from the Gardner. For information, call (617) 566-1401; for the box office, call (617) 278-5156.

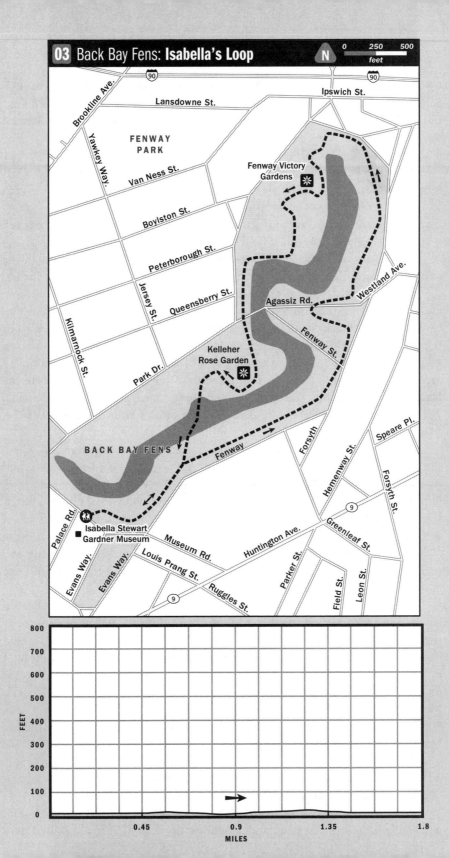

Charles and 3 miles north of the Merrimack River, John Winthrop Sr. arrived at Salem aboard the *Arbella* in a fleet of 4 ships soon to be joined by 13 more. What they found upon landing left Winthrop unimpressed, so days later, the *Arbella,* the *Talbot,* and the *Jewel* went farther south to Charlestown. Others dispersed to places they renamed Medford, Watertown, Rocksbury, and Dorchester.

Found to be sorely lacking in potable water, Charlestown proved even less hospitable than Salem. And in no time, the mood of Winthrop's company turned from disappointed to nothing less than desperate. Watching, or perhaps visiting from across the river, William Blackstone witnessed their misery and invited them to his fair and benevolent land on Shawmut.

This time John Winthrop liked what he found and quickly renamed the peninsula Boston. Three years later, after Blackstone had sworn loyalty and obedience to the newly founded Massachusetts commonwealth by signing the Freeman's Oath, Winthrop granted his gracious host 50 of the 800 acres he had long before claimed. Blackstone complied with the deal but promptly sold back 44 of the acres, keeping his 6-acre garden and orchard in case he should come to need it, and left town. By 1633, the population of Blackstone's peaceful Shawmut had grown to nearly 3,000 Puritans. In the month of June alone, 14 shiploads of the black-robed immigrants had arrived. Blackstone himself settled for good on a 200-acre farm in Old Rebohoth, Rhode Island, near a river that now bears his name. He called his new home "Study Hill."

Blackstone's farmstead was located between the Charles River and where the State House now stands on Beacon Hill. Beyond it, to the west, was a tidal estuary that the settlers called "Back Bay." As Boston's population grew and industry began to take hold, this marsh, naturally pungent without human input, turned septic. Still, nature's under-appreciated maid—the tide—came twice a day and kept conditions tolerable. But like most maids, the tide was denied the respect it deserved, and so in 1821 an entrepreneur named Uriah Cotting was permitted to build the Roxbury Mill Dam. The result was a stagnant 500-acre bay that stank beyond all imagination.

Desperate for an end to the perpetual offense of odors, the City of Boston resolved to bury the nuisance. The filling began in 1837, and in time Boston's citizens had their second park, the 24-acre Public Garden and Swan Boat lagoon. But much of the marshy tidal zone remained, spreading to Sewall's Point near Brookline. By 1858 the mounting pressures of a growing population prompted the State of Massachusetts to go for broke and hire the contracting firm Goss & Munson to relocate a sizable piece of Needham to the sludgy wasteland. It took 40 years, but somehow a total of 80 men moved what a glacier had deposited in Needham to the salt marsh of the Back Bay.

Incredibly, 35 car trains loaded with sand and gravel made 25 trips every day and night except Sunday. By 1890, the wetland was filled to Sewall's Point (Kenmore Square) to an average depth of 20 feet.

While the "Big Fill" was under way, many gave their two cents and more with regards to how the new land should be developed. Some, such as David

A glimpse of a footbridge at a bend
in the Muddy River

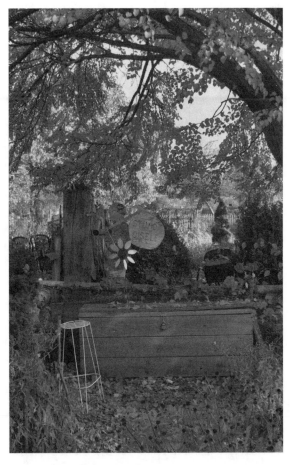

Stewart, the father of Isabella Stewart Gardner, seized on the opportunity and bought up lots; others passionately made the case for preserving some of the fast-disappearing open space for parkland. As of 1863, New York City had Central Park—designed by Frederick Law Olmsted—to boast of, and some Bostonians feared that in short time the possibility of having a park of equal stature in their city would be lost.

Responding to increasing public demand, the city passed a Parks Act, and three years later, faced with the task of proposing a parks system the city's commissioners turned to Olmsted. Most urgent was what to do about the Fens and the Muddy River, said to be "the foulest marsh and muddy flats to be found anywhere in Massachusetts, without a single attractive feature." Though Olmsted had suffered a great deal in seeing the Central Park project through, he accepted the challenge.

Cotting's attempt to turn the marsh into a mill-based center of industry had failed. Lacking even an ounce of doubt, Cotting estimated his project would result in 81 new mills, and from these, other businesses would blossom. Investment money blew in like a nor'easter, but in 1821, when the project was finished and Cotting was dead, his prediction proved off by 78. Only three mills took root—and the cost overrun was near 300 percent. Meanwhile, the 100 acres west of a second dam (which roughly followed the course of Massachusetts Avenue), being on the receiving end of Roxbury, Brookline, and Brighton sewers, had become a health hazard of alarming proportions. One glance and Olmsted knew the job would require a good deal more than planting tulips.

In addition to demanding a steady dose of imagination, it also called for terrific feats of engineering. Working with city engineers, Olmsted solved sanitary and drainage problems by redirecting the sewers and the freshwater Stony Brook

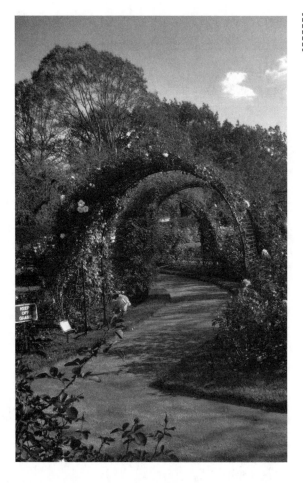

The Kelleher rose garden at the center of the Back Bay Fens

River for asthetic reasons rather than allow the Fens to remain brackish. Olmsted designed this section of the Muddy River to be entirely salt water. Anticipating freak storms, his design ensured that the Fens could absorb overflow from Stony Brook if necessary.

Once the engineering aspect of the job was completed, two thirds of the Fens was dredged and filled. Next, the entire landscape, including the river, was rebuilt. Nothing was as it had been when, as a last touch, the land was carefully graded and planted to create the naturalistic look Olmsted prescribed. Every inch of the Fens was planted from scratch.

Not fully confident in his own horticultural knowledge, Olmsted consulted botanist Charles Sprague Sargent and others for advice on plant selection. But it was the German-born horticulturalist William L. Fischer in whom he put his complete trust. Having become acquainted with Fischer's skills while working on New York's Central Park, Olmsted resolved to lure him to Boston. The Fens tree-planting plan was entirely Fischer's doing.

To give a sense of the scale of the plantings—more than 100,000 shrubs, vines, and flowers were planted on the 2.5-acre Beacon Street entrance. The reason for the enormous number was that much of the planting was experimental. Indeed Olmsted expected most specimens of the initial planting to die. In striving for a "wild" effect, Olmsted mostly used native species. But besides beach plum, bayberry, and other New England shrubs, he also included exotics like Oregon Grapeholly (*Mahonia aquifolium*), a native of the Pacific Northwest brought east by the Lewis and Clark expedition.

Starting from the mansion of the art collector and eminent Boston society figure Isabella Stewart Gardner at 280 on The Fenway, cross the street to reach the Fens. Make your way down a banking to the footpath that runs along the Muddy River, and bear right to continue southeast.

Sheltered by a veil of reeds and shrubbery, mallards paddle and bob along the rippled ribbon of water. The path passes a decommissioned footbridge as the stately granite Museum of Fine Arts and its school of art come into view. Beyond Forsyth Street, the path arrives at the second of the park's two gatehouses designed by H. H. Richardson. Just after a tremendous London plane tree (*Platanus acerifolia*), the path reaches Agassiz Road, named for the geologist and glaciologist Louis Agassiz.

Nearing the Boston Conservatory of Music, bear left at the fork to dip to a playground called "Mother's Rest," brilliantly designed as an escape from the city above. From this enclave, climb steps decorated with an ornate handrail to return to street level. After pausing to look at the view from H. H. Richardson's bridge, follow the path as it descends to the Fenway Victory Gardens. Established in 1942 in response to a wartime request by President Roosevelt, the victory garden was the first of its kind. It is also the only World War II–vintage victory garden still in existence.

Although not a part of Olmsted's design, the 500 individual victory gardens on the seven acres are well worth touring. Not a few have been in the same hands for many years and are fantastically elaborate. Continue straight to enter, then take the first left to stroll down one of the narrow avenues that runs between the rows of private gardens. Reaching the Muddy River again, bear right to pick up a paved path. A moment later, go left at a junction and weave amid fruit trees to head south once more. Indulge your senses and, when ready, locate the compost heap and, keeping it to your left, follow the path to another that parallels Park Drive.

Beyond Agassiz Road, a path diverges left to lead to a veteran's memorial and the Kelleher Rose Garden. A gorgeous destination in and of itself, the rose garden was designed by Olmsted's protégé Arthur Shurcliff and opened in 1930. Meticulously maintained, the garden shows off more than 200 varieties. Hike around to the western side to find the arched entranceway.

Leaving the rose garden, follow the path toward playing fields lying to the west, and, arriving at a T-junction, bear left. Sweeping toward the Muddy River, the path crosses a footbridge and rejoins The Fenway. Curve round an oxbow in the river to return to the home of Isabella Stewart Gardner.

NEARBY ATTRACTIONS

Adding a visit to the Isabella Stewart Gardner Museum is the perfect way to round out a hike in the Fens. The museum is open Tuesday through Sunday, 11 a.m. to 5 p.m. (the admission desk closes at 4:20 p.m.) and most holidays except Independence Day, Thanksgiving, and Christmas. Admission: $12 for adults, $10 for seniors, and $5 for college students with I.D.; for children under 18, admission is free. Check **www.gardnermuseum.org** for additional information.

04   MUDDY RIVER LOOP

KEY AT-A-GLANCE INFORMATION

LENGTH: 3.42 miles

CONFIGURATION: 2 linked loops

DIFFICULTY: Easy

SCENERY: Views along the Muddy River, and of woodland, ponds, and historic architecture

EXPOSURE: Mixed sun and shade

TRAFFIC: Moderate to heavy

TRAIL SURFACE: Clay, turf, and pavement

HIKING TIME: 1.5 hours

SEASON: Year-round, unrestricted

MAPS: Available through the Emerald Necklace Conservancy at 2 Brookline Place, Brookline, 2 blocks west of the park, off Boylston Street (MA 9), www.emeraldnecklace.org

FACILITIES: Restrooms are open to the public during the summer at Jamaica Pond, located adjacent to the Muddy River's southern end.

SPECIAL COMMENTS: For more information about the Emerald Necklace and Frederick Law Olmsted, stop by the Emerald Necklace Conservancy.

WHEELCHAIR TRAVERSABLE: The entire length of the Muddy River is wheelchair traversable; however, several paths chosen for this hike are not.

DRIVING DISTANCE FROM BOSTON COMMON: 3 miles

Muddy River Loop

UTM Zone (WGS84) 19T

Easting: 325435

Northing: 4687860

Latitude: N 42° 19' 24"

Longitude: W 71° 07' 07"

IN BRIEF

This hike follows the course of the Muddy River from the edge of Boston's Back Bay to Jamaica Plain through parkland designed by Frederick Law Olmsted.

DESCRIPTION

In 1881, with the monumental redevelopment of the Back Bay Fens three years along, Frederick Law Olmsted met with Boston's Board of Commissioners and presented his plan for a series of parks he described as a "green ribbon." It would take time and many patient conversations with commissioners, engineers, and gardeners, but Olmsted's vision prevailed. Once completed, the Emerald Necklace would make a 1,100-acre chain from the Boston Common to Franklin Park. The Olmsted plan for the Muddy River improvement won approval and, after a 10-year delay while the city searched for funding, workers hefted shovels and broke ground.

Locate the trailhead at the northeast corner of the parking lot, and hike up the western slope of the drumlin Nickerson Hill to enter woodlands. Reaching a U-junction, bear left and continue north on a path of packed

----

Directions ⸻⟶

To reach the parking area on Pond Avenue by car, take the Jamaicaway south to where it intersects with Perkins Street. Turn right onto Perkins Street and then right onto Chestnut Street, at the next intersection. Exit the rotary at the first right. The parking lot is immediately to the right on Pond Avenue. The Muddy River parks are easily reached by public transportation via the #39 bus that runs along Huntington Avenue and Center Street in Jamaica Plain or the Longwood train on the MBTA Green line.

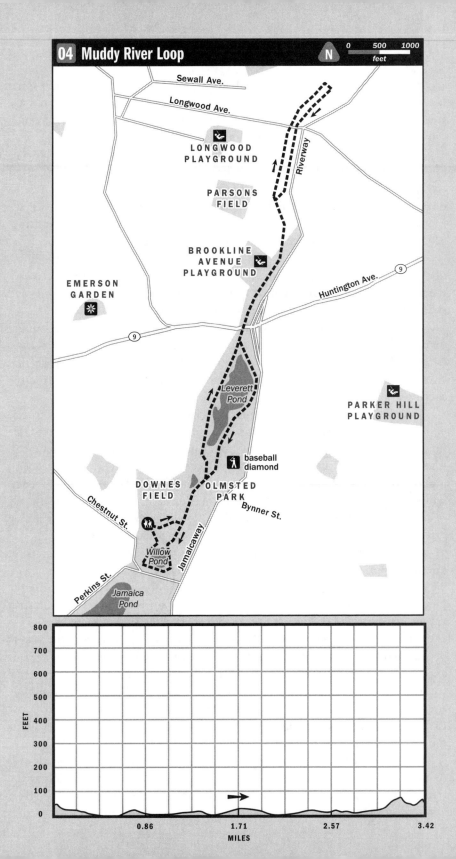

earth and loose stone above the Muddy River, following it down the hill's softly tapering northern side. At the split ahead, choose the path to the right and make your way past a mix of black oak, sweet gum, and beech to reach Spring Pond, a shallow "natural history pool" of Olmsted's design.

Surely a favorite spot for many who frequent the park, this shaded pool harbors the southernmost freshwater population of threespine sticklebacks (*Gasterosteus aculeatus*) in the country. If hiking through in spring, try to spot the males of this small species of fish building nests to impress eligible females. In that the Massachusetts Division of Fish and Wildlife lists them as endangered, it is astonishing that threespine sticklebacks live right in the heart of Boston.

Just past Spring Pond, the path crosses a stream that flows from the home of the stickleback to Willow Pond, which lies to the left. Several yards ahead, the path forks as it reaches Willow Pond Road. Opt for the left-hand route and stride across this lightly trafficked road to rejoin the footpath.

After scrambling up the gravel banking on the other side, continue straight on a narrow packed-earth trail to stay within Olmsted's planted woodlands. Arching over this gentle hill, the trail descends through trees to a path that sweeps east to west. Bear left and continue to a stone bridge built across the southern tip of Leverett Pond.

The far end of the bridge connects to two paths running parallel to one another and to the water; the nearer path is for pedestrians, and the farther one for bicycles. Bear right, following close to the pond's banking, to pass three small islands just offshore. Created by Olmsted to add visual interest, these peaceful islands are rich with wildlife. Each spring, pairs of Canada geese—likely themselves hatchlings of the islands—assert ownership of nesting sites on this lovely real estate. Despite dangers, including dogs, foxes, coyotes, raccoons, snapping turtles, and humans, a clutch or two of new goslings emerge every year.

This section of the hike—Olmsted Park—ends at the northern bank of Leverett Pond, where MA 9 interrupts the Emerald Necklace. To continue, you must either brave the traffic between lights or cross the busy road by taking the Jamaicaway bridge. If choosing the former, aim for the break in the median strip cut for bicyclists and pick up the worn path beyond the sidewalk opposite.

Flowing unseen below MA 9 (and other roads along its course), the waters of the Muddy River reappear once you are beyond the pavement. Keeping this gurgling brook to the right, continue on River Road past the home of Brookline Ice and Coal and a ramp to the Jamaicaway and travel alongside Brookline Avenue. Using the crosswalk at Aspinwall Avenue, cross Brookline Avenue and Parkway Road to reach another gem of the Emerald Necklace, Riverway Park as the Muddy River continues north towards the Charles River.

A short way in, the path crosses a broad stone bridge arching northward. As the path resumes its course over ground, it is embraced on either side by the river. Below steep bankings, ducks kick up ripples in the shade of beech trees. Olmsted created this and a second thickly planted island to hide the former

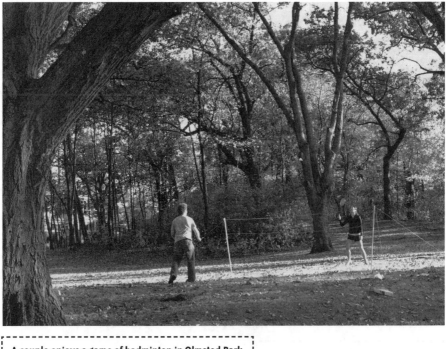

A couple enjoys a game of badminton in Olmsted Park

Boston and Albany Railroad (now the MBTA) and muffle the creaks and clangs of passing trains. A moment later, the lightly used (soon to be closed to cars) Netherlands Road breaks the path. After the interruption, the path approaches Brookline's Longwood neighborhood. Here Olmsted insulated the park from houses and other aesthetic and sensory disturbances by having earth mounded to the height of a man's head and planted with ornamental shrubs.

The Longwood neighborhood is rich in history and intrigue in its own right: Judge Sewall—of Salem Witch Trial notoriety—once owned a generous portion of the area; in fact, when Brookline succeeded (after its third attempt) in winning its independence from Boston in 1705, it took its name from that of the Sewall family farm, which bordered the Charles to the north and the Muddy River to the east.

Soon after Uriah Cotting and company built the Roxbury Mill Dam across a tidal estuary between Beacon Hill and Sewall Point (Kenmore Square) in 1821, David Sears II, one of Boston's wealthiest citizens, seized on what he recognized as a budding opportunity, and promptly began buying low-lying meadowland spread over 500 acres south and west of the Charles River.

In the same year that Cotting began constructing his dam, Napoleon Bonaparte died in exile. To honor Napoleon, or because he shared one or two of the general's most notable traits, Sears named his neighborhood "Longwood" after the Frenchman's final home on the island of Sainte-Hélène.

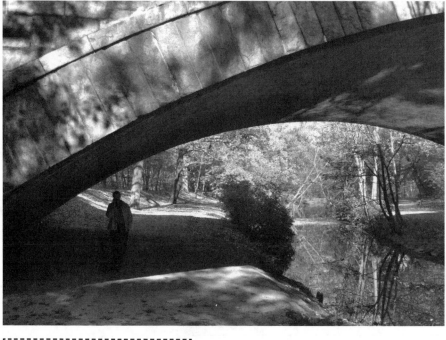

Passing under the Longwood Bridge, designed by Shepley, Rutan, and Coolidge and built in 1898, the path continues along the narrowest section of the park and widens as it reaches a smaller footbridge, the Chapel Street Bridge.

In total, the Muddy River park system includes 17 bridges, each painstakingly designed. It is all but forgotten now, but Olmsted had anything but an easy time getting his bridges built. One complicating factor was that some of the bridges lay on both Boston and Brookline land and were, therefore, joint projects. Another was that Olmsted had to dance a two-step to satisfy conflicting tastes. In keeping with his vision of creating a rustic, naturalistic landscape "slightly refined by art," Olmsted intended that the bridges be simple structures made of fieldstone. Others, like Charles Sprague Sargent, the director of the Arnold Arboretum, were aggressive in expressing opposing taste. They insisted that the bridges be more finished and ornate—that they include wrought-iron rails and details. The resulting bridges are therefore products of hard-won compromise.

To complete a tour of the park end to end, stay left, following the river's west bank; otherwise, turn right to hike across the Chapel Street Bridge and, once on the other side, bear right to hike back upriver.

The path runs the entire length of the river's east side, but because of heavy traffic on the Jamaicaway—a roadway that in Olmsted's time served horse-drawn vehicles but now serves speeding cars—it is best to return to the river's quieter west bank once you reach Netherlands Road.

From Netherlands Road, resume the path traveled earlier and retrace your steps to Leverett Pond and Olmsted Park. On returning to the pond, bear left to weave back to the greenway's east side to vary the view. The clay-surfaced footpath runs flush to the Jamaicaway and Leverett Pond before dipping away from the rushing roadway as the park widens. Ease right at the fork ahead to stay close to the ten-acre pond.

Before the Muddy River Improvement Project was under way, this was not so much a pond as a dense sewage-fouled cattail swamp. Before human tampering, salt water flowing into The Fens from the Charles River eventually mixed with freshwater from springs in Jamaica Pond. In drawing up his plan for the park system, Olmsted somewhat reluctantly decided that The Fens should be a purely saltwater park and that the Muddy River should be strictly freshwater fed. The wetland that became Leverett Pond was dammed, dredged, and finally contoured to a shape drawn by Olmsted. To make sure the pond was kept well fed, another wholly separate brook was diverted to it from Brookline.

Nine acres of hand-planted hardwood trees help make the city disappear again as the path passes alongside Leverett Woods. Continuing south to skirt a baseball diamond at Daisy Field, the path soon encounters Willow Road. Once across, pick up the footpath that travels between Willow Pond and the Stickleback pool, and bear right at the first fork to switch to a path not yet taken. Continuing south through a landscape designed by the Wisconsin Glacier and left all but untouched by Olmsted, take the second left to connect with a path shooting up Nickerson Hill.

After pausing at the fine vantage point of this stony knuckle, head down the hill's south side and take the path below clockwise around Ward's Pond. Left wild by Olmsted, this kettle hole harbors all sorts of wildlife, including birds, amphibians, and such fish as bluegill (*Lepomis macrochirus*), largemouth bass (*Micropterus salmoides*), and pumpkinseed (*Lepomis gibbosus*). After jumping the stream on the pond's northwest side, take the first path to the left to return to the parking lot.

NEARBY ATTRACTIONS

Both Brookline and Jamaica Plain offer a great assortment of restaurants, many within walking distance. If you have a hankering for coffee or ice cream, visit J. P. Licks (659 Center Street, Jamaica Plain). For a hearty, wholesome, and affordable brunch, lunch, or dinner try Center Street Café (669A Center Street, Jamaica Plain). For more exotic fare visit Bukhara (701 Center Street, Jamaica Plain) for its wonderful Indian cuisine, or J. P. Seafood (730 Center Street, Jamaica Plain) which serves excellent sushi and a full menu besides. Located at 7 Station Street across from the Brookline Village MBTA (subway) stop, Kookoo's Café serves up tasty robust coffee, a fine collection of teas, highly delectable sweets, homemade soups, sandwiches, and lunch dishes with a distinctly Persian touch. On Washington Street half a block away, Restaurant Stoli (213 Washington Street) and Café St. Petersburg (236 Washington Street) entice with authentic Russian entrées.

05   JAMAICA POND LOOP

KEY AT-A-GLANCE INFORMATION

LENGTH: 1.45 miles

CONFIGURATION: Loop

DIFFICULTY: Easy

SCENERY: Views from the banks of a kettle pond landscaped by Frederick Law Olmsted and a boathouse designed by the Dorchester architect William Downer Austin and built in 1912

EXPOSURE: Mixed sun and shade

TRAFFIC: Varies from light to heavy

TRAIL SURFACE: Choice of clay or pavement

HIKING TIME: 30–45 minutes

SEASON: Year-round sunrise–sunset

ACCESS: Free

MAPS: Not needed

FACILITIES: Restrooms, drinking fountain, and community boathouse offering rowboat and sailboat rentals and youth programs

SPECIAL COMMENTS: Each Halloween a Lantern Festival is held at the pond. Concerts are held at the pavilion next to the boathouse all summer long.

WHEELCHAIR TRAVERSABLE: Yes

DRIVING DISTANCE FROM BOSTON COMMON: 4.5 miles

IN BRIEF

This wonderful hike for all ages and abilities is located in a historic neighborhood right in the heart of Boston.

DESCRIPTION

In 1923, the Jamaica Plain resident Carl Anthonsen wrote in his journal, *"Tonight I fulfilled my vow to go skating. The weather being ideal, skated for several hours on Jamaica Pond. Paid little attention to the festivities and was quite oblivious of the 50,000 gathering."*

Two years later, having been at the same municipal skating festival when the weight and exuberance of tens of thousands of skaters caused water to surge through cracks in the ice, Anthonsen complained, "There are too many people in the world."

Incorporated into the Emerald Necklace in 1892, Jamaica Pond was, by the turn of the century, a favorite recreational destination for people from the neighborhood and far beyond.

The largest freshwater pond in Boston, at 68 acres, Jamaica Pond was, until the mid-1880s, Boston's primary source of drinking water. Incorporated in 1795, the Jamaica Plain Aqueduct Company laid 45 miles of pitch-pine pipes to convey the water. In addition, the frozen pond provided households the ice needed

---

Jamaica Pond Loop

UTM Zone (WGS84) 19T

Easting: 325216

Northing: 4687588

Latitude: N 42° 19' 15"

Longitude: W 71° 07' 16"

Directions ⟶

Jamaica Pond is located on the Arborway across from Pond Street in Jamaica Plain, Boston.

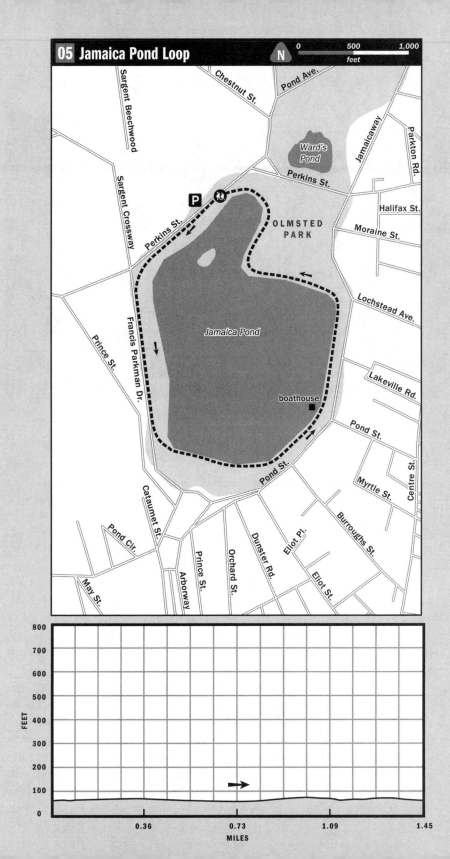

N

0　　　500　　　1,000
feet

Chestnut St.

Pond Ave.

Sargent Beechwood

Ward's
Pond

Jamaicaway

Parkton Rd.

Perkins St.

Sargent Crossway

P

Halifax St.

O L M S T E D
P A R K

Moraine St.

Perkins St.

Prince St.

Francis Parkman Dr.

Jamaica Pond

Lochstead Ave.

Lakeville Rd.

boathouse

Pond St.

Cataumet St.

Pond St.

Centre St.

Myrtle St.

Pond Cir.

May St.

Prince St.

Arborway

Orchard St.

Dunster Rd.

Eliot Pl.

Eliot St.

Burroughs St.

FEET

800
700
600
500
400
300
200
100
0

0.36　　　0.73　　　1.09　　　1.45

MILES

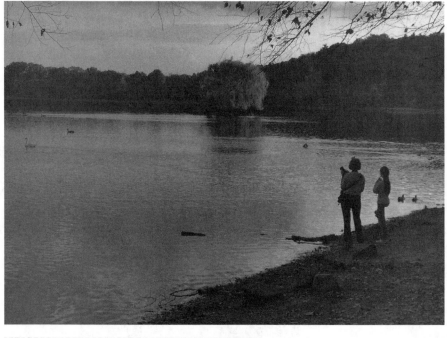

Shea's Island viewed across the waters of Jamaica Pond

to keep food from spoiling. The Jamaica Pond Ice Company, with its multiple icehouses, supplied Boston nearly all its ice for more than half a century.

Initially part of Roxbury, then West Roxbury, Jamaica Plain was settled in 1640 by the intrepid Curtis family. A century later, Joshua Loring, a commodore in the British army, kept a summer house less than a mile from Jamaica Pond. After spooking Loring back to England in 1774, colonial troops took the house over and made it their headquarters during the war for independence.

The question of how Jamaica Plain got its name may never be resolved. Some say that it is an Anglicization of Kuchamakin, the name of a chief of the Massachusett tribe; others say that the explanation lies in the involvement of some of its founding citizens in rum trade with Jamaica. However, it is also asserted that it was so named in 1677 to commemorate Cromwell's success at wresting control of Jamaica from Spain.

By the mid-19th century, Jamaica Plain had attracted many wealthy families, who built summer homes on or close to Jamaica Pond. Francis Parkman, the author of *The Oregon Trail*, spent summers in a large house outfitted with a dock extending into the water. Not a healthy man, despite his reputation as an adventurer, Parkman gave up writing and turned to horticulture in his later years. Said to be afflicted with a neurological disorder, Parkman liked to row on Jamaica Pond every day for exercise and relaxation. To keep his hour-long workout from getting dull, he named points along the pond after famous capes.

He called one jetty the Cape of Good Hope, and named a cove the Bering Sea. Out rowing on a Sunday in 1893, Parkman developed appendicitis and several days later died.

That Jamaica Pond was made a public park was to a large degree Frederick Law Olmsted's doing. With the construction of Franklin Park, the Arnold Arboretum, and the Muddy River Improvement Project well under way, by 1891 Olmsted's concept of a "green ribbon" around Boston was on the road to being realized. Advocates for the park needed only to point to concerns over population growth and the sorry condition of the icehouses to convince Boston's city officials to add the pond to what is now called the Emerald Necklace.

Unlike the other "jewels" designed by Olmsted, Jamaica Pond looks much as it has since the retreat of the Wisconsin Glacier. After several private homes were seized by eminent domain then moved or demolished, Olmsted's instructions dictated little more than what should be planted and where. As ever, his aim was to have the landscape look as natural and poetic as possible. As stated in his own words, he saw the pond as "a natural sheet of water, with quiet, graceful shores, rear banks of varied elevation and contour, for the most part shaded by a fine natural forest-growth to be brought out over-hangingly, darkening the water's edge and favoring great beauty in reflections and flickering half-lights."

The place to start a hike around Jamaica Pond is often dictated by parking opportunities. Being circular, the path has no start and no end. I chose to begin on its northwestern side, where, except for Perkins Street, Jamaica Pond connects with the Muddy River. Where a crosswalk meets the path, bear right and walk counterclockwise, passing a sandy beach dotted with fishermen. Rounding a turn, the path runs beside a stone wall bordering Francis Parkman Drive to the right, and the shore of the pond.

A hundred yards or so farther, Shea's Island obstructs the view across the water. Neither entirely natural nor entirely man-made, this island is said to have begun as a bump formed on the lips of the two co-joined kettle holes that make Jamaica Pond. Local lore has it that the island was first "improved" by Indians, who built it up with stones to create a fish trap. Before the start of World War I, the "island" showed itself only in hot, dry summer months. It was the wife of Charles Sprague Sargent, the first director of the Arnold Arboretum, who dreamt up the idea of making a more permanent island. Using her influence, and charm, Mrs. Sargent appealed to James Shea of the Parks Department. The plan was promptly approved, and construction commenced the following summer. Two years later, populated with half a dozen willows, the island stood soundly above the water. Today, flocks of Canada geese, mallard ducks, and American coot congregate around the hummock.

Halfway along this bank, part way up a gentle slope, the path passes an enormous plain tree. This tree and the tremendous beech trees growing to the right of the path ahead are likely among the few trees remaining from Olmsted's time. Beyond the beeches, the path approaches the junction of Prince Street and

Parkman Drive, the site of Francis Parkman's house, demolished near the turn of the century.

Rounding the pond's southern bank, recessed between the water and upland, the path climbs past land that, from 1760 to 1769, was owned by the royal governor Sir Francis Barnard. Under the later ownership of Captain John Prince, the acres supported fine orchards of pears, apples, apricots, plums, and grapes. Later, a Jamaica Pond Ice Company icehouse stood hereabouts.

On this turn, cut in away from the path, to walk along the water. This wide beach is a favorite for fishermen practicing fly casting. Looking north, on a summer's day you will likely see sailboats tacking lazily across the water.

From the beach, climb the granite stairs back to the path and turn left to walk toward the boathouse. Stout fruit trees, planted to replace Olmsted's originals, blossom along this stretch in the spring. Mighty, but now somewhat collision-weary red oaks fend off cars the length of the Arborway, once, but no longer a carriage road meant to be traveled by horse and buggy.

Reaching the junction at Pond Street, help yourself to a drink from the spring-fed fountain in front of the Tudor-style boathouse. Passing the bandstand and a row of benches to the left, note a young evergreen tree growing just in from the Arborway and the path. Not a species of Olmsted's choosing, the tree would please him nonetheless since it was planted to commemorate a successful campaign to keep the nearby Hellenic Hill free from development.

Continuing north, the path echoes the shape of the pond, traveling several feet in from the water behind the trees and shrubs planted along the bank. Mallard ducks paddle in the shallows, tipping tail up now and again to feed on submerged pondweed. Bending westward at a grassy passage to a kettle-shaped field, the path passes steep upland dense with trees and shrubs. Until recently, an estate named Pinebank, once owned by the Perkins family, sat upon this hill. Acquired by the Boston Park Department in 1891 on Olmsted's recommendation, the former mansion has since been used as a commissary. Curving around the base of this hill, the path returns to the hike's beginning at the crosswalk off Perkins Street.

NEARBY ATTRACTIONS

As many as 25 breweries operated in the area within a mile of Roxbury Crossing before national prohibition (1919–1933). One of these was Haffenreffer Brewery, at Stony Brook in Jamaica Plain. Today, the Boston Beer Company, makers of Sam Adams Beer, brews beer at the same location (30 Germania Street, Boston, 02130). The brewery offers tours to the public for a $1 donation; all the proceeds go to a local charity. Tours are offered Thursdays at 2 p.m., Fridays at 2 and 5:30 p.m., and Saturdays at 12, 1, and 2 p.m.; there is an additional tour on Wednesday at 2 p.m. from May through August. To reach the brewery, take the MBTA's Orange line, or call (617) 368-5080 for recorded directions.

ARNOLD ARBORETUM TOUR 06

IN BRIEF

The Arnold Arboretum is an urban oasis where you can take walks among botanicals collected from all over the world. With the plant life in constant flux, every day offers a different spectacle of beauty ranging from a hillside of blooming lilacs to great blue herons fishing in ponds ornamented with lilies, and the glow of a blue spruce in morning mist.

DESCRIPTION

Founded in 1872, Harvard University's Arnold Arboretum exists thanks to the generosity and vision of two men, New Bedford whaling merchant James Arnold (1781–1868) and businessman Benjamin Bussey (1757–1842). Alike in their love for and commitment to agriculture, each of these men donated their fortunes to Harvard so that the university might use the assets to advance plant science.

Shortly after the Arnold Arboretum was established, Charles Sprague Sargent was made its first director and given the title of Arnold Professor of Botany. Soon after, with

Directions →

From Boston, take Storrow Drive west to the Kenmore Square/Fenway. Bear left following signs for Fenway/US 1 south. Bear right onto Boylston Street, following signs for Boylston Street. Continue on Boylston 0.4 miles, after which it turns into Brookline Avenue. Stay on Brookline Avenue 0.5 miles. Take a left onto the Riverway (also called the Jamaicaway). Follow Riverway to a rotary at Jamaica Pond (on your right). Follow signs for South Dedham/ Providence. Enter the next rotary and take the second exit onto MA 203 east. The arboretum's main entrance is about 50 yards past the rotary, on the right.

KEY AT-A-GLANCE INFORMATION

LENGTH: 3.6 miles
CONFIGURATION: Loop
DIFFICULTY: Moderate
SCENERY: Tree and shrub species from all parts of the world; views of the Boston skyline and the Blue Hills
EXPOSURE: Shade and sun
TRAFFIC: Light on weekdays during business hours; heavy on weekends, especially during the spring and summer months
TRAIL SURFACE: Variable, including packed earth, grass, paved road, and gravel
HIKING TIME: 2.5 hours
SEASON: Year-round sunrise–sunset
ACCESS: Free
MAPS: Posted at each entrance
FACILITIES: Restrooms located inside the arboretum headquarters, accessible during business hours. Members of the public may use the arboretum's library by appointment.
SPECIAL COMMENTS: Free guided tours are available.
WHEELCHAIR TRAVERSABLE: Although the hike described is not wheelchair friendly, much of the Arboretum is traversable by wheelchair.
DRIVING DISTANCE FROM BOSTON COMMON: 5 miles

Arnold Arboretum Tour
UTM Zone (WGS84) 19T
Easting: 325266
Northing: 4686088
Latitude: N 42° 18' 27"
Longitude: W 71° 07' 12"

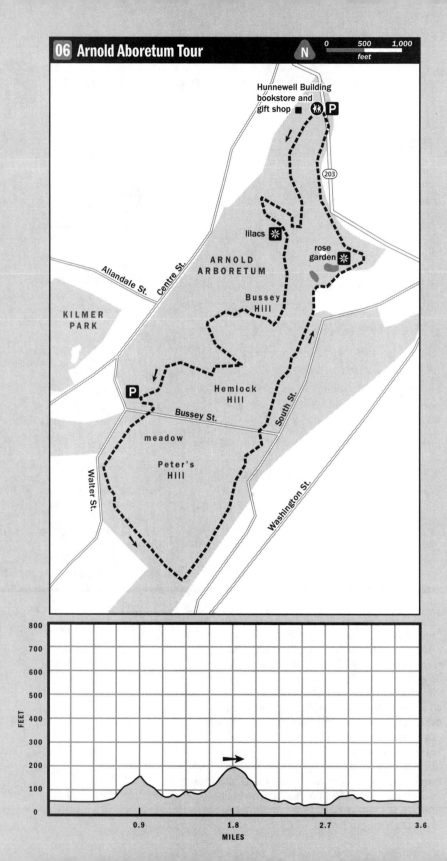

the help of the prominent landscape architect Frederick Law Olmsted, he laid out the road and pathways and planned distinct zones according to family and genus. Today the arboretum's 265 acres serve as a living classroom and research center for Harvard's students and professors as well as a link in Boston's park system known as the "Emerald Necklace."

After entering the Arborway Gate, begin walking on the paved road leading past a cattail-filled wetland to the left and the arboretum headquarters housed in the brick Hunnewell building to the right. On a day in March, your nose will likely draw your attention to the large Chinese witch hazel planted near the headquarters' steps.

Walking on, you will pass a pussy willow tree with branches reaching out into the road. In most seasons, this tree is hard to identify, but in March its velvety buds attract as much interest as any summer flower. Next, on the left, you will notice a particularly magnificent silver maple standing in a cork grove.

The arboretum is full of lovely and intriguing trees and shrubs from all over the globe. You may not recall any one tree in particular after just one visit, but as a frequent visitor, you are bound to develop favorites. One cork tree, in fact, was so roundly adored that the bark of one of its low-hanging branches was worn to a permanent shine.

Once you are past the wetland, leave the road and head into the maple grove to the left. Brushing beneath branches, you might startle mourning doves that favor this spot. Though established by Harvard University as a center for the study of trees, horticulture, and agriculture, the arboretum's 265 undeveloped acres attract a large number of migrating birds. In March, red-winged blackbirds and grackles liven the bogs and ponds. In summer, warblers, finches, and orioles flash their yellow and orange hues amid the bushes and trees.

Where the road reaches a hill, cross over and pick up a trail that curves to the right around the base of the slope. You will pass a vernal pool hidden behind a tangled thicket on the right then shortly come to a collection of chestnut trees and hickories. Ahead a dense growth of bamboo forms a rabbit's paradise on the edge of another slope. Walk straight back, heading northwest, and turn left behind the towering fronds.

Follow the base of this second hill, hiking south through linden woods back to the foot of the first hill then climb to a path that runs along the top and follow it southward.

If it is a day in May when you emerge from the woods to the paved road that winds up the hillside ahead, the purple haze of blooming lilacs you encounter will likely stop you in your tracks. In other months broad-leafed catalpas or delicate birches vie for attention. In any case cross the road and make your way up the hill, bearing left past mulberries of all shapes and sizes.

Once beyond the mulberries, aim for the stump of a tree cut into a sort of throne and upon reaching it stop for a breather, then continue uphill bearing left to an enormous black oak tree. Standing beside this tree and looking to the southern horizon, you can see the dark silhouette of the Blue Hills. From here,

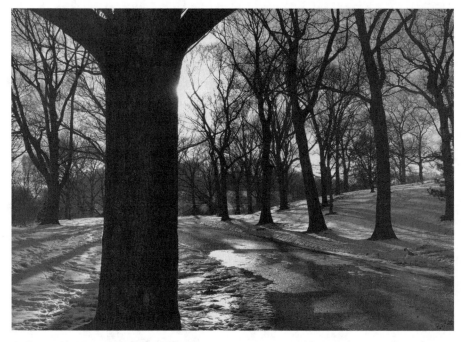

follow the path as it dips to the right of the oak then rises to an open lawn. This peaceful spot is rimmed with evergreens, Asian fruit trees, and ornamental bushes. Find the road to your right and follow it downhill several yards to where it meets a path descending a steep slope to the left. Head down into the deep oak grove below, bearing right. Cross the road curving in front of you and cut between the rocks and evergreens.

Arriving at a group of conifer cultivars, turn southeast and continue past a drooping Norway spruce and a graceful weeping hemlock to the right. Make your way straight downhill to a cypress grove to emerge at a small field then walk to a grand pine at the eastern edge of this grassy plateau and follow the path as it turns to the west.

Passing a row of beeches on the left, you will soon come to a boulder nested beneath pines near a stream outfitted with a picturesque footbridge. Keeping the stream to your left, hike up the slope littered with pine needles and cones then continue to the narrow stream welling from a spring marked by a blue atlas cedar, giant sequoia, and dawn redwood. Make your way across this wet zone taking time to marvel over this jaw-dropping triad, then duck beneath the sheltering boughs of Asian spruces beyond. Bear left on descending the hill and cross the field to a second footbridge. Once on the far side of the stream, turn left to follow the clay path to the Bussey Street Gate.

When the traffic permits, cross Bussey Street to the gate at Peter's Hill.

Where the steep grade begins to ease, look for a path to the right which leads in to a grove of evergreens.

In spring, the hill's orchard of crab apple and ornamental cherry trees fill the view with pink. When leafless the gray branches of these trees caste lovely silhouettes against the stark winter sky.

Follow the path as it arcs to the crest of the hill and, once at the top, leave the trail to steal a look at Boston's skyline couched in trees.

Return to the trail and follow it as it runs along the stone wall at this southernmost edge of the park. Passing the backyards of the arboretum's Roslindale neighbors, you will notice a small grave site to the left of the path.

Stay with the footpath as it rounds the perimeter of the property, paralleling the Boston–Needham commuter line on the eastern border. On the left, in a cleft of the hill, pass a vernal pool and several willow trees. Just ahead, the field forms a basin on the edge of South Street. Follow the path as it leads back uphill to the arboretum's paved road. Turn right to walk down an avenue of oaks heading northeast toward Poplar Gate at the corner of Bussey and South Street.

Because this intersection is often busy and has a tight curve, take extra care crossing back to the arboretum on the north side. Step up onto the low stone wall to find a path running along the base of Hemlock Hill. Follow this path as it reaches a stream and curves westward. After passing through a grove of rhododendrons rooted to the rugged face of Hemlock Hill, the path leads to a bridge on the right. Cross the stream then the paved drive beyond to reach a path that ascends between beech trees of tremendous scale and architecture. On reaching the gravel path at the top, continue northward, passing a century-old tulip tree on the left.

Trees and bushes on the right shield the concrete home of the Massachusetts State Laboratories. Though incongruous with its verdant surroundings, red-tailed hawks have made it their own. The path curves as it runs north then downhill toward two ponds. When you come to the end of the path, cross the paved road to the larger pond. In March, red-winged blackbirds sing from the larch tree on the bank opposite. In summer, you may see a great blue heron standing stock-still waiting to strike at hapless tadpoles.

Keep the pond to your left and hike ahead to the rose garden. Choose your own route through this gorgeous spot, meandering along its various paths invariably dotted with resident cottontail rabbits. The busy Arborway lies just north of this garden. When you are ready, pick up the trail that runs along the stone border between the Arborway and the arboretum and head northwest. Upon reaching the maple grove that lies ahead, you may recognize trees you passed earlier.

Bear right and follow the path beside the Arborway. You will soon pass the wetland crowded with cattails, and beyond it you will see the arboretum's brick headquarters. Continue a bit farther to arrive back at the main gate.

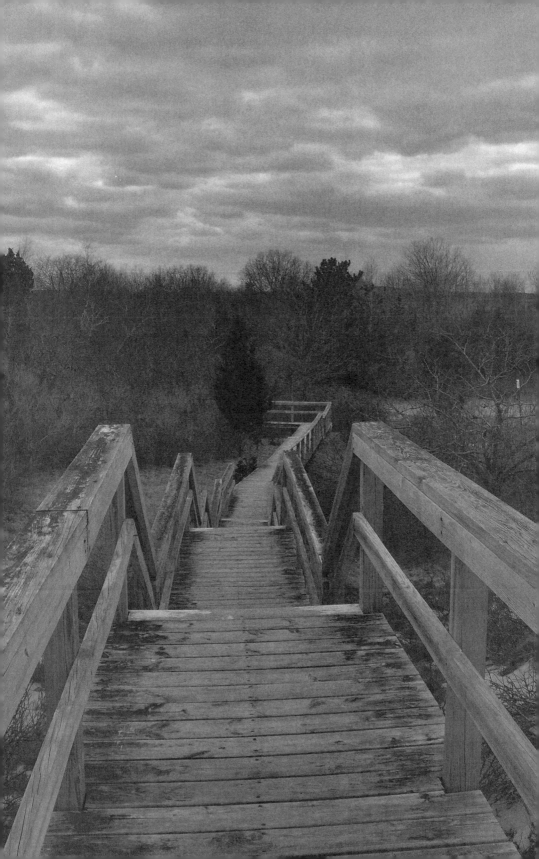

SEASIDE HIKES

07 CRANE BEACH: Dune Loop

IN BRIEF

On this hike—best done barefoot—you will follow lapping waves along the length of one of Massachusetts's most immaculate beaches. Approaching the marshes of Essex and the granite-littered coast of Gloucester, you will cross the high dunes of the inner beach, and upon reaching the peninsula's tip, hike ocean-side back to the start.

DESCRIPTION

In 1908, amidst a lively rumor that the brother of President Taft had bought "Castle Hill Farm" from the estate of the recently deceased Chicago railroad tycoon John Burnham Brown, the Crane Plumbing heir Richard T. Crane Jr. slunk in and bought the property outright with pocket cash. Or so it seemed. Regardless of the circumstances, the 36-year-old Richard T. Crane took possession of the 250 acres made up of bald drumlins and picturesque meadows flush to salt marsh for $125,000. Not one to stand still while the grass grew beneath his feet, Crane set to work building the first of his mansions at the crest of Castle Hill. By the first spring, the 65-room Italianate house was ready for habitation, its grounds reconfigured and primped by none other than the landscape design firm of Frederick Law Olmsted Jr. In

---

Crane Beach: Dune Loop

UTM Zone (WGS84) 19T

Easting: 355341

Northing: 4727302

Latitude: N 42° 41' 03"

Longitude: W 70° 45' 57"

Directions ————————————————➤

From MA 128 north (toward Gloucester), take Exit 20A (US 1A north) and follow it 8 miles to Ipswich. Turn right onto MA 133 east and follow it 1.5 miles. Turn left onto Northgate Road and follow it 0.5 miles. Turn right onto Argilla Road and follow that 2.5 miles to Crane Beach gatehouse at the end of the paved road.

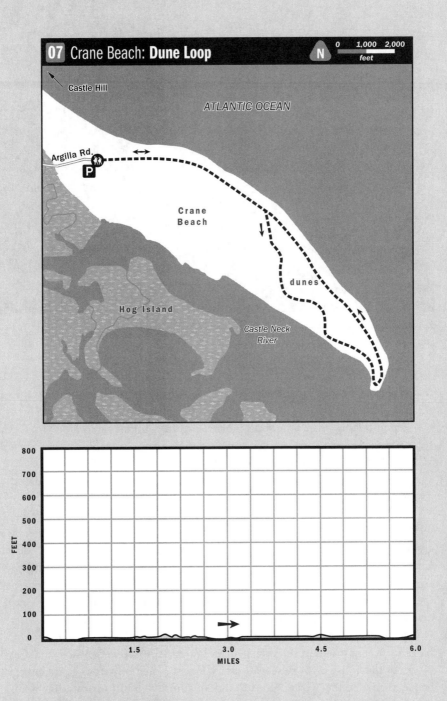

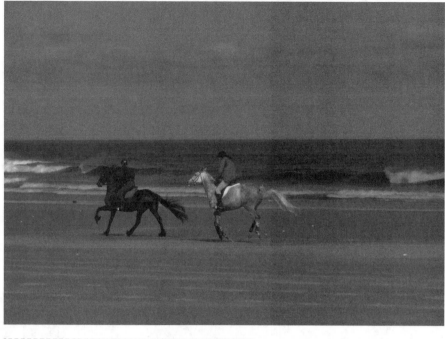

Horseback riders gallop beside the surf at Crane Beach.

1925, no longer enamored of the house, Crane had it demolished and replaced by the smaller but no less grand Georgian-style mansion that still looks down from the hill today.

Upon settling in, Crane soon fancied owning all that surrounded him. And so, turning desire to action, he bought up Wigwam, Sagamore, and Caverly Hills; Woodbury's Landing opposite Hog Island; both Hog Island and Patterson's Islands; and another farm across the creek. The sum total amounted to about 3,500 acres.

Miffed that the 5-mile Great Neck Beach had passed into Crane's hands with no review by the selectman, despite the town's claim of perpetual ownership, locals were not quiet about their resentment. But with an ear cocked, Crane heard their murmuring and responded affably by inviting the entire Ipswich school population of 900 to his son Cornelius's birthday party. Henceforth the outing became an annual event, and as time passed, people accepted Crane's ownership and gradually referred to the beach simply as "Crane's."

In 1945, fourteen years after her husband's death on his 58th birthday, Florence Crane gave 1,000 acres, including most of Crane's Beach and Castle Neck, to the Trustees of Reservations. When she died only four years later, she bequeathed also the "Great House" and an additional 300 surrounding acres.

From the out-of-town visitor parking lot to the right of the entrance, take the southernmost boardwalk to the beach. If it is a warm, clear day, you will want to free your feet from your shoes and socks, sink your toes in the sand, and feed your eyes on the Prussian blue sea before diverting your attention back to land.

When the air is particularly dry and particle free, you can see as far north as Maine's Mount Adamenticus. The Isles of Shoals lying off the coast of Portsmouth, New Hampshire, may also be visible as dark slivers on the horizon. On most days absent of heavy weather, Newburyport's Plum Island is visible stretching close to Ipswich's now thickly populated Great Neck and Little Neck, located on the left, opposite the mouth of Foxcreek and the toilet tycoon Cornelius Crane's grand estate at Castle Hill.

On a beach as beautiful and appealing to the senses as Crane's, to wander directionless, willy-nilly as your spirit wills, makes more sense than following a prescribed route. This hike therefore invites—even assumes—improvisation as it leads from the water-lapped tide line to the deep sands of Crane's highest inner dunes and back.

Having stretched driving muscles and exposed your pent-up thoughts to the robust winds ever reconfiguring the ground you stand on, turn to the right and lay footprints eastward. Though New England's beach season is understood to run from the first day of summer through Labor Day, a good many natives of towns such as Ipswich know that the beach is at its most sublime in the autumn and is certainly at its most dramatic during the frozen winter months. Swimmers should note that, though warmer than Plum Island, the water at Crane's Beach numbs limbs all months of the year but is tolerable in August, particularly at low tide, after sizzling sands have passed the sun's energy onto the retreating sea.

If the tide is high or rising fast, the path will lead across loose, finely ground granite sand sparkling with mica. In places, veins of feldspar color the sand a hard, heat-absorbing purple. Wriggle your heals in as you walk through these spots to make the beach squeak or "sing." At low tide, chances are the lively waves and the piping plovers sprinting between them on blurred spindle legs will lure you to the glistening packed sand in the intertidal zone.

Crane's is one of just three locations in North America where piping plovers are known to rear young. Reliant on undisturbed beaches, piping plovers lay their eggs directly on the sand in abbreviated nests. Where their traditional nesting grounds have been compromised by development and other human activity, breeding pairs have been known to try their luck in paved parking lots. Consequently, these small birds that subsist on aquatic and terrestrial invertebrates are several flittering heartbeats away from extinction. For this reason, the Trustees of Reservations ask beach visitors to help them protect their resident plovers by staying out of sensitive nesting areas.

Crane's, like any beach or natural coastal area, is highly plastic. Hurricane forces and each gentle afternoon breeze act to reshape the beach's contours. Generations ago, dunes cast deep shadows all along the peninsula from one end to the other. Today, the beach sands lie flatter, spreading to the east like the palm of a great, submerged hand. When gravitational forces tip the water toward Asia twice a day, pools form, adding exciting alterations to the beachscape. Crosscurrents furrow these flats in a wet, sandy corduroy, concealing razor clams and the beefier bivalve—the sea clam.

Should a stiff wind, the sight of a kite, or a like distraction bid you to turn and walk backward across this stretch, a half mile on you will find the Crane Castle hidden behind a bend. Looking ahead, you will see Cape Ann against the horizon. Following a trajectory of your own choosing, look to the dunes gaining in magnitude to the right and you will find a passage to the inner beach. Until this point, wire fencing restricts foot traffic to the seaweed-laced high-water mark and sands lying to the east.

Turn here and follow this wide, wire avenue westward into the muffled sands beyond. Knife-sharp blades of beach grass fall in wind-tussled waves over the banks alongside. Without this grass and its binding roots, there would be no dunes.

The trail's grade steepens to crest a dune several hundred feet in. Striding, half sliding, down the other side, you come to a level junction. Bear left to take the yellow trail south. Insulated by sand granules piled to great depths, the air in the still valleys is warmer and softer than the biting salt air blowing off the sea. In this unique microclimate, intriguing plants take root. Mushrooms—that when dry burst into star shapes—dot the trail amid bayberry bushes.

After winding along the rim of a bog lying to the right, the trail serpentines southeastward funneling through dune clefts before climbing to a sandy pinnacle overlooking the beach's southernmost tip. Pause here to survey Gloucester's Wingarsheek Beach on the opposite shore, the channel waters flowing past Conomo Point to Essex Harbor, and the uplands surrounding the Crane family's Great House to the northwest.

Continue following numbered yellow trail markers as they lead across Castle Neck and deliver you to a spot directly across from Choate, or Hog Island, as it is informally known. This beautiful island with a humble name has the distinction of being the birthplace of Senator Rufus Choate, the burial place of Cornelius Crane, and the setting for much of Nicholas Hytner's film *Crucible*.

This stretch of beach on a secluded cove receives more visitors by boat than by foot, and few at that. Occasionally, harbor seals swim ashore here to enjoy some sun or respite from life at sea. In certain months, vast numbers of romantically minded horseshoe crabs mingle in the shallow waters looking like armored military vehicles on reconnaissance.

Leave the yellow trail and make your own track southeast along the neck's thin fringe of beach. On the mild October afternoon I hiked these sands, game monarch butterflies fluttered northward, crossing the channel against a stiff breeze. Considering the size of their motors concocted of milkweed and hocus-pocus within cocoons, their quest to reach the dunes 100 yards beyond seemed disastrously quixotic. But milkweed, goldenrod, tansy, and asters must generate energy beyond the wildest dreams of oilmen, for these fire-colored bugs were achieving the impossible. Tossed in all directions by heartless gusts, they fluttered onward, making headway like battened-down beetle cats sailing seaward into heavy weather.

As you round the peninsula's tip, the wind will catch you at a different angle. Heading west with hair clutching at your face or blown straight out behind you, you'll see the beach broaden again. Catty-corner to Gloucester's Halibut Point, mixed flocks of gulls congregate where a foamy seam marks a crosscurrent. Soon, bending northwest, Plum Island comes into view, followed by the cottages and the water tower on Great Neck, and finally Crane's Castle nestled regally on its hill. Cut back into the loose sand of the seaweed-strewn upland to find the first of the two boardwalks when fading light, foul weather, or a growling stomach sends you back to your car.

NEARBY ATTRACTIONS

Any trip to Crane Beach should include a stop at Russells Orchard (phone [978] 356-5366), located enroute to the beach at 143 Argilla Road. From April 28 through November 25, this family-run business sells fresh fruits, vegetables, baked goods (including scrumptious cider donuts and delectable pies), hot and cold beverages, and fine fruit wines made on site. Between sips of coffee and tasty bites, there is plenty more to tempt or distract you, including a selection of books by local authors, potted perennials, pumpkins, and friendly farm animals.

Those looking for a hearty meal of local seafood might like to try one of the many restaurants located on MA 133 between Ipswich and Essex. To reach MA 133 from Crane Beach drive approximately 0.5 miles on Argilla Road, bear left onto Northgate Road, and continue to the end. At the intersection of Northgate Road and MA 133, turn left and continue 3 miles to Main Street in Essex.

If you trust local opinion, go no farther than Village Restaurant, located at 55 Main Street. Village Restaurant is open Tuesday through Sunday, 11:30 until 8 p.m., 9 p.m. on Friday and Saturday; call (978) 768-6400 for more information.

08 HALIBUT POINT: Quarry Loop

KEY AT-A-GLANCE INFORMATION

LENGTH: 2 miles

CONFIGURATION: Loop

DIFFICULTY: Moderate

SCENERY: Views of granite quarries and the magnificent Cape Ann coast

EXPOSURE: Mostly sunny; some shaded areas

TRAFFIC: Moderate

TRAIL SURFACE: Packed earth leading to the coast, and great granite boulders along the tidal zone

HIKING TIME: 1.5 hours, depending on weather conditions

SEASON: Year-round 8 a.m.–sunset

ACCESS: Parking $2

MAPS: Available at visitor center and at the ranger's booth at the entrance to the parking lot

FACILITIES: Restrooms and picnic tables

SPECIAL COMMENTS: Halibut Point is an excellent spot for bird-watching. In 1997, a renewable-energy demonstration center was constructed on site.

WHEELCHAIR TRAVERSABLE: The paths to the visitor center and to the main quarry are wheelchair accessible.

DRIVING DISTANCE FROM BOSTON COMMON: 32 miles

IN BRIEF

Shaped by geologic forces, glacial ice sheets, the chisels and sweat of quarrymen, and crashing waves off the Atlantic, Halibut Point is as variable as the weather. On warm summer days this knuckle of granite facing the sea offers a pleasant place to sunbathe and picnic. In less benign seasons the point is a terrific place to watch nature flex its muscles.

DESCRIPTION

Legend has it that the first house built on Rockport's hardscrabble turf was erected around the bend from Halibut Point in 1692. As told by authors Copeland and Rogers in their book *The Saga of Cape Ann,* the "Old House," as it is known locally, was built by two young men from Salem for their mother, who had been condemned at the Salem Witch Trials. Spared death because she was pregnant, the woman was expelled from the community and exiled to the wilderness of Cape Ann. Bears, wolves, and Agawam Indians accented the landscape, along with a handful of hunting shanties built by settlers of Ipswich.

In *The Town on Sandy Bay: A History of Rockport,* Marshall W. S. Swan writes that until 1840 when it was incorporated as an independent town, the vast acreage that is

---

Halibut Point:
Quarry Loop

UTM Zone (WGS84) 19T

Easting: 366357

Northing: 4727311

Latitude: N 42° 41' 12"

Longitude: W 70° 37' 53"

Directions

From Boston, take MA 128 north toward Gloucester. At the first traffic circle, go three quarters of the way around and take MA 127 toward Pigeon Cove. Continue 5 miles, passing through the villages of Annesquam and Lanesville. The parking lot is 1 mile into Lanesville on Gott Avenue, across from the Old Farm Inn.

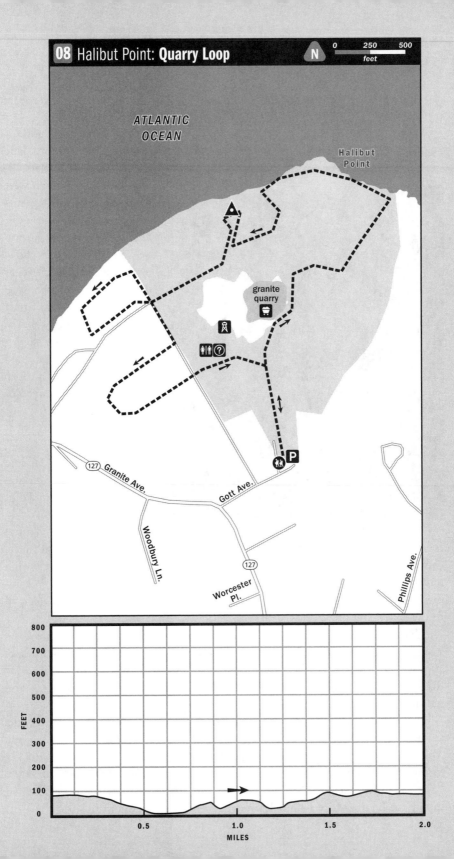

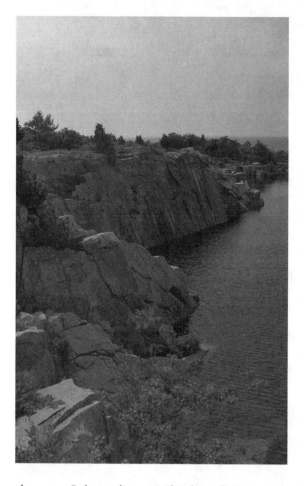

now Rockport was nothing more than commons land to Gloucester's settlers. Its woods and open fields were forage ground for dry milk cows, oxen on the dole, and horses unfit for harness or saddle. In time, however, the voting citizenry decided that all the land from Lane's Cove to Sandy Bay—as Rockport was first known—should be apportioned to qualified tax-paying householders born in Gloucester who were 21 years of age or older.

One qualifying beneficiary was John Babson, who was provided land to establish a fishing station southeast of Halibut Point at Gap Head. Soon after building himself a cabin at the spot, Babson discovered a bear living nearby. Uninterested in fostering a commensal relationship with the animal, Babson put an end to the bear with a hunting knife, skinned it, and strung its hide over a rock by the sea to dry. Passing fishermen caught sight of the bear's shaggy remains and henceforth referred to the rough spit of land as "Bearskin Neck."

The craggy coast north of Gloucester's Sandy Bay grew slowly through the 1700s. Characterized by thin soil rich in little besides granite and tiny harbors exposed to violent seas, the land lent itself to few lucrative enterprises. And yet Rockport's first families, the Tarrs, the Pools, and the Babsons, hung on and multiplied.

Driven from Saco, Maine, by warring natives, Richard Tarr moved his young wife and two sons from temporary safe haven in Marblehead to Cape Ann in 1695. A lumberman by trade, Tarr saw opportunity in the cape's thickly forested land. John Pool shared Tarr's vision and relocated his family to Sandy Bay from Beverly to establish the first sawmill. Together, they and others helped supply the boatloads of hemlock needed for wharf building in Boston.

As the trees dwindled, the fishing industry began to take hold and the shipping trade expanded. But the Revolutionary War, and the War of 1812, severely dampened the commercial vitality of Cape Ann. Many fishing boats were sunk and trade ships shackled, seized, or destroyed during these conflicts.

In the mid-1800s, Nehemiah Knowlton, another of Gloucester's enterprising men, introduced a new industry to Cape Ann—stone quarrying. Upon noting the success of Quincy's quarries, Knowlton took a chance and cut 500 tons of granite at Pigeon Cove and advertised it for sale in a Boston newspaper.

By 1860, the cape's quarries employed 450 workers, and 100 more manned the sloops that ferried the granite to ports as far away as San Francisco, Cuba, and South America.

The Chain Link Bridge that spans the Merrimac River near Maudslay State Park in Newburyport is constructed of Cape Ann granite, as is Boston's Post Office Building and Longfellow Bridge.

For nearly a century, men equipped first with hand tools and eventually steam-powered tools and dynamite cut stone from Babson Farm Quarry at Halibut Point. It was the crash of 1929 and the emergence of concrete that finally closed the industry down.

Cross Gott Avenue at the northwest corner of the parking lot to pick up a wooded path to the visitor center. Halfway along, you will pass two small quarries, with narrow trails leading to them to the right. Filled with rainwater and well camouflaged by vines and scrub, these excavations leave a great deal to the imagination. Not so the enormous quarry at trail's end.

Arriving at a broad T–intersection—you will feel the rush of bracing air and catch a view of the sea. Shifting your focus from the distant waves to the foreground, you will find an enormous water-filled cavity before you. Herring gulls and ducks now bob on thin ripples raised by wind gusting across this old work site where, men cut great slabs of rock, producing this enormous void.

Take the trail to the left to find the visitor center, or continue walking along the edge of the quarry on the gravel path past sparse woods of cherry, sumac, and blackberries. Markers along the quarry coordinate with a self-guided tour.

Heading northeast, you pass the quarry to your left as you turn toward the ocean. After walking a short distance downhill, you will find a narrow, packed-earth path leading off to the right. Leave the gravel trail and pick up this new path traveling northeast. At the next fork, take the right-hand path to continue eastward.

Close to the shore now, you will see wild beach roses which, when blooming in the heat of summer, give off a heady scent—stronger than that of any cultivated counterpart. Stay to the right at each of the next splits to reach the easternmost end of the reservation. At the border, the trail turns toward the sea. Here you will come to a sign that reads "Sea Rocks this way."

"Sea Rocks" refers to the enormous boulders lying along the shoreline of Halibut Point. Consisting of sheets of granite mixed with irregular orbs tossed into heaps by quarrymen and the thunderous surf, Sea Rocks offers a dramatic setting for picnicking, tanning, surf-casting, tidal-pool gazing, and especially rock hopping. If your inclination is to do nothing at all, there is always plenty to watch, from day-sailors tacking off the point to migrating birds and spectacular weather in all seasons.

To continue your hike, make your way northwest, keeping the breaking waves to your right. No walk along here is ever the same since the tide level determines one's route, length of one's stride and one's ability or inclination to leap across chasms. Beware of low tide, when kelp and sea moss clinging to rocks make for treacherous footing.

Looking ahead, you will see a mountain of granite blocks tapering steeply to the sea. Walk or rock-hop to the base of this granite behemoth for a good look to appreciate the hours of sweat and muscle strain represented by this pile of castoffs. Though forces of nature have reshaped the pile, it was quarrymen who heaved the stone here.

Once you have taken in this impressive sight backtrack to a broad sandy trail leading off to the right. The trailhead is not formally marked, but a sign warning of the dangers of swimming off the point alerts you to the turn, as does the miniature Stonehenge just inside the bend. Impromptu artists have arranged palm-sized quarry remnants into intriguing sculptures in a sandy enclosure just off the path.

Follow the gravel trail back uphill, and once at the top, bear right to walk to the lookout on the peak of the mountain of quarry debris. From this point, on a clear day, it is possible to see as far north as Maine's Mount Agamenticus, and in the nearer distance, Plum Island of Newburyport.

Leaving the peak, walk back toward the visitor center and the lighthouse. To tour the grounds, turn right and follow the wide path westward past birch, sumac, and cedar trees. A short way farther, turn onto the Bayview Trail to head back toward the sea. This trail descends steeply then rises again as it curves westward. Looking up, you're likely to see a flock of cormorants fly by, traveling from rookery to fishing grounds.

Curving back uphill, the Bayview Trail loops southwest past a grassy overlook. A small trail to the right leads to another lookout. Returning to the Bayview Trail, follow it to its end, then continue straight ahead on a wide gravel path.

Look for a sign for the Back 40 Loop, and take this grassy route westward, walking downhill before swinging left to head south once more on this peaceful "lane."

Closing the loop, you find yourself back at the clearing where you began. From this junction, continue straight to join the trail that leads to the rear of the visitor center. Keep left to pass in front of the visitor center and rejoin the path that leads back to the parking lot.

PLUM ISLAND: Hellcat Trail

IN BRIEF

This hike explores a once all but impenetrable swamp and night heron colony located at the midway point of Plum Island. Traveling over an elevated boardwalk, the hike surveys the freshwater marsh of the Parker River Wildlife Refuge, passes through Plum Island's inner beach, then crests enormous dunes to reach a lookout over the Atlantic Ocean.

DESCRIPTION

In days long gone, there was not a more remote and forbidding place on Plum Island than Hellcat Swamp. Marm Small harvested cranberries and provided board to "Gundalow men," (those who shuttled salt hay from the marsh to Newbury's Old Town on flat-bottom barges) at Halfway Farm located just across the mouth of the Parker River; and duck hunters set up camps farther south at a beach in a cove called The Knobbs—but few passed through the swamp that lies between.

Tides, terrain, and weather have long conspired to make the center of the island inaccessible at best and deadly at worst. Newburyport's

---

Directions

From Boston, take Storrow Drive East, following signs for US 1 north. Merge onto US 1 north toward Tobin Bridge/Revere. At 15.1 miles, merge onto I-95 north. From I-95, take Exit 57 and travel east on MA 113 to MA 1A south to the intersection with Rolfe's Lane; continue 0.5 miles to its end. Turn right onto Plum Island Turnpike and travel 2 miles, crossing Sergeant Donald Wilkinson Bridge to Plum Island. Take the first right onto Sunset Drive and travel 0.5 miles to the refuge entrance. Continue 3.5 miles to the Hellcat Wildlife Observation area on the left.

KEY AT-A-GLANCE INFORMATION

LENGTH: 1.84 miles
CONFIGURATION: Double loop
DIFFICULTY: Easy to moderate
SCENERY: Salt marsh, the inner beach, sand dunes, and the Atlantic Ocean
EXPOSURE: Equal parts sun and shade
TRAFFIC: Moderate
TRAIL SURFACE: Packed earth
HIKING TIME: 30–45 minutes
SEASON: Year-round sunrise–sunset
ACCESS: The daily entrance fee is $5 per car, $2 for people on foot or bicycle.
MAPS: Available at the Parker River National Wildlife Refuge headquarters and visitor center (6 Plum Island Turnpike, Newburyport, MA 01950), at the gatehouse, and at the trailhead, while supplies last.
FACILITIES AND COMMENTS: See longer note at end of description.
WHEELCHAIR TRAVERSABLE: A small section of trail located off the southernmost parking area (7) is specially designed for wheelchair users. In addition, Pines Trail (located at parking area 5) and many of the wildlife-observation areas are wheelchair accessible.
DRIVING TIME FROM BOSTON COMMON: 38 miles

Plum Island:
Hellcat Trail
UTM Zone (WGS84) 19T
Easting: 353028
Northing: 4733673
Latitude: N 42° 44' 29"
Longitude: W 70° 47' 44"

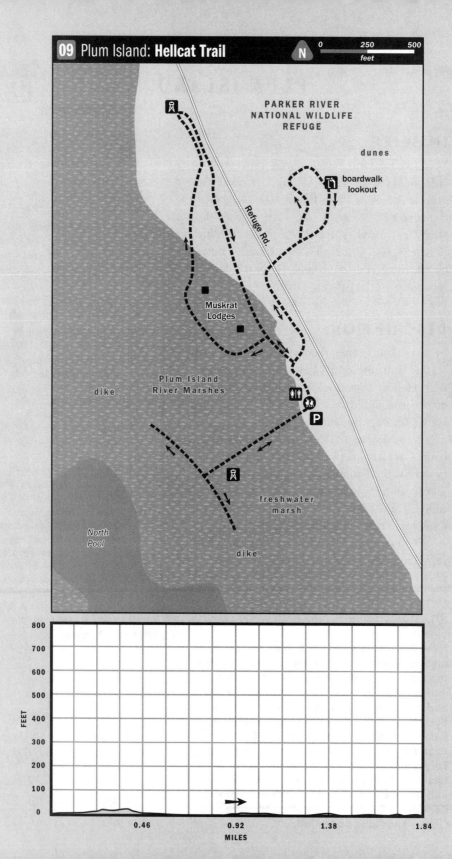

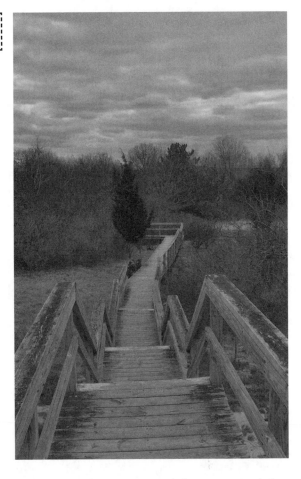

Crossing the inner beach, the boardwalk scales lofty dunes.

town records document more than one unfortunate episode involving Plum Island's marshes and beach. One such story is that of Richard Jackman and his young son who, in the winter of 1798, made a trip to the island for wood and, on heading for home the following day, succumbed to the elements after being forced from their boat and trying to continue on foot.

Before 1942, when Audubon turned over its Annie H. Brown Wildlife Sanctuary to the federal government, allowing it to become part of the Parker River National Wildlife Refuge, there was no way of reaching Hellcat Swamp other than by boat or by foot. After acquiring the land, the government constructed the access road that now runs the entire length of the island. Tragically, in building the road workers inadvertently destroyed an enormous black-crowned night heron rookery at Hellcat Swamp.

Today, thanks to an elevated boardwalk, it is possible for nearly everyone to venture into the farthest reaches of the swamp and the inner beach that insulates the swamp from the sea.

Begin at the trailhead located north of the parking lot beside the path that leads northwest to a wildlife lookout tower. Step up onto the boardwalk and follow it south through bayberry bushes to a junction where the trail divides in two. To start the hike with a tour of Plum Island's dunes, bear right and continue east.

Ahead, where the boardwalk bends north to cross the island, the trail passes through woodland where black oak and red maples grow in an oasis created by the weather-shielding dunes and marsh. Farther along, the boardwalk reaches an area where freshwater vernal pools form when hard-hitting storms bore craters in the sand. As sources of rain fed fresh water, these pools are critical to the

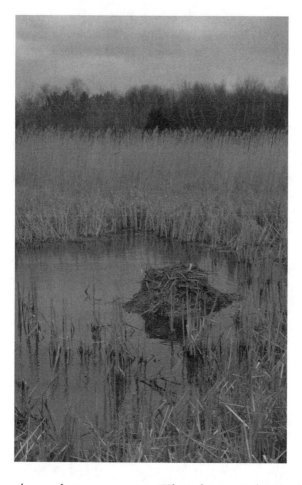

Several muskrat families live in Hellcat Swamp.

island's mammals and the amphibians that inhabit them.

After bearing east once more, the trail is bisected by the access road. Cross carefully, then take up the boardwalk again as it climbs into the beach's back dunes. Little besides tenacious black cherry trees (*Prunus serotina*) and cedars grow here.

In the interest of observing the island's distinct ecological zones in the sequence in which they were formed, continue left at the split beyond the road. As the trail emerges from the shelter of the inner dunes and proceeds through the more exposed territory of secondary dunes, botanical changes become apparent. Where fierce wind and salt spray are able to penetrate, only specially adapted plants such as beach heather (*Hudsonia tomentosa*) manage to survive. They, in turn, function to stabilize the ever-shifting sands by holding the dunes with a netting of dense roots. On the western slopes of the next dunes, bayberries and beach plums (*Prunus maritima*) grow in sheltered niches.

An incongruous stand of black pine (*Pinus nigra*) adds a thick wedge of trees ahead to the northeast. Native to Austria and other parts of Europe where conditions approximate the austerity of a New England beach, these trees were planted as part of a dune-stabilization effort in 1953. Although the black pine took hold successfully, the project was of dubious merit. What scientists understand now but didn't then is that barrier islands quell forces—such as hurricane winds—by deadening them with the drag of sand and waterlogged marsh peat. Tampering with this natural system does nothing but impair its performance.

Bearing right at a memorial to conservationist Ludlow Griscom, the trail travels eastward, crossing a lull in the rolling dunes where breeze-blurred footprints of small animals mark the sand among tufts of heather. The Joppa Flats and the Merrimack River are visible to the left across a landscape dominated by sky. Sound-swallowing walls of sand block sight of all but a sliver of Prussian-blue Atlantic to the east.

Sloping uphill toward primary dunes that sit like sand-castle replicas of Everest beside the ocean, the trail scales neat sets of stairs to reach a final climb to a lookout constructed behind one last great dune. On a clear day, Cape Ann takes the form of a solid purple-brown bar on the eastern horizon. To the right, the pale band of Crane Beach stretches south to Essex.

From the lookout, the trail descends steep stairs as it retreats back under tree cover on its return southwest. After recrossing the access road, retrace steps over the boardwalk to the trail's initial fork, and this time bear right onto the Marsh trail.

Where the trail splits a short way in, follow it left as it departs high ground dense with bayberry and beach plum for open marsh thick with cattails.

Though once part of the Great Salt Marsh stretching up the Parker River and beyond, the freshwater marsh immediately surrounding Hellcat Swamp is man-made. In the 1940s and 1950s, the Fish and Wildlife Service created the marsh to aid the recovery of populations of waterfowl species and other native and migratory birds. By building an enormous dike around it, they cut the marsh off from the sea's tidal currents.

Elevated about three feet above the floodplain of the marsh, the boardwalk bears west then eases north to circle territory claimed by two families of muskrats. The tops of their lodges of woven reed stalks rise a foot or so above the pool.

In winter months all is quiet except for the eerie sounds of the wind whistling through weather-bleached reed stalks, and a marsh hawk's occasional call. But as early as March, migratory birds arrive and fills the silence with a symphony of honks, screeches, and chirps. Upward of 350 species have been sighted on the island, and Hellcat Swamp is a favorite viewing location. Purple martins arrive in mid-April as do hundreds of American kestrels, sharp-shinned hawks, and other raptor species. Come the waning days of spring, waves of warblers, thrushes, vireos, fly-catchers, and other songbirds arrive and settle to rejuvenate and nest.

After arching out to a lookout station that provides a view over the northern freshwater pool and the town of Newbury beyond, the trail aims east and returns to high ground. Upon reaching a junction, bear left to access a wildlife lookout.

Returning by the same path, bear left at the next fork in the boardwalk and continue south through the shrub land that borders the marsh. Sharp white birches lean into the breeze above an otherwise tangled thicket. In August ripening beach plums add a fruity scent to the air, mixing with the smells of salt water and sunscreen. Continue straight at the next fork then bear right at the last to arrive back at the trailhead.

Extend the hike by following the trail to the right of Hellcat Trail to a lookout tower positioned beside the dike and the freshwater pools.

Note about facilities: There are no concession stands on the reservation; however, there are several restaurants and shops located where the Plum Island Turnpike ends just outside the reservation entrance. Facilities at Hellcat Swamp include restrooms, an information center, a public boat launch, and many wildlife observation areas.

Special comments: Although Plum Island's 6.3-mile beach is closed from April 1 to August 31 to allow piping plovers to nest and rear their chicks, the Hellcat Trail remains open all year. Also, being an interpretive trail and entirely boardwalk, it is convenient for less able-bodied lovers of the outdoors and for families with small children. For those interested in increasing their hiking time, options include adding the Pine Wood Trail, located south of the Hellcat Trail and/or the Sandy Point Trail that loops around the southern end of the island opposite Ipswich Bay (see hike number 10).

NEARBY ATTRACTIONS

Newburyport boasts an assortment of attractions, including many historic homes listed on the National Register of Historic Places. An historic locale of unique appeal to boat lovers is Lowell's Boat Shop, located in nearby Amesbury. The boat shop opened for business in 1793 and has been producing dories continuously ever since. For information about the boat shop, call (978) 388-0162. For information, schedules, and listings of special events, visit Historic New England's Web site, **www.historicnewengland.com.** Though steeped in history, Newburyport is a vibrant commercial and cultural center with many excellent restaurants. The town's independent cinema, The Screening Room, shows films frequently overlooked by mainstream megaplexes. To check show times, call (978) 462-3456 or consult the Web site: **www.newburyportmovies.com.**

PLUM ISLAND: Sandy Point Loop 10

IN BRIEF

On this exploration of the southernmost tip of Plum Island you will forge your own trail around a drumlin known as Bar Head to reach Ipswich Bluffs (Stage Island). From Stage Island, the Sandy Point Trail leads into the shelter of dunes and salt marsh to complete the loop.

DESCRIPTION

An exclamation point is nothing without the dot below the vertical slash; similarly, Plum Island would not be the 8-mile-long barrier beach it is today without the drumlin poised at its southern tip. Without this static, rounded mound and the several others lined up north of it, the sand and silt caught in the riptides and weather would not have settled here crystal upon crystal to form the island's silica snake of dunes.

Planetary forces conspired to shape Plum Island 6,000–7,000 years ago. Along with unrelenting wind and waves and earthquakes along the Parker River fault line, subsiding

KEY AT-A-GLANCE INFORMATION

LENGTH: 2.38 miles
CONFIGURATION: Loop
DIFFICULTY: Easy to moderate
SCENERY: Beach and views of the Atlantic Ocean, Ipswich Bay, and salt marshes adjoining Plum Island Sound and the Parker River
EXPOSURE: Full sun
TRAFFIC: Moderate
TRAIL SURFACE: Sand, packed earth, and a short section of paved road
HIKING TIME: 1 hour
SEASON: Year-round sunrise–sunset
ACCESS: Entrance fee is $5 per car, and $2 for people on foot or bicycle.
MAPS: Available at the information center located at the gatehouse; more information and resources are also available at the refuge headquarters, located on Rolfe's lane just off Plum Island Turnpike.
FACILITIES: Restrooms, information center, public boat launch, and many wildlife observation areas. There are no concession stands on the reservation; however, there are several restaurants and shops located where Plum Island Turnpike meets the northern end of the island.
DRIVING DISTANCE FROM BOSTON COMMON: 38 miles

Directions

From Boston, take Storrow Drive east, following signs for US 1 north. Merge onto US 1 north toward Tobin Bridge/Revere. At 15.1 miles, merge onto I-95 north. From I-95, take Exit 57 and travel east on MA 113 to MA 1A south to the intersection with Rolfe's Lane and continue 0.5 miles to the end of that road. Turn right onto Plum Island Turnpike and travel 2 miles, crossing the Sargent Donald Wilkinson Bridge to Plum Island. Take the first right onto Sunset Drive and travel 0.5 miles to the refuge entrance.

Plum Island:
Sandy Point Loop
UTM Zone (WGS84) 19T
Easting: 353037
Northing: 4733665
Latitude: N 42° 44' 29"
Longitude: W 70° 47' 44"

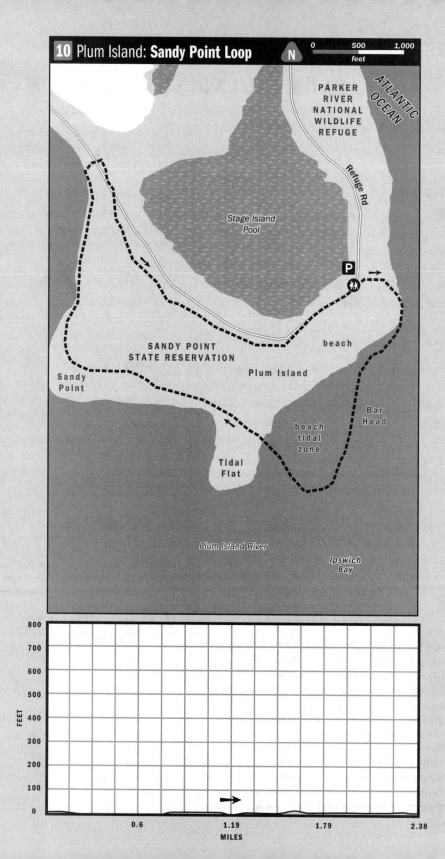

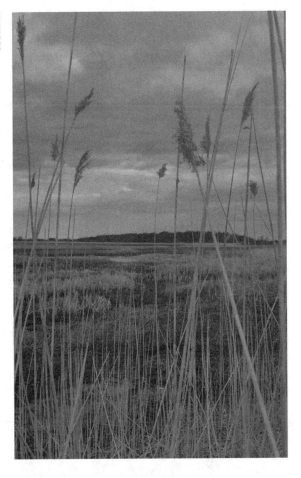

Looking across the Great Marsh to Rowley

earth and a rising sea level contributed to the island's creation. Once the beach materialized, the growing gap between the belt of sand and shore gradually filled to form freshwater marsh. Three thousand years ago, the sea level stabilized and for the most part, the island and its beach looked much like it does today—notwithstanding periodic rearrangement by hell-bent nor'easters.

As the area became populated in the decades following the 1635 arrival of Reverend Thomas Parker and company—and as wolves, bears, and Indians grew scarce—settlers ventured to the island with their rifles and cattle. Besides good grazing, thatch for their roofs, and teeming waterfowl, they discovered enormous quantities of beach plums. These they must have been especially happy about—despite the fruit's near mouth-blistering tartness—as they immediately came to call the sliver of land Plum Island.

Though apparently of little consequence to citizens of Ipswich and Newbury, Plum Island and all the land along the Atlantic from the Naumkeag River (Salem) to the Merrimack had in 1621 been granted to Captain John Mason by the president and council of Plymouth. Regardless, from the earliest days, Plum Island ("Isle Mason," to the Plymouth officials) was viewed as common land by the General Court and was made available to settlers of Ipswich, Newbury, and Rowley.

Captain Mason, it seems, was too distracted to notice or care. When Reverend Parker and company were investing their hearts and souls in their new settlement upriver from Ipswich, Mason was at work securing his right to an even larger territory north of the Merrimack, a holding he christened New Hampshire.

In any case, settlers were soon squabbling over their own rights to the land.

On March 15, 1649, acting on concerns for the economic viability of his settlement, Parker petitioned the General Court to grant all of Plum Island to Newbury. After eight months of rumination, the court finally ruled that the island should be divided into fifths, two fifths went to Ipswich, one to Rowley, and two fifths to Newbury. The island's fertile southernmost end and Sandy Point officially became part of Ipswich.

In the early days, aside from free-range pigs and other assorted livestock, Plum Island had few year-round residents. However, as is frequently the case with remote places, the island attracted seasonal hunters as well as those on the fringe.

At the end of the 1600s, a certain Elizabeth Perkins and her husband, Luke, settled around the bend from Bar Head on Grape Island to escape persecution from Ipswich mainlanders. The couple's ordeal began when Elizabeth was taken to court for accusing their minister of immorality and for speaking unflatteringly of her parents; for this, she was accused of being "a virulent, reproachful and wicked-tongued woman." Though the sound whipping to which she was sentenced was commuted to a three-pound fine, the Perkinses found that they had had enough of town life and set off for the island.

In 1769 Newbury and Newburyport combined resources and built a hospital, or "pest house," on the northern end of the island so that ships could drop off sailors stricken with smallpox or yellow fever before sailing on to Newburyport's harbor. Effectively quarantined, ill sailors were ordered to bury their clothes and other "soft goods" in the sand for nine days and to stay out of town until they either succumbed or were declared rid of disease.

As told by Nancy V. Weare in *Plum Island: The Way It Was,* besides the farmers who set up homesteads on such fertile glacial deposits as the Knobbs, Grape Island, and Cross Farm Hill, day-trippers and summertime vacationers populated the southern end of the island in increasing numbers from the late 19th century to the end of the 1920s. And all the while there were plenty of "gunners" getting away from it all as they set up in camps and bagged rack after rack of waterfowl. In 1881 Mr. Emerson, the proprietor of the Ipswich Bluffs hotel, claimed he killed 40 birds with just two shotgun blasts.

The place of many a grand plan, it is as much by luck as by sheer good sense that rather than being developed as a resort or residential community, the bulk of Plum Island was conserved as a wildlife refuge and park. By the 1890s the bird population was clearly in freefall as a result of year-round hunting and the loss of nesting grounds to development. So, in 1929, when a Stoneham woman named Annie Hamilton Brown willed a hefty sum to the Federation of Bird Clubs of New England the federation set to work purchasing tracts of Plum Island.

Working in tandem with the Massachusetts Audubon Society (with which it eventually merged) the federation succeeded in acquiring all the southern end of the island but Grape Island and Sandy Point (which is now state owned).

By offering $5 an acre for adjoining marshland, they managed to expand their holdings westward as well.

Regretably, Annie Brown's tremendous foresight and generosity are unknown to most because in 1943 Audubon sold the 1,600-acre Annie H. Brown Wildlife Sanctuary to the federal government, allowing it to merge with the Parker River National Wildlife Refuge.

From the Sandy Point Reservation parking area behind Bar Head, set out hiking east on the wide path that leads through dunes to the beach. With the ocean in full view, bear right and choosing a course through the many boulders, tree trunks, and other often curious tidal detritus, hike south toward the drumlin of Castle Hill, across the bay.

The boulders protruding from the sand and sea on the beach east of Bar Head are known as Emerson's Rocks. Being encrusted with barnacles and slick with seaweed, the exposed rocks are menacing enough, but when hidden by surf at high tide they are positively murderous.

Between 1772 and 1936, no fewer than 55 ships wrecked off Plum Island. Of these, 10 were dashed to pieces at Emerson Rocks. At least 27 more vessels—schooners, trawlers, and steamers—went down near the mouth of the Merrimack River. The treacherous Ipswich Bay channel claimed at least eight ships as they tried to enter Plum Island Sound from Ipswich Bay. Indeed, Newbury native Samuel Sewell (of Salem Witch Trail fame) wrote in his journal of getting stranded overnight at Sandy Point when he attempted to sail the strait against the wind in an ebbing tide.

Where the slope of Bar Head slides to meet marsh and dune on the neck's western side, ships, or "sand droghers," once loaded sand to be used for mortar in Boston. In the late 1800s, when this industry was at its height, each man of the three- to five-man crew was expected to move 50 tons of sand in the space of two tides.

When bearing west round the 'point, take care not to get trapped on the wrong side of a channel as the tide pours in—otherwise, be resigned to getting wet feet and possibly a drenching.

Documented finds along this stretch where the wind howls over the finger of upland called Ipswich Bluffs add credence to legends that pirates buried treasure in these parts. In 1907 the islander Albert Leet, of the lifesaving team stationed at the Knobbs made two exciting finds—the first was a silver coin dated 1749, then several days later more silver. Another summer resident found silver buckles apparently of ancient Spanish design close to where Leet had discovered the money.

Where the tree-covered upland of the Bluffs begins, a sign sends hikers north, away from the beach, to Stage Island. Take this turn and follow the lightly worn footpath into the shelter of brush. The trail is vague in places but generally cuts a line between the Stage Island estuary and dunes drifted against the western side of the Bar Head drumlin.

Although the wolves that once denned here are gone and the cacophony of honks and quacks from inconceivable numbers of game birds has been hushed, the wildness of the place is largely restored. Ancestors of the fox that darted away as British troops fighting in the War of 1812 came ashore to butcher an islander's cow live on, hunting voles and field mice at dusk; but barely a hint remains of the soldiers and farmsteading sea captains.

Where the Sandy Point Trail reaches the iron gate by a parking area beside upland and beach, cross the pavement, bearing left to follow the drive back to the entrance of the Sandy Point Reservation.

Note: Due to efforts to save the piping plover from extinction, nearly all of Plum Island's beach is closed every year from April 1 to August 31, but Sandy Point State Reservation remains open year-round. A hike on Sandy Point begins with the 8-mile drive from the reservation's entrance gate to the trailhead. Though slow, and dusty during dry summer months, the drive can be something of a safari—those on the alert are likely to spot a good deal of wildlife, some of it quite rare, such as the snowy owls which sometimes stop by in the spring, fall, and winter.

Wheelchair Access: A small section of trail located off the southernmost parking area (7) is specially designed for wheelchair users. In addition, Pines Trail (located at parking area 5) and many of the wildlife observation areas are wheelchair accessible.

NEARBY ATTRACTIONS

The town of Newburyport boasts an assortment of attractions, including many historic homes listed on the National Register of Historic Places. An historic locale of unique appeal to boat lovers is Lowell's Boat Shop, located in nearby Amesbury. The boat shop opened for business in 1793 and has been producing dories continuously ever since. For information about the boat shop, call (978) 388-0162. For information, schedules, and listings of special events, visit www .historicnewengland.org.

Though steeped in history, Newburyport is a vibrant commercial and cultural center with many excellent restaurants. The town's independent cinema, The Screening Room, shows films frequently overlooked by mainstream megaplexes. To check show times call (978) 462-3456 or consult the Web site: www .newburyportmovies.com.

NASKETUCKET BAY STATE RESERVATION HIKE 11

IN BRIEF

Once open grazing land for sheep, the Nasketucket Reservation now offers wooded trails and access to a beach on historic Buzzards Bay.

DESCRIPTION

By the time the burly *Acushnet* glided downriver from Fairhaven to Buzzards Bay breasting waves soon to break on Sconticut Neck and Nasketucket, the 21-year-old Herman Melville was sobering to the reality of life on a whaling ship. Describing the event through Ishmael, Melville, wrote, "As the short northern day merged into night, we found ourselves almost broad upon the wintry ocean, whose freezing spray cased us in ice, as in polished armor. The long rows of teeth on the bulwarks glistened in the moonlight; and like the white ivory tusks of some huge elephant, vast curving icicles depended from the bows."

Shipbuilding began in Mattapoisett in 1740, and by 1800 with four shipyards in operation, it was one of the East Coast's primary shipbuilding towns. When Fairhaven's whaling ship, the *Acushnet,* pulled anchor

KEY AT-A-GLANCE INFORMATION

LENGTH: 2.78 miles

CONFIGURATION: Double loop

DIFFICULTY: Easy

SCENERY: Woods, former farmland, and views of Nasketucket and Buzzards Bay, and on clear days Martha's Vineyard

EXPOSURE: A mix of sun and shade

TRAFFIC: Light

TRAIL SURFACE: Packed earth and beach sand

HIKING TIME: 1–2 hours including idle time on the beach

SEASON: Year-round sunrise–sunset

ACCESS: Free

MAPS: Posted on a kiosk in the parking lot

FACILITIES: None

SPECIAL COMMENTS: A great family hike, consider bringing bathing suits and a picnic to enjoy the rocky but pleasant beach

WHEELCHAIR TRAVERSABLE: Wheelchair users can access the full length of Bridle Trail.

DRIVING DISTANCE FROM BOSTON COMMON: 60 miles

Directions

From Boston take I-93 south. At Exit 4, merge left onto MA 24 south. After 18.3 miles, take Exit 14A toward Cape Cod, continue 19.7 miles, and at Exit 1 merge onto I-195 west. After 9.1 miles, take Exit 19A toward Mattapoisett, and at 0.3 miles merge onto North Street. After 0.9 miles, turn right onto US 6. Continue 1.7 miles on US 6 to a left turn onto Brandt Island Road. Follow Brandt Island Road, bearing left at the fork, then bear right at the sign for Brandt Beach Road. Park on the right at the Massachusetts Department of Environmental Management (DEM) sign.

Nasketucket Bay State
Reservation Hike
UTM Zone (WGS84) 19T
Easting: 346992
Northing: 4610931
Latitude: N 41° 38' 08"
Longitude: W 70° 50' 13"

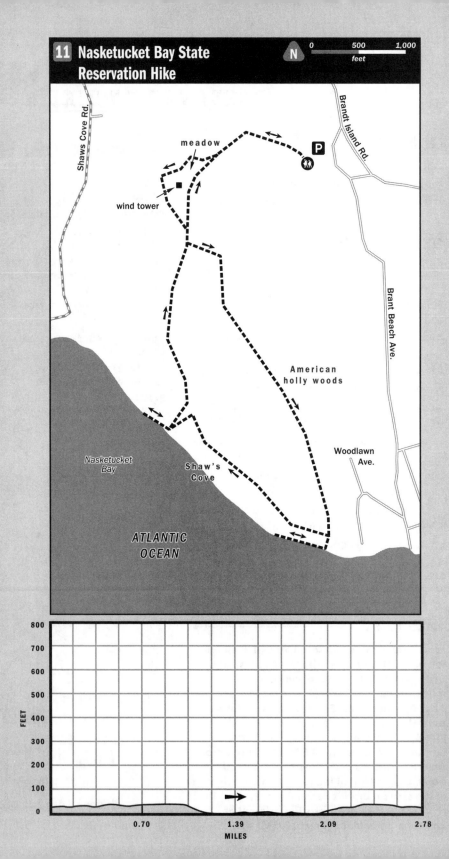

N

0   500   1,000
feet

Shaws Cove Rd.

Brandt Island Rd.

meadow

P

wind tower

Brant Beach Ave.

American
holly woods

Woodlawn
Ave.

Nasketucket
Bay

Shaw's
Cove

ATLANTIC
OCEAN

800
700
600
500
400
300
200
100
0

FEET

0.70   1.39   2.09   2.78

MILES

and set course for the waters off Polynesia, it had 16 or so sister ships to keep it company, though hundreds of miles often separated them.

From the kiosk at the head of the parking lot, follow a short connector path to the start of the Bridle Trail. Rolling wide and flat over a swath cut through woods and weeds, the trail bends farther west to meet the Meadow Trail just ahead. Bear right here and follow this narrower, somewhat overgrown path a few hundred yards behind wetland to another split. Keep left to step out from the dense thicket of blueberry bushes and tangled shrubs and proceed across the open grassland toward the needle-thin tower at the center. Because of light traffic and infrequent mowing, this path can be difficult to discern, therefore feel free to improvise.

Once part of a farm, this open meadow is now a refuge for flora and fauna, birds and insects. Fruit trees lean on the breeze to the north. The tower topped with propellers was erected by the state to collect wind data as part of an alternative-energy initiative. If the data shows the site to be suitable, wind turbines may eventually be installed.

South of the tower, the trail becomes more distinct. Hike along the meadow as it tapers to a point along the edge of woods to the right. Prickly blackberries reach through the grass and grab at pants cuffs as the trail filters into the Bridle Trail by a posted marker. Resuming this track, continue southeast several feet to where it meets the Holly Trail. Leave this sandy belt and turn left into the woods. Passing by white pines and sassafras over level ground, the path curves eastward. On the right, a stone wall fades behind tree limbs like a half-forgotten thought. And in the later part of summer, if the days have been hot but the air not too dry, you may spot frothy cream-colored cauliflower fungi (*Sparassis crispa*) erupting from the loose weave of pine needles and decaying deciduous tree leaves.

With plenty of maples, oaks, and basswood trees growing along the trail, it takes some time to notice the first of the holly trees. But as the trail continues south toward the seashore, the angular trees with elephant-gray limbs and tough, crinkled leaves soon become ubiquitous. Beyond a stretch where the trail dips and mud puddles form even in dry months, past a grove of beech trees, the trail surfaces from the woods to cross the sun-bleached tail of the Bridle Trail. Beyond this junction, the Holly Trail then continues on to Buzzards Bay. Silvery birch, oak, and sassafras mix with increasingly impressive hollies. A glance to the right over the stone wall running alongside the trail catches sharp slivers of light flashing off the water less than a mile away. Shooting like an arrow to the sea, the trail passes several minor paths cut by bushwhackers of the human or animal kind.

Sloping gently downhill, the trail soon arrives at a rocky beach and just before it, a right turn to the Shore Trail. Unless weather is gnashing its teeth, ditch plans and watches and head for the water. The fist at the end of a scrawny arm of rocks to the east is Brandt Island; Mattapoisett Neck and Antassawamock reach beyond

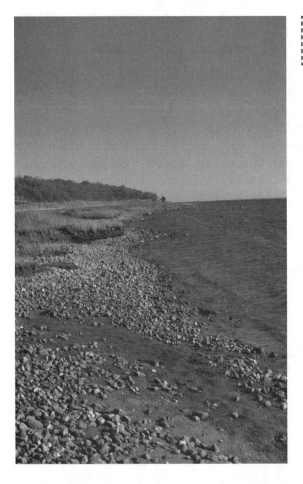

> With a sharp eye you might spot a seal in the bay or a hawk soaring over the marsh.

to Buzzard's Bay, Woods Hole lies approximately 11 miles farther south as the crow flies, and 6 miles farther still lies Vineyard Haven of Martha's Vineyard. When the heat of the sun abates, the wind picks up, or the last sandwich is eaten, quit the beach and backtrack to the head of the Shore Trail.

As you travel west 0.4 miles along the edge of land nibbled by storm surges, a thin canopy of trees grown in since farming days shelters the trail. Tipping to wetland, the path has some muddy patches where logs laid flat improve footing. After brushing past a boggy meadow, the trail snakes past an uncommonly large sassafras tree and a pine grove. More hollies of slight and mammoth girth follow, and after a swing to the left and another to the right, the trail spills into a grassy clearing. At this three-way junction, bear left to take up the Salt Marsh Trail, and head southwest back to the seashore.

Approaching the beach, this former cart road encounters a substantial stone bridge built over a channel. The view straight on is of Nasketucket Bay, with Sconticut Neck lying prone on the horizon. The tidal zone of the Nasketucket River lies to the right, and just before it is Shaw's Cove. Shallows behind the strip of sand left in a glacier's wake has filled in over the ages to form salt marsh. Vastly important to a panoply of endangered species, the marsh lying to the west is part of the South Shore Marshes Wildlife Management Area. If you harbor any lingering beach craving, hike to the right toward Shaw's Cove. A 5-foot granite spike jutting from the sand a hundred yards along serves as a handy destination point. After looping around this odd protuberance, head back to the Salt Marsh Trail.

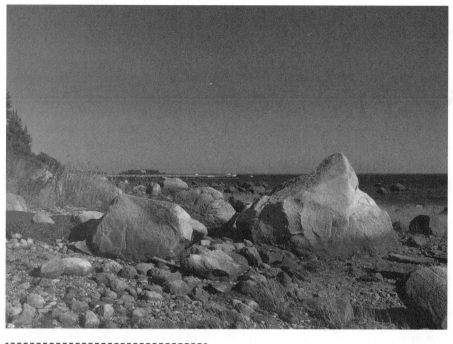

The fist of rock to the east is Brandt Island.

Passing blackberry bushes and beach roses, return to the grassy junction visited earlier and continue straight on the Salt Marsh Trail heading northeast. Starting wide and becoming narrower, the trail travels through woods. Climbing a subtle incline as it nears the Bridle Trail. At this split, keep to the left, beside the salt marsh. The Salt Marsh Trail soon turns to upland and once more crosses paths with the Bridle Trail. Appearances suggest that this trail once continued north, however the remainder of this old cart road is now overgrown, therefore bear left onto the tried-and-true Bridle Trail and follow it back to the parking lot.

NEARBY ATTRACTIONS

Any trip to the area ought to include a visit to the New Bedford Whaling Museum at 18 Johnny Cake Hill, New Bedford, (508) 997-0046. Admission is $10 for adults, $9 for senior citizens and students, $6 for children age 6 to 14, and free for children under 6. The museum is fully wheelchair accessible.

12 WORLD'S END TOUR

IN BRIEF

On this tour you will explore a spectacular peninsula, following its outer rim. Once a proposed site for the United Nations, landscaping touches of Frederick Law Olmsted are still apparent as are signs of the peninsula's agricultural past.

DESCRIPTION

World's End has always been associated with grand ambitions. Under the management of its longtime owner, John Brewer, the land supported a flourishing farm complete with its own blacksmith shop, greenhouses, smokehouse, windmill, and homes for the many farmhands. In 1889, Brewer's vision for the property changed, and he hired the landscape architect Frederick Law Olmsted to draw up a design for an elegant subdivision, one with 163 house plots, cart paths, and tree-lined roads. Yet the plan never developed past the drawing board. Later, in 1945, officials from the town of Hingham made a bid to have World's End selected as the site of the United Nations headquarters. Though town residents still boast that Eleanor Roosevelt exclaimed at the beauty of Hingham, planners of the United Nations passed it by. In 1965, the lovely World's End experienced another close call. In the year of

---

World's End Tour

UTM Zone (WGS84) 19T

Easting: 345622

Northing: 4680257

Latitude: N 42° 15' 33"

Longitude: W 70° 52' 18"

Directions

From Boston, take I-93 south to MA 3 (to Cape Cod). Take Exit 14 and follow MA 228 north 6.5 miles toward Hingham. Turn left onto MA 3A and follow it 0.4 miles. Turn right onto Summer Street and continue straight through a major intersection with Rockland Street. The road becomes Martin's Lane. Follow Martin's Lane 0.7 miles to its end.

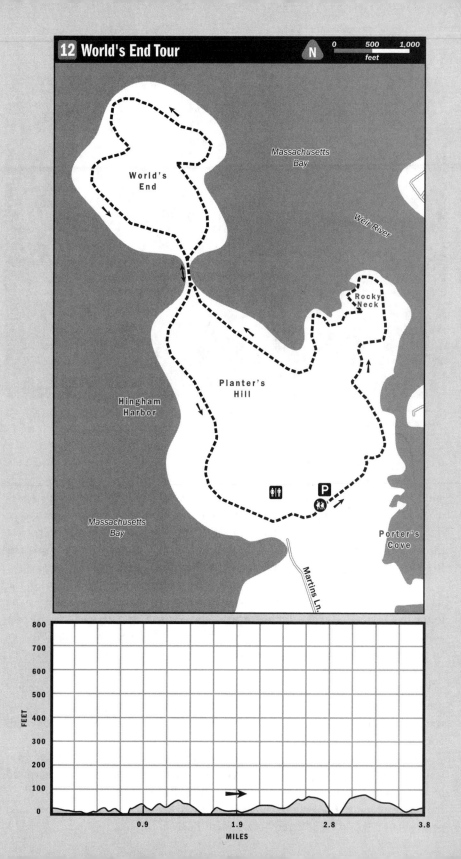

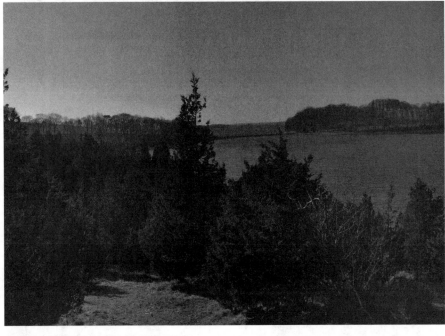

World's End as viewed from Rocky Neck

the most widespread blackout in history, World's End almost succumbed to a surging interest in nuclear power. Turf formerly trod by showy thoroughbreds and prizewinning Jersey cows nearly became the foundation for a nuclear power plant. In the end, Hingham's residents, rumored to be feverishly protective of their environment, thought better of this idea and voted down the plan. This last threat to this fantastic peninsula proved fortuitous as it prompted the Trustees of Reservations to insure its preservation by buying it two years later.

The trail begins at the northeast end of the upper parking lot. This path, the width of a carriage, heads directly into woods of oak and pine. Down a rocky slope to the left, you will catch a glimpse of a marshy bog and an open meadow. Farther along on the right, the trail opens to a marshy shore and a waterway called Porter's Cove. Houses dominated by porches sit close together on the opposite shore.

The path bends to the left after the water view and meets a trail splitting to the right. Take this narrower trail and looking through the eastern-side underbrush, you will see waves lapping at the rocky coast. On the left, pass a freshwater bog populated by ducks. Another fork and a small pond lie just beyond. Stay to the right, keeping with the water. The woods are dense here.

Circumnavigating this small outcropping, the trail undulates gently as it leads to tiny beaches hidden in the curve of the land. As the trail comes around to face north, you get a clear view of the Weir River and the town of Hull on the opposite bank. Looking to the west, you will see the great hourglass-shaped peninsula of World's End stretching toward Boston.

On Fourth of July weekend, scores of boats tie up here, one to another, displaying scantily clad revelers draped over their decks. In winter, on February's chilly President's Day weekend, the waters are empty except for a smattering of eider ducks and seagulls.

The trail comes back around, heading southeast as it reaches the base of Rocky Neck. At each of three forks, bear right, to head south. Dipping through a cedar thicket, the trail soon opens to meadowland. Leave the woods behind and walk uphill to the carriage road. Stepping onto this level, gravel path, head north, keeping the Weir River over your right shoulder.

In John Brewer's day, horses drew carriages along this route as dark-eyed jersey cows grazed on either side. Today there are no grazing herds, but, for the benefit of raptors, bluebirds, and bobolinks, the fields are mowed to keep them as they were when farmed. Under Olmsted's direction elm trees once draped branches over the avenue, however, since the Dutch elm disease epidemic, ashes now stand in place of the fabulous shade tree.

Follow the road as it eases downhill and arrives at sea level. Ahead, look for the glacial isthmus linking Planter's Hill to the northern tip of World's End. This spit of gravel and ground shells serves as a handy causeway.

Cross here, taking time for sun and maybe a swim, then follow the carriage road uphill, bearing right. Continuing northward, the carriage road soon reaches a split. When the road forks, proceed straight. This option takes you into what's referred to as the Valley. Shortly, this path reaches another junction. Turn sharply right and follow the trail as it circles the land counterclockwise. The road rises out of the dark woods of the Valley to lead back to a domed meadow. From here, Hull's waterfront homes look almost close enough to touch.

Upon reaching the end of the island, the road curves sharply south. This point affords a clear view of Boston. A wedge cut in the tree line and a bench invite hikers to stop for a good look at the city's skyline and smudged halo.

Continue along the road as it heads south along the western side of the reservation. Hingham Harbor lies to the right through the trees, at the bottom of a steep embankment. Listen for waves washing against the coarse boulders at the waterline. Keep walking beside the harbor when the trail merges with each of two routes coming from the east. Sitting well below the top of a meadow to your left, the trail gradually climbs as it approaches a northern lookout above the causeway.

Having completed the loop around World's End, make your way downhill to "The Bar" and cross back over to Planter's Hill. Unless the footpath etched into the face of this steep hill lures you, stay with the carriage road as it continues right. On the peak of the hill, you can find the site of one of the grand elms that once stood in Brewer's Grove. A stone memorial was placed at the spot to honor F. Arthur Edwards, the last of the Brewer's farmhands, who died in 1967.

As you gain elevation, the wind eases, and on a biting winter day, the sun suddenly feels a great deal warmer. Approaching the mainland, the road again eases downhill. Ashes tilt across from both sides interspersed with the occasional larch, oak, or linden. Soon, you will see a stone wall on the left, paralleling your

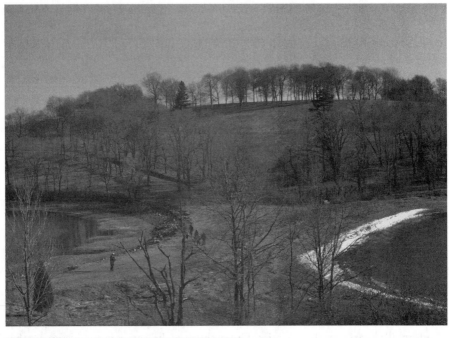

A glacial isthmus links Planter's Hill to World's End.

path. A little farther along, another stone wall picks up on the right, delineating fields that once held livestock. A few old apple trees hint at what were once productive orchards.

Quiet Martin's Cove bends in around Pine Hill to the left, and to the right you will see Damde Meadows. A project is under way to restore the meadow to the salt marsh it once was. Walking downhill to a causeway, you will see the tide spilling through from one side to the other. This wetland was previously dammed to add acreage to the farm's hay fields.

Straight ahead up a rise, you can spot the reservation's entrance. After the trail splits to the left, leave the cove and climb the granite steps. At the top, you'll find picnic tables set in a clearing overlooking the salt marsh estuary. Not far beyond, you will pass two outhouses before reaching the lower parking area.

Note: The Trustees of Reservations organizes occasional special events, such as evening owl watches. Horseback riding is allowed; the annual permit costs $100. Leashed dogs are welcome.

NEARBY ATTRACTIONS

Camping is available at Wampatuck State Park, in Hingham. You can help yourself to the healthy waters of Mount Blue Spring, located inside the park. To get there from World's End take, MA 128 west toward US 3 and turn left onto Free Street.

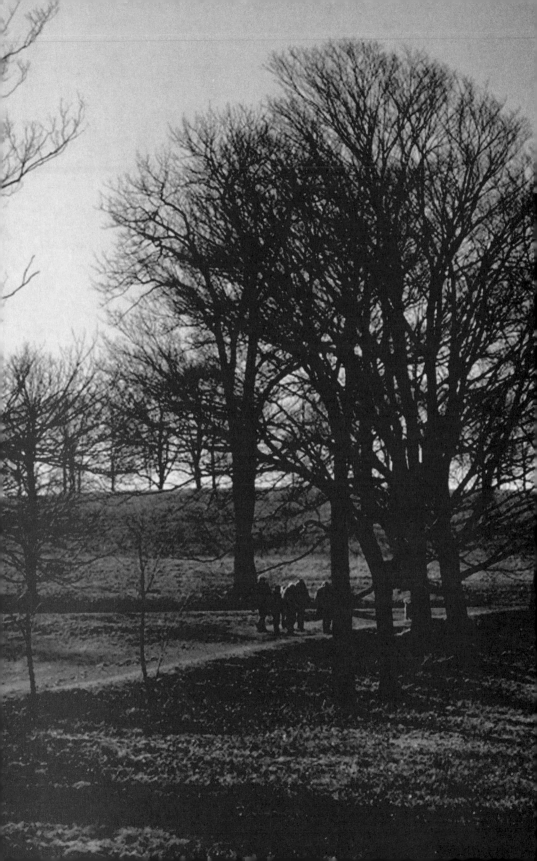

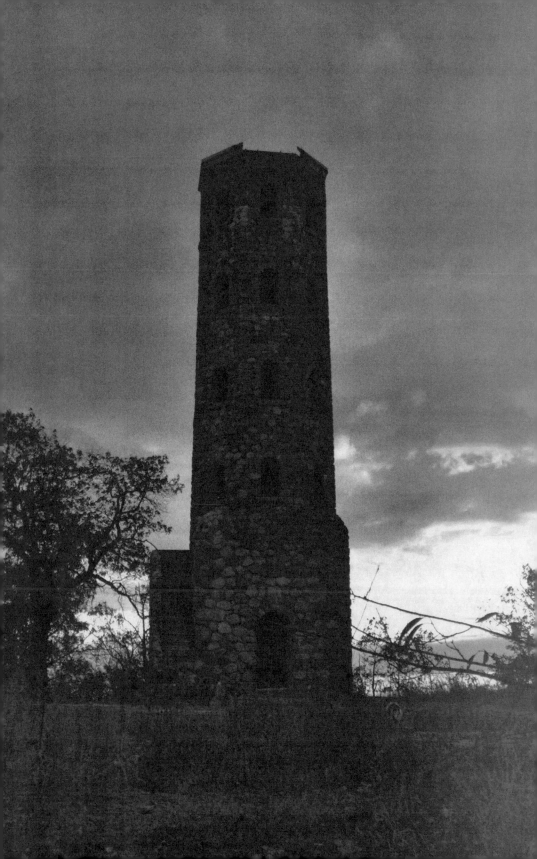

NORTH OF BOSTON

13 THE MIDDLESEX FELLS RESERVATION WEST: Skyline Trail

KEY AT-A-GLANCE INFORMATION

LENGTH: 7.21 miles
CONFIGURATION: Loop
DIFFICULTY: Moderate to strenuous
SCENERY: A landscape composed of granite outcrop, hemlock forest, and hardwood stands surrounding a chain of ponds. Two peaks traversed on the hike offer views of Boston.
EXPOSURE: Mostly shade
TRAFFIC: Moderate
TRAIL SURFACE: Gravel, packed earth, rugged boulders, and sheets of granite
HIKING TIME: 3.5–4 hours
SEASON: Sunrise–sunset year-round
ACCESS: Free
MAPS: Available from the Friends of the Middlesex Fells, www.fells.org, friends@fells.org, (781) 662-2340
FACILITIES: No
SPECIAL COMMENTS: Prepare for a hike in the Middlesex Fells as you would for a hike in remote mountain regions. Wear sturdy shoes and bring plenty of water and a flashlight in case the sun goes down midhike.
WHEELCHAIR TRAVERSABLE: Reservoir Trail (orange) is recommended for wheelchair users.
DISTANCE FROM BOSTON COMMON: 10 miles

IN BRIEF

Setting a course over jagged upland surrounding wetland and three enormous reservoirs, Skyline Trail circles the entire 2,060-acre Middlesex Fells Reservation.

DESCRIPTION

Unbeknownst to Captain Myles Standish and the Pilgrims he served, war and disease had decimated the native tribes of New England well in advance of the *Mayflower's* arrival. What the Pilgrims found when they first set foot on shore in the winter of 1620, were mounds entombing human remains and stashes of corn. As described by their first governor, William Bradford, what the Pilgrims discovered was, "death, and, by God's good providence, their (own) salvation."

On into March, the English struggled against winter's brutality, and with fear of Indians who now and again revealed themselves, though only fleetingly. The Pilgrim's first face-to-face interaction with an Indian came on March 16th when, as Bradford described in his journal, "a lone, tall, straight" man walked boldly into their settlement.

Introducing himself in English, "Samoset" handily eased the Pilgrims' fright and, despite their reluctance to have him, stayed

---

Middlesex Fells:
Skyline Trail
UTM Zone (WGS84) 19T
Northing: 4700605
Easting: 325659
Latitude: N 42° 26' 18"
Longitude: W 71° 07' 10"

Directions

From Boston, take Storrow Drive east to the ramp for I-93 north toward Concord. Take I-93 north 5.2 miles to Exit 33 toward Winchester. Stay straight to access MA 28 north. Enter the next roundabout and take the second exit, onto South Border Road. Continue approximately 1.3 miles to the parking area on the right.

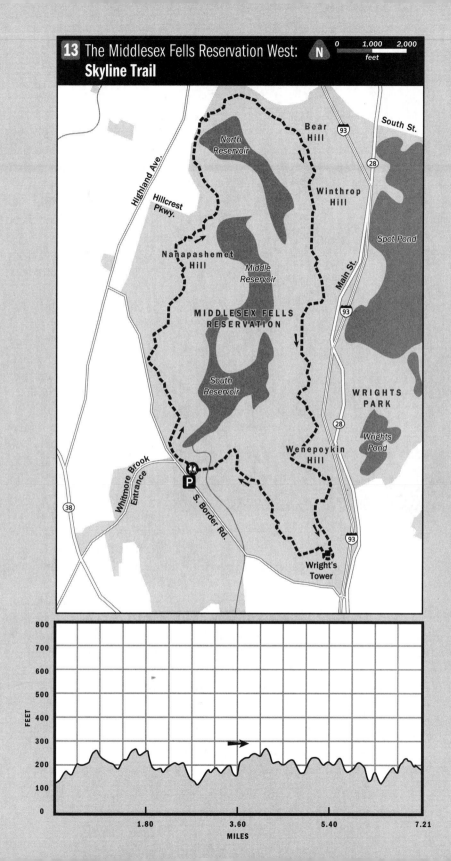

N

0   1,000   2,000
feet

North
Reservoir

Bear
Hill

93

South St.

28

Highland Ave.

Hillcrest
Pkwy.

Winthrop
Hill

Nanapashemet
Hill

Middle
Reservoir

Spot Pond

Main St.

MIDDLESEX FELLS
RESERVATION

93

South
Reservoir

WRIGHTS
PARK

Wenepoykin
Hill

Wrights
Pond

28

Whitmore Brook
Entrance

P

S. Border Rd.

38

93

Wright's
Tower

800

700

600

500

FEET 400

300

200

100

0

1.80   3.60   5.40   7.21

MILES

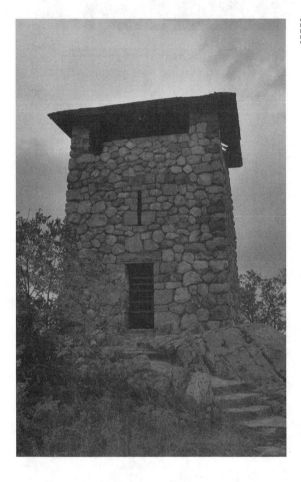

Wright's Tower atop Pine Hill

all day and night. Over a meal of "strong water and biscuit, and butter, and cheese and pudding, and a piece of mallard," he explained that, like them he was an outsider, being Monhegan and hence from a place far north of where they now resided. He also informed the English that the land they had settled was called "Patuxet," and that, four years earlier, all of the inhabitants had died of an extraordinary plague.

Six days later, Samoset returned, this time accompanied by another who spoke English with even greater fluency. This second man was Tisquantum of the Patuxet tribe, who, due to having been kidnapped, enslaved, and sent to England by George Weymouth in 1605, on returning to America found himself the lone surviving member of his people.

The two men came with word that the great Wampanoag leader Massasoit, his brother Quadequina, and 60 tribesmen were nearby. Serving as a neutral envoy, Tisquantum conveyed the goodwill of each side to the other and brokered sufficient trust between them that Massasoit ventured alone to the Pilgrim's settlement for a meeting with their governor.

Documenting the event in his journal, William Bradford wrote:

[Massasoit] was conducted to a house, then in a building, where [the Pilgrims] placed a green rug and three or four cushions. Then instantly came [Governor Williamson] with drum and trumpet after him and some few musketeers. After salutations, [Governor Williamson kissed Massasoit's hand] and the king kissed him, and they sat down.

With niceties done, they shared a toast of "strong water" and signed a treaty detailing six terms for peaceful relations.

The following year, Captain Myles Standish, his crew of ten English soldiers, Tisquantum, and four Wampanoag men canoed up the coast to the Mystic River to establish friendship and trade relations with the new leader of the Massachusetts, "Squaw Sachem."

Two years earlier—while the Pilgrims were arranging to lease the *Mayflower* and the *Speedwell* for their escape across the Atlantic, the Massachusetts, led by Grand Sachem Nanapashemet, were desperately trying to hold off attack from the Tarrentine. Forced from territory that covered the New England coast from the Charles River to Salem and area extending many miles to the west, the Massachusetts retreated to a fortresslike hill in the Middlesex Fells. Wise to their whereabouts, the Tarrentine warriors pressed harder and, in the course of a merciless battle, assassinated Nanapashemet and decimated his tribe.

When the dust had settled and the dead buried, Nanapashemet's widow assumed her husband's position and become the queen of the Massachusetts, or simply the "Squaw Sachem."

There was little to no fight left in the Massachusetts when Myles Standish and company found them at their camp on the Mystic River. Seeing the English approach with muskets and Indian allies, they braced themselves for more horror. But none came, and so the Massachusetts welcomed Standish forthwith and soothed anxiety and hungry stomachs with a tremendous feast for all—except the conspicuously absent Squaw Sachem.

Over the next three decades, the Massachusetts and the whites had many dealings. With the help of her three sons, Sagamore John, Sagamore James, and Sagamore George, Squaw Sachem continued to preside over the Massachusetts' territory, which rapidly shrank as John Winthrop and others persuaded her to deed it away to the whites. After giving up a large parcel to the settlers of Charlestown, she and her son John visited often. Far from showing any animosity to the newcomers, they extended friendship. John, a true admirer of the whites, adopted Christianity.

Within three years of the whites' arrival, John and James were dead of smallpox. Their other brother, Wenepoykin, "Sagamore George," lived on, but less and less peaceably. In time, the groundless lynching of his father-in-law curdled the last of his goodwill, and though nearly 60 years old, Wenepoykin joined King Philip's rebellion.

In the midst of the war, Wenepoykin was captured, sent to Barbados, and sold into slavery. Driven like a draught animal for eight years, he was finally rescued and returned home, thanks to Reverend John Eliot. One year later, he died. Defeated, his family deeded his territory in Marblehead, Lynn, and Salem to the settlers.

Begin by setting out on the gravel fire road heading northwest. Several hundred yards in, a tree decorated with colorful trail blazes, including white for Skyline Trail, marks where several trails run concurrently up a hill to the left. Single out Skyline's markers and leave the fire road here to hike north.

Set back in the woods away from South Border Road, the trail sets a rugged course from the outset due to the Fells' glacier-hewn topography. Following unsubtle undulations, the trail soon arrives at a small pond at the tip of a tree-hidden reservoir contained deep within the reservation. Cross the gravel access road on a diagonal to the left and resume Skyline Trail.

Climbing an easy uphill grade, the trail of compounded routes briefly passes close to the reservoir then tunnels back under tree cover. Long-established hemlocks, oaks, and maples stand their ground, though the occasional stand of pine indicates periodic clear-cutting—some of which was done under General Washington to provide timber to fortify Dorchester Heights.

Making its way north, now and again joining a cart road named for Nanapashemet, Skyline Trail passes over Nanapashemet Hill then dips within sight of the second in a chain of three reservoirs that lie at the center of the Fells.

After crossing Willow Spring Path, Skyline Trail clings to the westernmost edge of the fells, squeezing between North Reservoir and the houses of a Winchester neighborhood before bearing east back into woods a hair short of the reservation's northern boundary.

Sloping into wetland on the outskirts of the reservoir, the trail navigates a series of small bridges then climbs sharply as it meets the base of Bear Hill. Beyond Bear Hill Trail, joining in to the left and marked with blue, Skyline Trail drops straight south, narrowing to something like a goat path as it edges up the grizzled face of Winthrop Hill.

Proceeding from Winthrop Hill—named for John Winthrop, who in his journal described an exploratory expedition to the fells by the governor, the Reverend John Eliot, and others in 1632—the trail leads to a large meadow called the "Sheepfold," where, in the park's early years, a herd of sheep added a pastoral touch. The curious paved road beside the sheepfold is a soapbox-derby track built by the Metropolitan District Commission after World War II.

Arriving at a parking area, follow the white and orange trail markers right, onto Chandler Road. Skyline Trail soon diverts sharply left; take this turn onto a rocky slope and resume hiking south, to ascend Gerry Hill.

At the foot of the hill's western slope, after being bisected by Brooks Road, Skyline Trail takes on another hill, this one named Silver Mine Hill for the efforts of F. W. Morandi, who, with pickaxes and drills, went after precious metals here between 1881 and 1883.

The next more rock-strewn peak is Wenepoykin Hill, which offers an exhilarating vantage point. Bearing west and descending back into woods, the trail arrives at a junction in a clearing. Here Skyline Trail meets Cross Fells Trail, marked with blue. If the moon is rising and the daylight fading to silver, forsake Skyline Trail and continue straight on Cross Fells Trail—the parking lot on South Border Road is less than a mile away.

The next leg of Skyline Trail is marked, as always, with white blazes. Starting with a lengthy downhill over loose granite rubble into dense woods of pine

A dog stands on rock bearing glacial scarring.

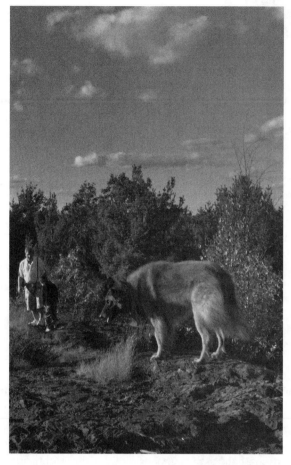

and hemlock, the trail twists its way to the top of twin peaks—Little Pine and the stone knuckle of Pine Hill, where it arrives at Wright's Tower.

From this stone tower, Skyline Trail slithers generally westward, clambering up sheets of granite grooved from the wear of glacial action and easing along placid stretches of cool, packed earth, passing the cave of a long-gone panther to rejoin Cross Fells Trail.

To stay with Skyline Trail to the end, bear right for one more climb and descent before rejoining the orange and green trails and concluding the hike with an easy amble back to the fire trail that leads to South Border Road.

NEARBY ATTRACTIONS

The Stoneham Zoo, founded in 1905, is located close by at Spot Pond on the Fells' eastern side (149 Pond Street, Stoneham, [781] 438-5100). Those interested in learning more about Native Americans of the Middlesex Fells are encouraged to visit Harvard's Peabody Museum of Archaeology and Ethnology, located at 11 Divinity Avenue on the campus of Harvard University in Cambridge. The museum's information line is (617) 496-1027.

14   LYNN WOODS HIKE

KEY AT-A-GLANCE INFORMATION

LENGTH: 4.96 miles

CONFIGURATION: Loop

DIFFICULTY: Easy to moderate

SCENERY: Miles of woods, scores of vernal pools, pristine Walden Pond, and view of Boston from a rocky peak

EXPOSURE: Mostly shaded except on peaks, where the trail is in full sun

TRAFFIC: Light to moderate

TRAIL SURFACE: Packed earth, some rocky slopes

HIKING TIME: 2.5–3 hours

SEASON: Year-round sunrise–sunset

ACCESS: Free

MAPS: Available on a first-come, first-serve basis at the reservation; Friends of Lynn Woods also provides maps on the organization's Web site, www.flw.org.

FACILITIES: Picnic tables and an amphitheater where open-air concerts are held in the summer

WHEELCHAIR TRAVERSABLE: Pennybrook Road and the many other gravel cart roads are traversable by scooters and other motorized wheelchairs; however, the other trails included in this hike are not.

DRIVING DISTANCE FROM BOSTON COMMON: 11 miles

IN BRIEF

In the course of circumnavigating the Lynn Woods Reservation this hike travels over rugged hiking trails and 17th-century oxcart roads to the top of Mount Moriah, the sweeping shore of Walden Pond, and the fault zone of Tomlin's Swamp.

DESCRIPTION

A glorious 2,200-acre oasis within the built-up City of Lynn, these woods were declared common land by English settlers in 1629. Turned over to private ownership in 1702, when the townspeople voted to divide the land among the town's landowners, the woods were gradually made public again after 1881 when a group of activists intent on creating a park organized to purchase lots.

From the parking lot, hike up the driveway to the special-needs camp. A blue arrow painted on a rock points to the trailhead to the right of the cul-de-sac located behind the buildings. At the immediate fork in the woods, take the green trail to the left and continue westward up a rocky slope.

Widening as it rounds Cedar Hill, the trail passes a granite outcropping just before a short path to the hilltop. Have a look, or better yet, pass this detour by, since the view

---

Lynn Woods Hike

UTM Zone (WGS84) 19T

Easting: 336703

Northing: 4704645

Latitude: N 42° 28' 37"

Longitude: W 70° 59' 12"

Directions

From Boston, take US 1 north to the Walnut Street exit in Saugus, then head east on Walnut Street into Lynn. After 2 miles, at a blinking light turn left onto Pennybrook Road. Follow Pennybrook Road to its end to reach the parking area.

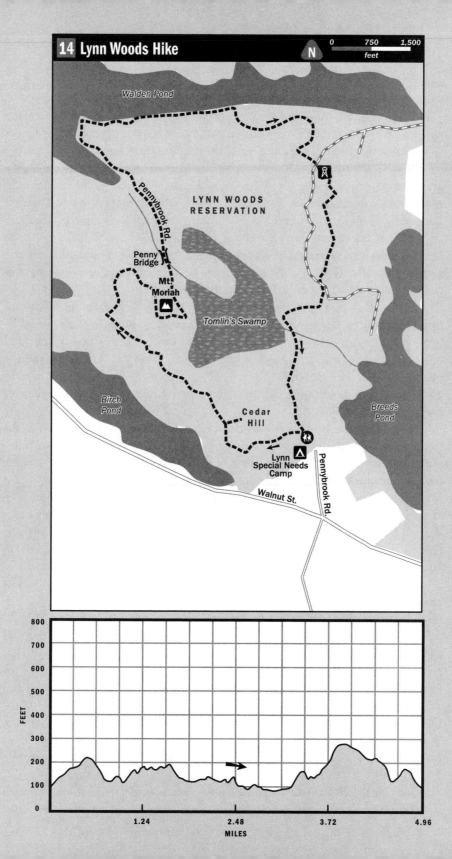

14 Lynn Woods Hike

0   750   1,500
feet
N

from Cedar Hill is of nothing but trees. To reach a superior view, proceed northwest from intersection B7-5.

Where Cedar Hill meets Mount Moriah, stay to the left to continue on the green trail heading north. After crossing a ridge strewn with rock cut, carried, and spewed by glacial action, the trail bears left at a two-way split.

Beyond a basin piled high with blocks of granite, the trail ascends up a gravel-laced incline. Surfacing on flat ground once again the trail then runs relatively free of stone cover to another two-pronged fork marked B6-3. Together these paths form a ring around Mount Moriah. To reach the hilltop by the more circuitous of the routes, opt for the path to the left.

Making its way around the peak, the trail dips to wetland then levels at a sort of causeway. Granite cliffs loom from one side, and blueberry bushes concealing bog and vernal pools, from the other.

Descending past oaks interspersed with white pine and tender birch saplings, the trail swings east at junction B5-4, bending around a tree charred by lightning. On the right, Mount Moriah stares down like a Cheshire cat, and blueberry bushes chilled to purple by autumn air crowd in. Arcing around the peak, the trail, now marked with blue, crosses a sheet of granite then rises to a plateau where, in autumn, oak trees the color of flames all but singe the soft green of pine and moss.

Beyond a pool, the trail splits in two yet again. At this junction, AB5-2, the dark-blue trail veers to the left, and the (reappearing) green trail curves right. Follow the green trail through a grove of spindly beech to junction B5-3, which lies just beyond. This section of trail, which winds south along the side of Mount Moriah is edged with carefully laid stone and, being well above treetops, provides an excellent vantage point. Birders will lose all sense of time as they catch sight of hooded warblers, golden crowned kinglets, and other less-seen species. During fall migration, from late August to early December, raptors coast by taking advantage of powerful wind currents.

For a 360-degree view of the surroundings, turn right on a short path ahead and scale the last few yards to the top of Mount Moriah. Boston's skyline on the northwest horizon is hard to miss.

To continue the hike, double back to the green trail, bearing right to descend southward. Upon reaching an intersection, turn left and follow this short linking trail to its end on Pennybrook Road. Leaving rocky elevations for a spell, turn left to pick up this centuries-old cart road.

Built for draft animals to haul out timber, this wide road tips gently toward the bridge for which it was named. About 0.25 miles on, at a broad intersection, Walden Pond Road departs to the left, heading for Saugus. Continue straight, following Pennybrook Road to where it meets a stream spanned by a fieldstone bridge. Long ago, all who crossed were charged a fee of one penny.

Stay on the cart road as it travels along Pennybrook's tall banking beneath the overreaching branches of maples, hickories, and hemlocks. In 1634, after

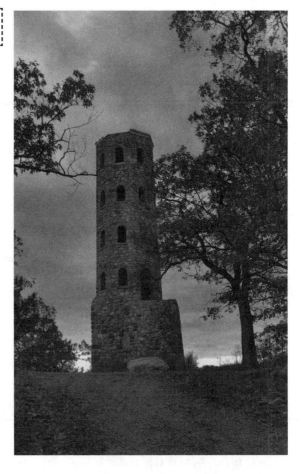

A fire lookout built in 1936 by the WPA

an exploratory trip to the New World and Lynn, in particular, an Englishman named William Wood published a book recounting what he had found. In this book, titled *New England Prospects,* Wood writes exuberantly about Lynn's water and forests. By his description, the water from the streams was "far different from the waters of England, being done so sharp but of fatter substance, and a more jettie color, it is thought there can be no better water in the world." Enraptured by the trees in the forests, he recorded, in a cheerful rhyme, both the name of each species and its attributes or uses. Noting more than oak and pine, Wood wrote, "Within this Indian Orchard fruits be some, The ruddie Cherrie and the jettie Plumbe, Snake muthering Hazell, with the sweet Saxaphrage."

Farther along the brook, the road's grade steepens. Soon, hemlocks gripped tight to a precipitous slope hide the water below. Shortly, however, the magnificent Walden Pond comes into view.

Before meeting the water, Pennybrook Road bends eastward. Where it commits to the new direction, a sign alerts visitors to dos and don'ts and arrows point left and right. Here take the Pennybrook Trail (B4-3), marked with blue, which dips immediately to the pond. Clear across, far enough off to look like a toy, a railroad line makes a silhouette against the sky and water.

Lightly enscribed, as if made by a wandering deer, the slender Pennybrook Trail traces a sketchy route beside the pond. Blue markers are at times hard to find, but with the water's edge to guide, there's no losing the trail. At a little over 0.5 miles, diagonally across from a water tower protruding from trees on the opposite bank, Tracy Trail diverts to upland. Leave the lapping waters of

Walden Pond here and follow this new route south to where it soon joins Great Woods Road. Turning left onto this cart road, hike on to the second path to the right, D5-6.

Zigzagging west to east, navigating Burrill Hill's granite ghosts of the last Ice Age, the trail emerges after 0.25 miles at the foot of a 48-foot tower. Although it looks medieval, this fieldstone fire lookout was built in 1936 under the auspices of the Works Progress Administration (WPA). At 285 feet, Burrill Hill is Lynn's highest point.

With the tower to the left, hike 0.1 mile downhill on the cart road (Cooke Road) to Boulder Trail. For 0.36 miles, this sliver of a trail meanders through a garden of granite vagrants dropped here by the Wisconsin ice sheet. At the trail's end, bear left back onto Cooke Road, then right at junction C6-3. From here, hike left, traveling downhill to pass the Undercliff Path before reaching a stream trickling toward Tomlin's Swamp. Climbing from the wetland, the trail traverses Waycross Road to connect with Pennybrook Road. Follow the cart road 100 yards or so south to return to the parking lot.

Note: Many seasonal events are hosted at the reservation. Program information is provided at **www.lynnma.net/community/lynnwoods**; additional information can be found at **www.flw.org**.

NEARBY ATTRACTIONS

A hike at Lynn Woods combines wonderfully well with a visit to Salem. Three attractions especially worth visiting are: The Salem Witch Museum (19-1/2 Washington Square, Salem; [978] 744-1692); the House of Seven Gables, made famous by Nathaniel Hawthorne's book by the same name (115 Derby Street, Salem; [978] 744-0991); and the Peabody Essex Museum (East India Square, Salem; [978] 745-9500 or [866] 745-1876; hearing impaired [978] 740-3649; program reservations: ext. 3011).

AGASSIZ ROCK HIKE 15

IN BRIEF

This short, rugged hike tours a hillside made spectacular by the handiwork of the Wisconsin Glacier. Two granite monoliths are the stars of the show, but wild flowers, streamfed pools and colorful birdlife add plenty of additional interest.

DESCRIPTION

From the gate at the trailhead, follow the broad stony path as it climbs abruptly into the woods. Sweeping southeast, the path meets a stream running from a source high on the hill. A wooden-plank bridge keeps you clear of the wet as you pass a vernal pool sided with granite rubble and adorned with ferns and luxuriant moss. Nestled in a cleft between hills, the trail runs on level ground briefly before beginning its climb. Switching east and northeast over protruding rocks and roots, the path eases downhill and soon arrives at a short causeway with a small pool to the right. Immediately ahead, a sign directs you left to "Big Agassiz" and right to "Little Agassiz." I chose to take the path to the left.

Heading north under overhanging branches, the trail passes another pool. Continuing on flat ground, step around a grand orb of granite on the right, brushing bayberry bushes as you go.

KEY AT-A-GLANCE INFORMATION

LENGTH: 0.77 miles

CONFIGURATION: Out-and-back with small loop

DIFFICULTY: Moderate

SCENERY: Woods with astonishing glacial erratics and a view of Gloucester from the hilltop

EXPOSURE: Mostly shaded

TRAFFIC: Light

TRAIL SURFACE: Packed earth with exposed roots and stones

HIKING TIME: 40 minutes

SEASON: Year-round 8 a.m.–sunset

ACCESS: Free

MAPS: Posted at the entrance

FACILITIES: None

SPECIAL COMMENTS: Swiss glaciologist and Harvard professor Louis Agassiz was the first to reason that enormous boulders often caught in precarious positions like those found on this hike were moved and arranged on the landscape by sheets of glacial ice.

WHEELCHAIR TRAVERSABLE: No

DRIVING DISTANCE FROM BOSTON COMMON: 30 miles

Directions

From Boston, take Storrow Drive East and merge onto US 1 north. Continue on US 1 for 13.6 miles. Merge onto I-95/MA 128 north. Drive 1.3 miles to MA 128 north. Take Exit 15 north and travel 0.5 miles. The entrance is off Southern Avenue on the right. A roadside pull-off will accommodate 10 cars.

Agassiz Rock Hike
UTM Zone (WGS84) 19T
Easting: 355035
Northing: 4717726
Latitude: N 42° 35' 54"
Longitude: W 70° 46' 01"

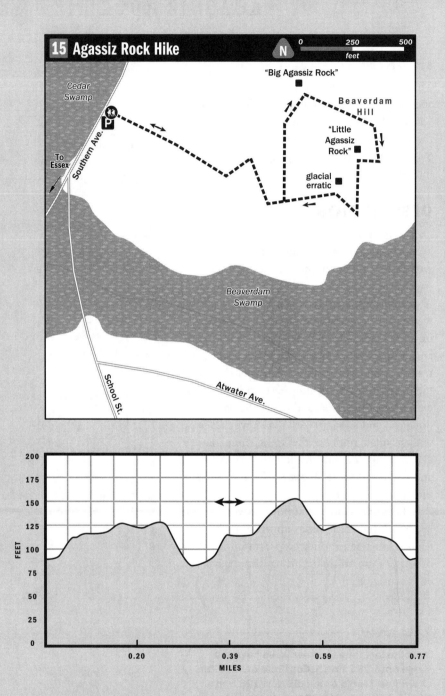

Curving northward, the slender trail runs downhill through a thick growth of bushes on either side. On the afternoon of my hike, steel-hued thunderclouds rolled onto each other like fighting dogs as heavy weather set in. Word has it that the top of this hill provides an excellent view of Cape Anne firework displays on the Fourth of July. Although Independence Day was weeks away from the look of the sky, I fully expected a brilliant light show within minutes, yet under the trees I felt safe and well-sheltered.

Tumbling through tangled brush, the trail suddenly emerges at a bog. Look to the left and you will see "Big Agassiz" submerged like a happy sow in the soggy ground. Resting in this spot for thousands of years, the rock is said to be far more massive than it appears. Like the iceberg that sank the *Titanic,* most of Big Agassiz lies hidden.

Through the ages, the curious placement of Big Agassiz and other such boulders was believed to be the work of God, but in the 19th century, Swiss-born geologist Joseph Agassiz convinced his peers and the general populous that ice, not God, was the force at work. By his explanation, this boulder and the others like it that litter New England, are "glacial erratics," the stranded victims of ice long melted away.

From Big Agassiz, return to the trail, taking it east as it continues upward from the edge of the wetland. Along this part, the trail is surfaced with coarse grit; not yet sand but finer than gravel, that may once have been a part of the famous boulder.

Passing a grove of beeches to the left and hemlocks to the right, the trail steepens as it bends south. Along here, you will see one or two lichen-bedecked boulders; though also glacial erratics, they are not Little Agassiz. Continue until you reach a flat expanse of granite to the left at the top of the hill. Walk out onto this for a look southeast over the tree line to Cape Anne.

Resist thoughts that you have seen all that there is to see, and walk to the right to find Little Agassiz behind another unnamed, but impressive boulder. Propped precariously on a tilted triangular stone, Little Agassiz seems to pulse with potential energy.

After spending some time surveying the view and taking in sun, cloudscapes, or fireworks, pick up the path just below Little Agassiz to the left. Checking the ground, you might spot the tiny columbine that grows from the gritty soil. Blooming in June, its minute flowers are pink with yellow pistils.

After a steep pitch, the trail eases as it returns to the shaded woods. Wintergreen grows profusely along the mossy path's edge. Soon the incline levels, and the walking gets easier as you arrive back at the junction, where the path bears right to Big Agassiz. Keep left to return to the trailhead at Southern Avenue.

16 MANCHESTER-ESSEX WOODS:
Cedar Hill–Pulpit Rock Hike

KEY AT-A-GLANCE INFORMATION

LENGTH: 4.75 miles

CONFIGURATION: 2 linked loops

DIFFICULTY: Easy to moderate

SCENERY: Cedar and maple swamps, vernal pools, and hemlock woods

EXPOSURE: Mostly shaded

TRAFFIC: Moderate

TRAIL SURFACE: Packed earth with rugged areas of loose gravel and exposed rock

HIKING TIME: 2.5–3 hours

SEASON: Year-round sunrise–sunset

ACCESS: Free

MAPS: A map is posted at a kiosk at the parking area. Maps can also be obtained from Manchester–Essex Conservation Trust, P.O. Box 1486, Manchester, MA 01944, (978) 526-1695 or (978) 526-7692; conserve@mect.org.

FACILITIES: None

SPECIAL COMMENTS: Beware of biting insects from spring until the first frost. Saxifrage, spicebush, marsh marigold, goldthread, bluets, and hepatica all begin blooming in early spring.

WHEELCHAIR TRAVERSABLE: No

DRIVING DISTANCE TO BOSTON COMMON: 30 miles

IN BRIEF

Beginning with a 0.15-mile-long boardwalk across a cedar swamp teeming with life, this hike explores granite hills, an old cart road, and bogs dense with bayberry, maples, and blueberries.

DESCRIPTION

From the parking lot, set out on the dirt road (Old School Road) heading southwest beyond a metal gate barring car access. Running along the edge of wetland past glossy ibises watching from the bleached branches of trees that have long since given up the ghost, the road reaches the trailhead of the Cedar Swamp Trail at 0.1 mile.

Crossing this spectacular bridge you'll see a rich array of species buzz, flit, or paddle by. Close to the opposite bank, the boardwalk widens to include a lookout platform and, below it, steps to a dock at water level. After taking in the sights, continue west to the boardwalk's end. Along the trail gnawed stumps chiseled to points, and nibbled trunks swaddled in chicken wire tell of an ongoing battle of man versus beaver.

After stepping off the boardwalk at a

Manchester–Essex Woods

UTM Zone (WGS84) 19T

Easting: 312811

Northing: 4679843

Latitude: N 42° 14' 54"

Longitude: W 71° 16' 09"

Directions

From Boston, take Storrow Drive east to the exit for US 1 north. Merge onto US 1 north toward Tobin Bridge/Revere. After 13.6 miles, merge onto I-95/MA 128 north toward Peabody/Gloucester and continue 1.3 miles to Exit 45 toward Gloucester. At 13.2 miles, take Exit 15, School Street, toward Manchester/Essex. At the end of the ramp, turn left onto Southern Avenue. Parking for the Manchester–Essex Woods is 0.56 miles ahead on the left.

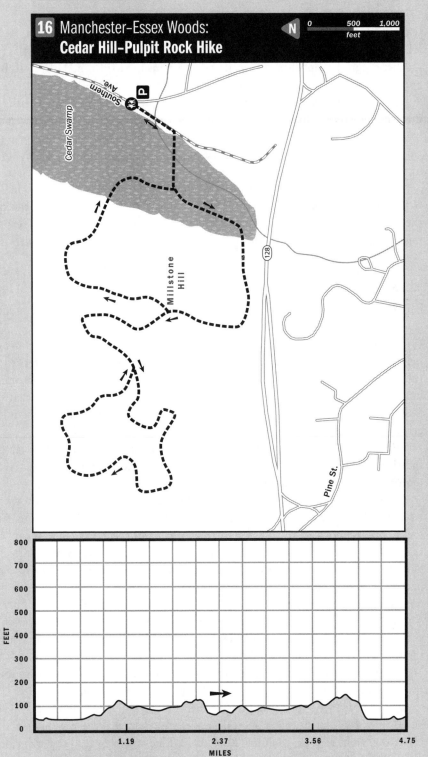

16 Manchester-Essex Woods:
Cedar Hill–Pulpit Rock Hike

well-marked junction, continue left to hike south flush to Cedar Swamp below a heavy brow of granite and lashes of hemlock. A short distance ahead, the trail reaches a sign that appears to identify two trails as the Millstone Hill Trail. Both are coded with orange. Pursue the left route, staying with the swamp.

On a summer's day, after a warm rain, the atmosphere is heavy with life-infusing moisture. Mosses and ferns pulsing with chlorophyll contrast with the black-brown mud underfoot and the purple-gray feldspar-blended granite that riddles the hillside. In early spring, when the day's sunlight temporarily melts the night's freeze, blossoms of spicebush (*Lindera benzoin*) add a zing to the air.

Continuing southwest toward the sound of cars whooshing by on MA 128, the trail sidles up to a stone wall. Bearing left to pass through, the trail then reaches a sign on the right which states "Private Property—No Trespassing." Regardless, stay with the trail as it climbs a rise and soon meets Old School Road.

Leaving the woods and swamp behind, take up the dirt road once more and travel west. After paralleling MA 128 for approximately 0.3 miles, the trail curves north to cinch the base of Millstone Hill. Follow as it ascends a rocky slope, and on reaching a split, bear left onto a wide gravel trail.

Passing an adjoining path on the right, the trail retreats gently downhill next to a stone wall. A hundred yards or so farther, another path splinters to the right, reconnecting with the Millstone Hill Trail. Continue straight to promptly intersect Ancient Line Trail, marked with both a red blotch and a wooden sign posted high on a tree. Bear left here, traveling northwest into a stand of hemlock growing in a cleft between two hillocks.

Just as the trail gets under way, it comes upon a detour sign. Here, arrows redirect hikers north. Habitat restoration or erosion mitigation sometimes require that routes be temporarily altered.

Well away from MA 128 and any other road, the immaculate woods feel wonderfully remote. Beech and linden trees stir the quietude of ubiquitous hemlocks. Bog reappears, and with its great density of water, mosses, ferns, and regenerative rot, softens the hard edges of dissonant sound waves. Grit and half-chewed chunks of granite bespeak the glacier that left nearby Agassiz Rock perched at a teasing tilt. Like a riotous crowd, the ice came, hung around, then quit the place, leaving behind a great quantity of granite litter.

Following a course that may as well have been determined by a myopic skunk on a slug hunt, the trail zigzags in all directions. Heading southeast, then west, the trail rounds upland, passing a good many birches, though the ground glows orange with pine needles. Arrhythmic boulders and pools of water trapped in basins of woven tree roots keep mind and feet occupied.

At the next junction, a sign for Ancient Line Trail Detour points east. From here follow red blotches west several hundred yards to a three-way intersection. Here, stay right to pick up Pulpit Rock Trail. Blue splotches lead the way northward along the edge of a hill. Ahead, a spring marks a junction where Grassy

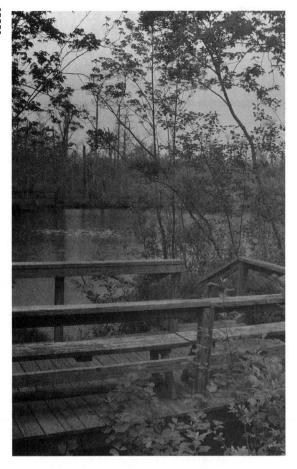

A view of Cedar Swamp

Ridge Trail bears right and Pulpit Rock Trail keeps left on its northwest trajectory.

In this region of hillocks sitting amid bogs, maples are abundant—fittingly, as this wetland is called Maple Swamp. Being perpetually damp, this area fosters an abundance of mushrooms. In June especially, delicious oyster mushrooms spread like meaty cream-colored fans from the sides of dead and dying hardwoods.

Climbing uphill over gravel, the trail parts woods that in days gone by were cut for lumber and fuel. Because of scant topsoil and unyielding ledge trees remain small, which lends the place an intimate feel. Gaining elevation, the trail reaches open areas with stretches of exposed bedrock. On reaching the pulpit the view opens to become panoramic and vast.

Rounding to the southeast, the trail follows blue markers back downhill toward wetland in a valley below. The double leaves of pink lady's slipper are easy to spot here. Those hiking between April and July might be lucky enough to catch these extraordinary orchids in bloom.

Reaching the center of a dell, the trail traipses over logs tossed together to bridge mud then climbs west to the relatively dry flank of another hill. After some twisting and turning, the trail bends decidedly south on upland, passing a pool and stream. On arriving at a junction, continue left bearing away from Pulpit Trail and another route climbing steeply to the right. Ahead, partly hidden by hemlock boughs, a sign for the Ancient Line Trail points southeast. Two junctions lie ahead, one following the other. Bear left at the first, then left again at the second, hiking northeast and away from the Cheever Commons Loop Trail, which is marked with light blue.

A stone wall beside the trail confirms that these were once grazing grounds,

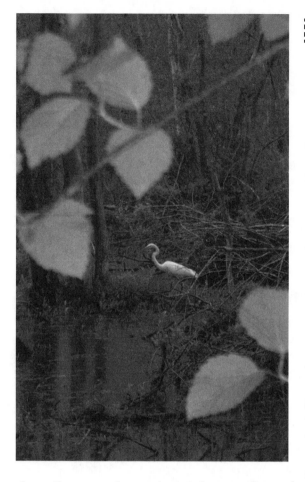

though not particularly nourishing ones, judging from the grit underfoot and the general paucity of both grasses and pioneer shrubs and trees. Bearing east, the trail climbs steadily uphill, keeping flush to the wall before splitting off. Scruffy feral meadowland lies to the right. Stand quietly for a moment and you might spot a napping fawn, a clutch of turkey chicks or a fox on the hunt.

Turning southeast, the trail meets up again with the Cheever Commons Trail, but stay with Ancient Line Trail as it cuts tightly left, tucking under the steep upland banking. Running northwest again, making an elongated loop, the trail enters a herpetologist's heaven of vernal pools and cavernous spaces made by lichen-encrusted boulders heaved together. Continuing on nearly level ground, the trail weaves its way northeast 0.2 miles to return to the start of Pulpit Trail. Stay with Ancient Line Trail to double back to where it began.

Upon returning to the Millstone Hill Trail, turn left and follow what used to be the north–south track of Old Manchester Road. A granite town-line marker carved with the letter "M" stands erect on the Manchester–Essex border. Continuing north, the trail grows narrower and looks less and less like a road as hemlocks and birches crowd in. At 0.26 miles Old Manchester Road reaches a fork where the Cedar Swamp Trail diverts eastward. A moment later, this pleasant way leads to a two-way split. Both routes lead to evocative rock formations, one called Baby Rock and the other Ship Rock. If swayed by curiosity, hike left; otherwise, bear right to follow blue markers east.

Proceeding down a gentle grade, the trail passes through a dramatic rockscape fringed with hemlocks. Gradually oaks and beech fill in, and before long

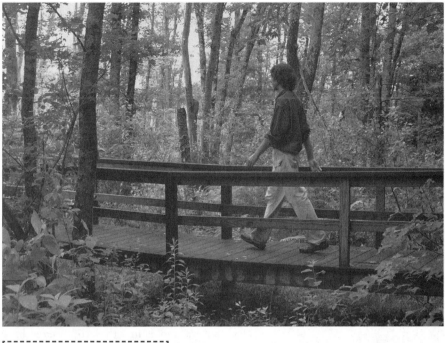

A boardwalk spans Cedar Swamp.

the trail arrives at Prospect Ledge Trail. At this and the next junction, Ship Rock Trail jogs this way and that. Keep an eye out for blue markers to stay on track to reach Cedar Swamp. Clutching the firm ground on the swamp's perimeter, the trail winds back to the boardwalk.

NEARBY ATTRACTIONS

If you have a taste for fried clams, oysters, lobster, chowder, or just superb onion rings; plan your hike around lunch or dinner at J. T. Farnham's in Essex. Farnham's is located 4 miles from the trailhead at 88 Eastern Avenue. From the parking area at the Manchester–Essex Woods, drive 2.5 miles north on Southern Avenue and turn right onto Eastern Avenue (MA 133). Farnham's is 0.6 miles ahead on the left, overlooking the salt marsh.

17 RAVENSWOOD PARK HIKE

IN BRIEF

Tucked into a corner of Gloucester, Ravenswood Park offers miles of hiking through a landscape left largely untouched since mass transit came in the form of a stagecoach. Following centuries-old footpaths, carriage roads, and a boardwalk through a magnolia swamp, this hike rambles through woods to reach Fernwood Lake before passing the cabin site of "The Hermit of Ravenswood" and two granite quarries.

DESCRIPTION

As rich in history as in rare and beautiful species of flora and fauna, these 600 acres have been maintained in their natural state thanks to the inspired vision and generosity of the Gloucester businessman Samuel Elwell Sawyer.

Gloucester's Ravenswood Park would never have been had the City of Boston not foiled Sawyer's original plan of establishing the park in Boston's neighborhood, West Roxbury. In 1853, Sawyer and his business partner James Haughton, purchased a 73-acre parcel known as "Old Sumner Farm," quickly registered the land as "Monteglade" and set to work realizing their vision of 22 houses situated on a wooded park called Ravenswood after the castle in Sir Walter Scott's *The Bride*

Ravenswood Park Hike

UTM Zone (WGS84) 19T

Easting: 360639

Northing: 4716890

Latitude: N 42° 35' 31"

Longitude: W 70° 41' 54"

Directions

From Boston, take Storrow Drive East, following signs for US 1 north. Merge onto US 1 north via the ramp on the left to cross the Tobin Bridge. From US 1 north merge onto I-95 north. Take Exit 14 (MA 133) and follow it 3 miles east toward Gloucester to MA 127. Turn right onto MA 127 and follow it 2 miles to the entrance.

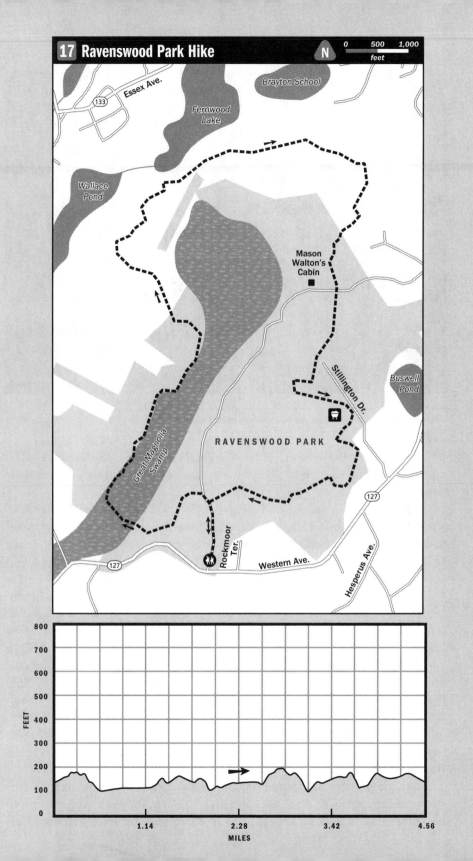

17 Ravenswood Park Hike

N

| 0 | 500 | 1,000 |

feet

Essex Ave.

133

Brayton School

Fernwood
Lake

Wallace
Pond

Mason
Walton's
Cabin

Buswell
Pond

Stillington Dr.

RAVENSWOOD PARK

Great Magnolia
Swamp

127

127

Rockmoor
Ter.

Western Ave.

Hesperus Ave.

FEET

800
700
600
500
400
300
200
100
0

1.14   2.28   3.42   4.56

MILES

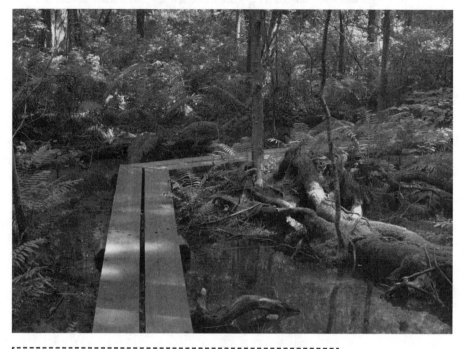

Magnolia Swamp is named for the rare and beautiful Sweetbay Magnolia.

of Lammermoor. But in short order Boston claimed rights to the property by eminent domain and with strokes of a pen Sawyer and Haughton's Monteglade was lost.

Shocked by the seizure and what they felt was grossly insufficient compensation, Sawyer and Haughton sued the city. Subsequently, the court ruled in Boston's favor, virtually bankrupting Haughton. Defeated but not deterred, Sawyer turned his sights from Boston to Gloucester, where he quickly set about acquiring land near his family's homestead at Freshwater Cove.

Sawyer recognized opportunity in the vast acreage to the west of the town center. Made up of woodlots grown in since the adoption of coal furnaces, the region included an old stagecoach road that has long since been replaced by the Eastern Railroad, the cellar remains of a slaughterhouse, and a 1777 vintage "pest house" built to curtail repeated outbreaks of smallpox. Negotiating deal after deal, Sawyer acquired a total of 205 acres for what amounted to $2,969. But, as Sawyer's holdings grew, so too did his frustrations. When the town's fire department failed to adequately respond when fire consumed his woods, and his cousin stonewalled him, by demanding an exorbitant price for a lot, Sawyer halted his campaign. The shooting of his dog in an altercation was the final straw.

Yet, despite his disillusionment, Sawyer's altruistic passion remained as strong as ever. When he died suddenly two years later, the town's paper featured his will in its entirety on its front page. In it, Sawyer instructed that nearly his entire fortune of $350,000 was to go to charity. Of this, $60,000 was to be held in trust to provide for the maintenance and expansion of Ravenswood Park. In 1993, the park trustees entrusted the property to the Trustees of Reservations. An ongoing success, the park continues to grow.

From the parking lot, hike northwest on Old Salem Road—the gravel road that bore Lowe's stagecoaches traveling to and from Boston in the 1700s. Running parallel with stone walls, the path soon meets Magnolia Swamp Trail on the left. Follow this narrower trail west under hemlock boughs, uphill to start, then downhill as it winds southwest.

If hiking in June, you will find the mountain laurel in full bloom. Heavy with white blossoms touched with pink, these elegant bushes dress the woods as if for a formal occasion. As the trail descends to wetland, the density of laurel increases.

Arriving at Magnolia Swamp, the trail transitions to boardwalk as it continues across the wetland. Lush moss grows on the edges of the narrow path, and thick shrubs close in on the sides. After taking you a fair distance through this wet zone alive with butterflies and frogs, the boardwalk terminates at the southeastern end of the swamp. Here you step onto earth again and continue along the granite ledge rimming the wetland.

A short distance ahead, the ledge gives way to an obstreperous chunk of granite protruding from the upland. The only way around is to ford the swamp or take the boardwalk built to accommodate the rock's complex contours and the trees growing from its crevices.

Reconnecting with the ledge, the trail continues below hemlocks and beeches. Blue jays flit in the foliage, scolding as you pass. Looking to your right, you may notice nylon netting enclosing a section of greenery. This fencing protects the tender shoots of sweetbay magnolia (*Magnolia virginiana*) from grazing deer. Undulating northward, the trail reaches a junction where the Magnolia Swamp Trail turns to the right and the Fernwood Lake Trail starts on the left.

Pick up the Fernwood Lake Trail, hiking northeast, and leave the wetland behind. Following blue markers, this trail passes through property outside Ravenswood's borders.

Crossing hillocks dotted with granite boulders of every shape and size, the trail passes through young beech groves varied by sassafras and laurel. Shortly, the narrow path spills into a wide clearing where trails radiate in all directions. Looking across to the right, you will see a bold blue dot marking the way. Continue on the Fernwood Trail to, travel east on what is an old carriage road.

Passing abandoned farmland on the left reclaimed by oaks and maples, the carriage road rolls on to soon reach a T-intersection. Blue arrows painted on a beech point east and west. Follow the right-pointing arrow and hike eastward. Through woods to the left, you will see the waters of Fernwood Lake. On this stretch of road, keep an eye out for exposed stone worn by the horse-drawn traffic of Jonathan Lowe's stagecoach company which by 1805, ran multiple trips daily to Boston and Gloucester and stops in between.

Turning east, the trail bends away from the lake, which is still visible to your left. Aside from some dips and short climbs, the trail follows a level route, usually paralleled by ramshackle stone walls. Several paths split off on either side, but follow blue markers to stay with the Fernwood Lake Trail. After passing a path that bears uphill to the left, you will notice that the trail is marked with both orange and blue; pay this no mind.

Arriving at a clearing, hike left onto a dirt road to pass great piles of granite before crossing to the right where blue markers point the way to Ravenswood's border.

Back inside the park, the trail descends a hill thick with slender birch and beech saplings. Reaching lower ground, you will encounter patches of mud and giant lichen-covered boulders.

Before long, the Fernwood Lake Trail comes to a four-way intersection where it meets Old Salem Road and Evergreen Road. It was near here that Mason A. Walton, better known as "The Hermit" kept house in a small log cabin he built with the landowner's permission in 1884.

A most gregarious hermit, Walton was highly educated and, prior to moving to the woods of Gloucester for health reasons, fully engaged in civic matters. Until the death of his wife and only child in their home state of Maine, Walton had campaigned vigorously for the Democratic Party and Maine's "Greenbackers." Far from reclusive, he sought communion with all walks of life. Every morning for the 33 years he spent living in these woods, Walton walked to town for breakfast and to sell goods he made from woodland plants.

He welcomed all visitors and received literally thousands, as is documented in the guest book he kept. Two of his most notable callers were a black snake that he fed saucers of milk, and Concord native Henry Thoreau. He and Thoreau had much in common, both being naturalists and writers. Two of Walton's published books are *A Hermit's Wild Friends* and *Proof That Animals Reason*.

From the intersection, continue hiking southeast on Evergreen Road. This broad gravel route, like Old Salem Road, once served horse-drawn carriages. Sweeping through hemlock woods, this elegant way soon leads to Quarry Road. Turn left here to take up this new route eastward. Pass the Ledge Hill Trail and continue a short distance farther to arrive at the quarry and another entrance to the park. Long abandoned, the water-filled quarry now functions as a grand home to rare amphibians.

Follow the narrow Ledge Hill Trail as it traipses up the left side of the man-made pool then makes a southern retreat into the woods. At the next junction, marked 9, turn left to follow a somewhat vague trail running downhill through a madness of glacial waste.

Reaching the bottom of the hill, the trail bends right to head south. Here, the way becomes more distinct as it approaches the park boundary and a house to the left. When you come to marker 8, bear right to head back uphill. Winding north and northwest on this narrow path, you pass more gray boulders, freakishly

In June, mountain laurel is in full bloom.

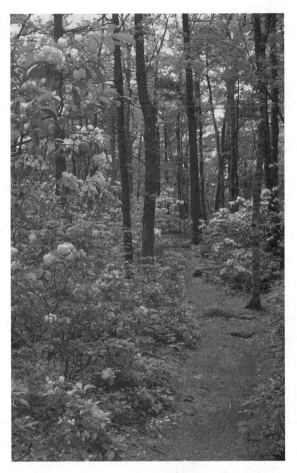

festooned with enormous ear-shaped fungus.

Soon the path joins the Ledge Hill Trail at a particularly massive rock. Turn left at this juncture to hike gently downhill. Following the route edged with small stones, you promptly come to a boulder that looks as soft and inviting as a worn sofa. Beyond this odd furnishing, the trail descends past a vernal pool. After rising again and easing by another small pond, the trail emerges from the woods at Old Salem Road just opposite the start of the Magnolia Swamp Trail.

NEARBY ATTRACTIONS

Hammond Castle, one of Cape Ann's most celebrated attractions, is located almost immediately across the street (MA 127) from the entrance of Ravenswood Park at 80 Hesperus Avenue. Built in the 1920s by inventor John Hays Hammond ("The Father of Remote Control"), the medieval-style castle offers for self-guided and prearranged tours. The castle is open seven days a week from 10 a.m. to 4 p.m. June 23 through Labor Day. Visit **www.hammondcastle.org** for a schedule of special programs and events. To book a tour, call (978) 283-7673.

If you are interested in great theater, you might want to coordinate an afternoon of hiking at Ravenswood with an evening performance at the Gloucester Stage Company. The theater's season runs from May to September. For information on its current productions, schedule, or to purchase tickets, visit **www.gloucesterstage.org** or phone (978) 281-4433. The Gloucester Stage Company is located at 267 East Main Street in a one-story brick building.

18 DOGTOWN COMMONS HIKE

KEY AT-A-GLANCE INFORMATION

LENGTH: 5.25 miles

DIFFICULTY: Moderate

SCENERY: Woods of oak, pine, and beech, ancient cellar holes and granite boulders inscribed with words of inspiration

EXPOSURE: Mostly shaded

TRAFFIC: Light

TRAIL SURFACE: Varies from packed earth to rough rocky spots

HIKING TIME: 3 hours

SEASON: Year-round dawn–dusk

ACCESS: Free

MAPS: Available at parking lot

FACILITIES: None

SPECIAL COMMENTS: Because of Dogtown Common's rugged terrain and interweaving trails both named and unnamed, it is a good idea to pack a compass and plenty of water.

WHEELCHAIR TRAVERSABLE: No

DRIVING DISTANCE FROM BOSTON COMMON: 30 miles

IN BRIEF

This hike tours historic Dogtown, a settlement abandoned nearly two centuries ago. After an inauspicious start, the hike gains interest as it follows a trail marked by boulders engraved with words of inspiration. Meandering footpaths lead to forsaken cart roads as the hike weaves through beech woods piled high with granite rubble, skirts swamp, and passes overgrown cellar holes while completing a circuit.

DESCRIPTION

Named for the many dogs that watched over the women and children of the village while the men were at sea, Cape Ann's Dogtown is as benignly mysterious as its name. In the 1600s, subsistent farmers built modest single-story homes here and spent their days striving to eke a living from the most ungiving land. Stone after stone was pulled from the ground to clear it for tilling and grazing. With ocean waters thick with fish just over their aching shoulders, it's no wonder Dogtown's men saw the folly of their labor and one by one took to the sea. By the mid-1800s, Dogtown was completely abandoned. The last to leave was a former slave named Cornelius "Black Neil" Finson. In the winter of 1830, Finson was found nearly frozen in a cellar and taken to

Dogtown Commons Hike

UTM Zone (WGS84) 19T

Easting: 363364

Northing: 4721527

Latitude: N 42° 38' 02"

Longitude: W 70° 39' 59"

Directions ⟶

From Boston, take MA 128 north to Gloucester. At the large traffic circle, exit left onto MA 127 toward Annisquam and follow it 0.5 miles, crossing a small bridge. Turn right onto Reynard Street. Follow Reynard Street to the end and turn onto Cherry Street; soon after, turn up a steep road to the right, marked with a sign for Dogtown Common.

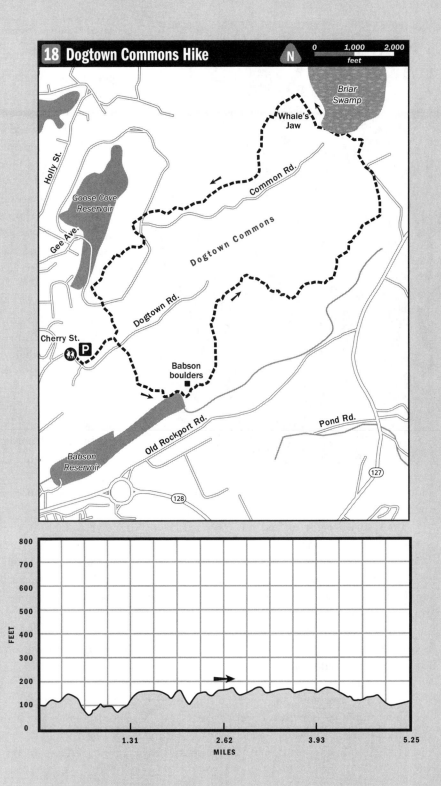

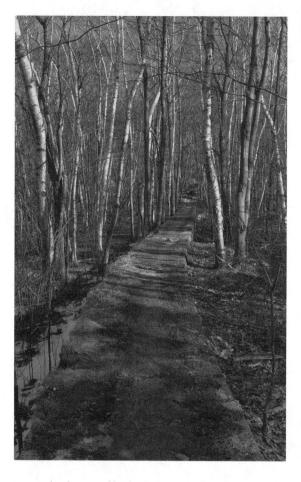

A causeway passes Briar Swamp

the poorhouse, where he died soon after.

In time, philanthropist Roger Babson, a descendant of one of Gloucester's oldest families, donated much of Dogtown's 3,000 acres to the City of Gloucester. Nature has all but reclaimed Dogtown which is now held in trust by Gloucester and Rockport to be preserved in perpetuity.

From the parking area, walk along Dogtown Road, heading southeast a short way to where it curves left and the pavement cedes to gravel. Here, you will encounter a gate limiting access to pedestrians and bicycles. Continue until the path dead-ends. Ahead, the tremendous mound of cast-off Christmas trees and other organic waste you see is not the town dump but Gloucester's new composting facility.

Look to the right to find the trailhead. Once you have walked in a few yards, notice a tree marked with the letter "G" and a sign that reads "Public Watershed," with a list of rules and regulations. The trail winds gently through woods, first uphill then down. Boulders of all sizes and weatherworn shapes lie amid spindly oaks and cedars stunted and stooped due to scant nutrients and the granite ledge at their roots.

After passing a stand of birch, you will see the Babson Reservoir at the bottom of the slope in front of you. Here, glacial erosion stripped away topsoil, leaving massive chunks of rock.

Make your way down the embankment 100 feet or so to the water, following the trail as best you can. Evidence suggests that the course of the trail has been interpreted in many ways over the years, and as a result no one way is the right way. Once at the water's edge, bear left. At the lake's eastern end, the trail regains definition and heads uphill to a clearing above the water. A passing train on the Boston–Gloucester line may draw your attention to the train tracks running along the opposite shore.

Continue northeast, through a split in a stone wall, and straight ahead you will see a large stone inscribed "Truth." This startling find confirms that you have reached the Babson Boulder Trail. During the Great Depression, millionaire Roger Babson hired stonecutters to carve words of inspiration into 23 boulders scattered along this route.

Stay to the left of "Truth" and follow a rocky stretch along an esker. You will come to a large thermometer nailed to a tree partway down the left-hand slope. Next to this piece of hardware is a sign marked 22. Another trail forks left here, but stay on the esker as the Babson Boulder Trail heads on to the right.

Peering between beech limbs, you will notice a neat network of stone walls laid out in a tumbling grid. Like a Scottish fairyland, the place has a mystical feel. Leathery ear-shaped fungi fastened to nearly every stone seem to listen for secrets. A little farther along, you will find another of Babson's boulders, this one inscribed "Work." Continuing eastward you will begin to notice mountain laurel adding softness to the hardwood forest. A water tower is just visible in the distance to the right, and a bit farther along, you will encounter a boulder carved with the word "Courage."

Note that several colors seem to denote the same trail; follow the blotches without concerning yourself with a particular color. After cutting through a gap in a stone wall, bear left. The other route leads across the railroad track to the Babson Museum.

Hiking northward takes you to the "Loyalty" boulder. The trail then becomes narrow and winds like the cow path it may once have been. One supposes this rugged terrain crippled more than one milk-heavy cow. Farther along, heading northwest while stepping among stones, keep an eye out for what looks like a large fossil not far from a boulder on the left with the inscription "Kindness."

At this point, the trail levels and begins to smooth. The beeches thin, making way for blueberries. Up ahead, you will find two more Babson stones, the first marked "Ideas," the second "Industry." Just beyond these, the trail forks right to take you to the enormous Uncle Andrew's Rock, bearing the words "Spiritual Power."

Make a semicircle around Uncle Andrew's rock and rejoin the Babson Boulder Trail. From here, the footing becomes grassy and flat, and the tangled thickets give way to pretty stands of birches. A short distance ahead, the path leads into a circular clearing with a large tree at the center. As trails radiate seemingly from all points, walk across the circle to a path slightly to the left of a large cedar tree. When this trail forks, bear right. A little farther along, look for a sign marked "10," denoting Art's Trail. Rather than taking this route, pick up the Tarr Trail, which heads right to another gathering of dwarfing boulders. Tarr Trail immediately turns squirrelly, becoming narrow and winding as it heads southeast. Coming to the end of a tricky downhill, the trail arrives at a wide intersection. A tree standing directly ahead is marked with red, white, and blue. Turn left here and ascends the facing slope. Here, again, you will see spots of all colors marking the way; turn a blind eye to all but lime green. The trail then weaves erratically northward as ragged rocks heaved together by glacial force make forging a straight route impossible.

As you twist through crevices to make your way along this goat path, listen for a stream to the west. The volume of both sound and water increase as you reach a wetland at the foot of the Tarr Trail esker. Red pine replaces beech as the dominant tree in these parts. Several big pines disgorged by lightning stand like atrophied corpses near the trail.

Reaching another clearing, you will notice a sign marked "13," denoting an old gravel pit. Continue to the left to hike northwest. Young beeches crowd out pines, and barbed-wire fencing subdued by rust lines the path.

Arriving at a rise called "Raccoon Ledges," the trail splits to the left and right. Choose the lefthand route, and continue northeast. Following the groove of the trail—not the color blotches—you'll soon come to a small vernal pool on the left. You may even see an abandoned off-road bike marked "For sale by owner."

After turning northwest, the trail runs downhill to the boardwalk at Briar Swamp. Be careful not to be lured off to the right by another trail running southeast. Look north to see a stone dam or causeway. The boardwalk is to the right, hidden in reeds. If you like, split off here for a short walk through the briar; otherwise, hike across the causeway. Up ahead, you come to a broad intersection where the boardwalk ends and Luce Trail starts. Continue walking northwest, passing trails heading sharply left.

Leaving the wetland, the trail becomes wider and much easier to follow. Passing another trail heading to the right, continue as the trail bends distinctly westward. After running southeast for a stretch, the trail passes to the right of Peter's Pulpit, another extraordinary boulder. Beyond, the gravel route veers west along woods of cedar.

Pass another trail heading left and continue on what is now called "Common Road." Looking into the woods, you might spot a stone carved with the number 34. This and others like it mark where Dogtown homes once stood.

On arriving at junction "2" turn left onto Adams Pine Trail. When you come to a split, continue left, to head southeast. The trail makes a loop then bisects another path. Cross this intersection and continue straight, to travel west. Before long, the trail ends at the service road for the Goose Cove Reservoir. Follow this paved road downhill to the right, keeping an eye out for a trail heading left back into the woods.

Follow this trail as it turns southwest, climbs past a pond, and continues over a narrow concrete dam. Winding on further, the trail converges with a stone wall, crosses a boardwalk, then comes to an end directly across from where the hike began.

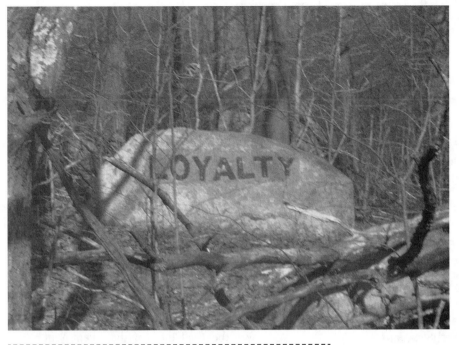

During the Depression philanthropist Roger W. Babson hired immigrant workers to carve boulders with words of inspiration.

NEARBY ATTRACTIONS

If sightseeing interests you after your hike, one destination to consider is Rockport's Bearskin Neck. This small peninsula located at one of Cape Ann's easternmost points has been the center of activity since settlers arrived in the 1600s. Once a busy docking area for fishing boats and the ships that ferried Cape Ann's granite to Boston and ports as far away as South America. Bearskin Neck is now a bustling artist colony with galleries, bookstores, boutiques, and eateries. From Cherry Street drive south 0.5 miles, turn right onto Poplar Street. At 0.2 miles turn left onto Washington Street/MA 127 south, and take the third exit from rotary onto MA 128 north. Turn left onto MA 127 and continue 2.8 miles. Turn right onto High Street, then turn left onto MA 127A north to Bearskin Neck, Rockport.

19 GREAT MEADOW– GERRISH'S ROCK HIKE

KEY AT-A-GLANCE INFORMATION

LENGTH: 0.8 miles

CONFIGURATION: Out-and-back

DIFFICULTY: Easy

SCENERY: Meadows bordered by woods overlooking the Parker River

EXPOSURE: Mostly sun, some shade

TRAFFIC: Light

TRAIL SURFACE: Grass, earth

HIKING TIME: 30 minutes

SEASON: Open year-round sunrise–sunset

ACCESS: Free

MAPS: Not needed

FACILITIES: None

SPECIAL COMMENTS: As part of the Great Marsh, the largest salt marsh in New England, Great Meadow is recognized internationally as an important birding area.

WHEELCHAIR TRAVERSABLE: No

DRIVING DISTANCE FROM BOSTON COMMON: 33 miles

IN BRIEF

If measured in feet or minutes, this hike across a 17th-century farm's meadows to salt marshes cleaved by a tidal river could be described as short; but if measured in beauty or ecological and historical relevance, it is boundless.

DESCRIPTION

In 1705, a newly married couple received this property as a wedding gift from an adoring aunt and uncle, Samuel and Hannah Sewall. Thirteen years earlier, the same Samuel Sewall, having been appointed by Governor Phips to the High Criminal Court, presided over the final days of the Salem Witch Trials. Perhaps because he, like the others on the court lacked legal training and was devoutly Christian, Sewall chose to believe the accusers. By September 22, 1692, about 100 men, women, and children had been jailed and 19 others executed by hanging.

Five years later, moved by the 12th verse of Matthew read to him by his son Sam on Christmas Eve, which in his journal the judge confessed "did awfully bring to mind the Salem Tragedie," Sewall resolved to publicly repent for his involvement in the horrible events. In church, on January 14, the day

---

Great Meadow–
Gerrish's Rock Hike

UTM Zone (WGS84) 19T

Easting: 342824

Northing: 4735473

Latitude: N 42° 45' 20"

Longitude: W 70° 55' 15"

Directions ———————→

From Boston, take Storrow Drive east to US 1, then head north toward Tobin Bridge/Revere. Continue 15.2 miles. Merge onto I-95 north and drive 15.4 miles to Exit 55 (Central Street). Head 0.3 miles toward South Byfield/ Newbury, then bear right onto Central Street. After 0.6 miles, turn left onto Orchard Street. Look for the entrance to the Great Meadows parking area on the right.

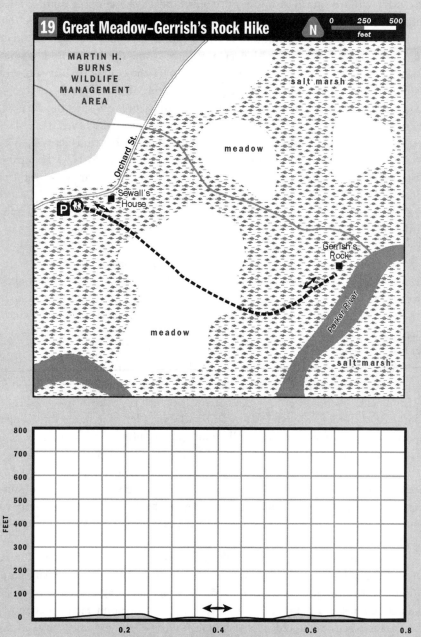

chosen by the General Court as "a day of fasting and prayer on account of what might have been done amiss in the late tragedy," Sewall handed a prepared "bill" to a Mr. Willard and had him read it out loud to the congregation. Notably, Judge Sewall was the only public official to offer such an apology.

Anne Longfellow Sewall and her new husband, Captain Abraham Adams, no doubt received their gift with deep gratitude. Anne, their first child, was born on April 29, and ten more children followed over the course of 16 years. Abraham, an enterprising sea captain, set about building ships on the property.

This salt marsh that fed the Adams' cattle in winter and fills the air now as then, with a briny scent, is part of what is now recognized as the Great Marsh, a tract of 20,000-acres that includes salt marsh, barrier beach, tidal rivers, estuaries, mudflats, and upland islands across Massachusetts to New Hampshire. Priceless ecologically speaking and otherwise, the Great Marsh has rightfully received a healthy amount of attention from environmentalists and land preservation groups. Because it is both a breeding ground and refuge for migratory birds, the Great Marsh—hence the Parker River—enjoys international renown as an important birding area.

In the late 1970s, thanks to a small group of people and a fledgling organization called the Essex County Greenbelt, the 100 or so acres that make up Great Meadow were saved from development. Some of the acres were donated, others purchased with money raised by tireless fund-raisers. A single driving force behind the project was my mother, Sally Lunt Weatherall. Today, the property is public parkland held by the Town of Newbury.

After parking, walk east on the dirt drive to the trailhead at a metal gate. Immediately ahead, past a fringe of woods, lie two sprawling fields separated by landlocked wetland. Follow the narrow footpath over the grassland, heading southeast. After a swale where a tractor path bears left, the path climbs steeply up the side of a softly contoured hill. MIdway, you'll find there is little to see but acres of hay fields rolling beneath the sky like great ocean swells.

As you crest the hill, the peaceful grassland falls away and the Parker River becomes the focus. Seen through a buffer of trees, the slender waterway snakes east to west through rich salt marsh looking much as it did in 1635 when Henry Sewall, (Samuel's father, Anne's grandfather), established one of Newbury's first plantations.

From this first lookout point, the path curves eastward along the topmost edge of the field then leaves the grassland through a split in a stone wall hidden by bushes. Continuing several hundred yards farther along a narrow peninsula, the path comes to an end at Gerrish's Rock, a narrow point facing a channel of the Parker River. Sheltered by salt marsh, the bowl-shaped creek just off Gerrish's Rock has been a favorite swimming spot for generations of hearty locals.

In 1681, Henry Sewall bought 160 acres of land near the Falls of Newbury from the family of an American Indian known as "Old Will," as well as their rights to other acreages in Newbury. That the land of Great Meadows was the

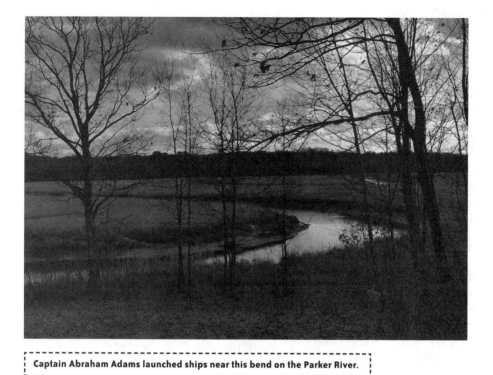

Captain Abraham Adams launched ships near this bend on the Parker River.

old camping and fishing grounds of American Indians is therefore uncontestable. Old Will and the other American Indians of Newbury were the people of the Pawtucket sachem Masconomo.

Like Massasoit, who befriended the Pilgrims at Plymouth, Masconomo was a peaceable man and as such accommodated the settlers who set up camp in his territory. When Governor Winthrop anchored off Cape Ann in June 1630, pausing on his voyage to what would become Boston; Masconomo and one of his men boarded Winthrop's ship, the *Arbella*, for a day-long visit. Fourteen years later, Masconomo became a Christian by his own volition. Never hostile to the colonists, he was in fact considered their friend until his death in 1658.

After taking in the landscape and all that inhabits it, particularly the rich diversity of bird life, meander back through the woods and over the meadow to return to the parking area.

20 MAUDSLAY STATE PARK HIKE

 KEY AT-A-GLANCE INFORMATION

LENGTH: 3.92 miles

CONFIGURATION: Loop

DIFFICULTY: Moderate

SCENERY: The grounds of a 450-acre estate designed by the landscape architects Charles Sprague Sargent and Martha Brooks Hutcheson, with views of the Merrimack River

EXPOSURE: Mostly shaded

TRAFFIC: Moderate

TRAIL SURFACE: Packed earth

HIKING TIME: 3 hours

SEASON: Year-round dawn–dusk

ACCESS: Parking $2

MAPS: Available at parking lot

FACILITIES: Restrooms and picnic tables

SPECIAL COMMENTS: The park hosts a full schedule of cultural events in the summer months.

WHEELCHAIR TRAVERSABLE: The path known as the Main Road accommodates wheelchair users; the other trails in this hike do not.

DRIVING DISTANCE FROM BOSTON COMMON: 38 miles

Maudslay State
Park Hike

UTM Zone (WGS84) 19T

Easting: 342546

Northing: 4742821

Latitude: N 42° 49' 19"

Longitude: W 70° 55' 34"

IN BRIEF

On this hike you will explore the former estate of one of Newburyport's most prominent families. Following trails and carriage roads, the hike takes you through meadows, woodlands, and formal gardens. From the site of the Maudslay mansion, the hike tracks the handsome Merrimack River, following its fast flowing waters north through hemlock woods where bald eagles roost in winter.

DESCRIPTION

From the parking lot entrance, cross Pine Hill Road to the start of Pasture Trail. Hike over the arc of the open field, keeping to the left when the slender path splits. On meeting a gravel carriage path, follow as it descends to the left off a hammock. In summer, yellow splashes against blue as goldfinches dart among lilting blossoms of black-eyed Susan and Queen Anne's lace growing in the meadow beneath open sky.

Where the trail turns to the northwest, the sun-drenched pasture meets shady woods. On the right is a stand of white pine planted by Frederick Moseley; to the left is a deciduous wood of shagbark hickory, beech, and various

Directions ⟶

From Boston take Storrow Drive east and drive 1.8 miles on I-93 north/US 1 north, then take Exit 27 toward Tobin Bridge/Revere. Drive 0.4 miles and merge onto US 1 north. After 13.9 miles, merge onto I-95 north. Continue 19.9 miles to Exit 57, toward MA 113 west. After 0.3 miles, turn left onto MA 113 (Storey Avenue). Drive 0.7 miles and turn right onto Gypsy Lane/Hoyts Lane. Drive 0.5 miles and turn right onto Curzon Mill Road. Parking is ahead on the right.

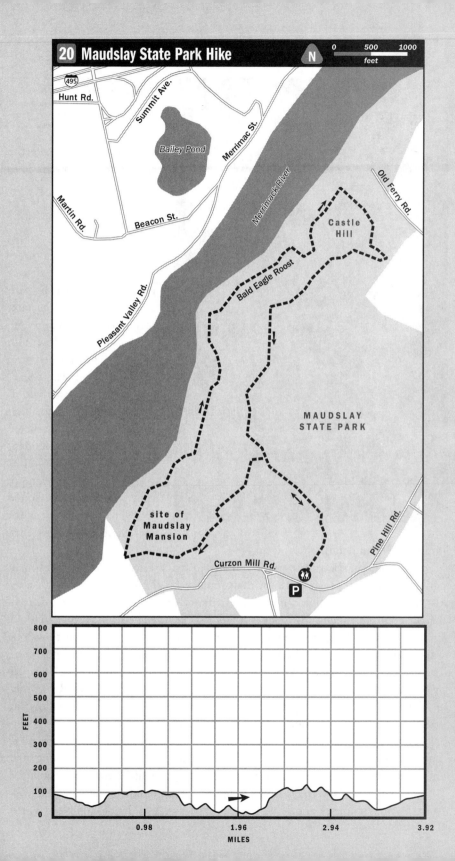

N

0   500   1000
feet

Hunt Rd.

Summit Ave.

Merrimac St.

Bailey Pond

Martin Rd.

Beacon St.

Pleasant Valley Rd.

Merrimack River

Old Ferry Rd.

Castle Hill

Bald Eagle Roost

MAUDSLAY
STATE PARK

Pine Hill Rd.

site of
Maudslay
Mansion

Curzon Mill Rd.

P

FEET

800
700
600
500
400
300
200
100
0

0.98   1.96   2.94   3.92

MILES

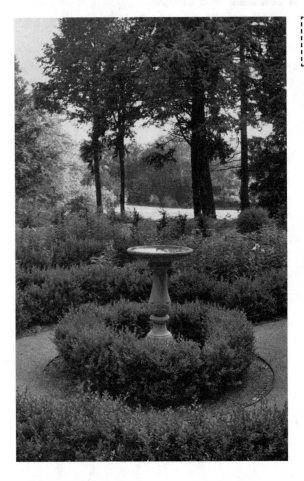

> The Garden Conservancy is working to restore this formal garden to its original splendor.

species of oak. Where the trail levels, another, less-pronounced path breaks off to the right. Bear left to enter the woods.

Before long, this broad trail reaches a three-way intersection; detour here onto a narrow path sweeping left. At the next fork, bear left again and follow the path downhill, brushing by bushes and sassafras saplings. Ahead, you come to a small foot-bridge, one of three that Moseley had constructed in 1915. The rhododendrons that envelop you as you stand in this tranquil spot were likely planted in 1926. A diary kept for the estate documents each improvement in detail.

In 1903, married four years and off to a lucrative career in investment banking, Moseley began work on the property he christened Maudsleigh after his family's ancestral home in England. Intent on replicating the grandeur of British country estates, Moseley turned to the esteemed landscape architect Charles Sprague Sargent of Harvard's Arnold Arboretum. The men took long walks together to survey the property and discuss its attributes and potential. Then, with a plan in place, Moseley set about reshaping the landscape. He began by planting thousands of white pine on the banks of the Merrimack River, then an avenue of maples along the main road, hedges of spruce and willow, an orchard, and a stand of rhododendrons on the hill behind his home.

Formerly known as Swann's Cottage, the house and the 11 acres surrounding it was Moseley's first purchase. Four years later, he bought an adjoining farm and transformed the cottage into a puritanically opulent 72-room mansion.

Traveling as if secretly through boughs of rhododendrons half a world away from the trees' country of origin, one feels closer to Asia than to the New World.

Bit by bit, the dark, fingerlike leaves of the rhododendrons give way to lighter foliage as the path ascends to a fork within a beech grove. Bear left here climbing ascend stone steps to emerge at the eastern end of the Garden Walk.

After his initial consultation with Charles Sprague Sargent, Moseley hired Martha Brooks Hutcheson to design the grounds around the house and several formal gardens. Chances are Hutcheson was responsible for the dramatic border hedge that demarcates this walk.

At the end of this lovely path, you come to a gravel drive and an entryway through an imposing hedge. Slip into the peaceful garden through this passage to reach the spot where Maudslay Hedges, the home of Moseley's daughter Helen C. Moseley Jr., once stood. Erected by Helen in 1939, the house mysteriously burned to the ground in 1978, four years after her death.

Exit through the hedge and turn right on the gravel drive and right again onto a path heading southeast through an orchard that provided fruit for Miss Moseley's pies.

Past a spruce hedge, you come to a small granite building that is now shuttered and bears a sign warning of feral honeybees. Ahead, the path leads to the shattered shells of the greenhouses and cold frames F. S. Moseley had constructed in 1900.

Continue on the gravel road as it curves sharply to the right to reach a formal garden currently being rehabilitated with help from the Garden Conservancy. After taking in the neatly geometric perennial beds and imported marble ornaments, depart through the gate at the far end of the garden. A meadow lies off to the left, as does the well for which the path is named. At the next junction, the path to the left leads to the site of the coachman's house and barn. To reach the site of the Moseley mansion, continue straight through to a yard of several barns in disrepair and, beyond these, to a sprawling lawn overlooking the Merrimack River. Nothing is left of the house but its lovely view.

In the wake of Helen Moseley Sr.'s death, years after the death of her husband, not one heir was prepared or willing to assume responsibility for the mansion, and so, on the orders of an impetuous son, the fine house was razed.

Having surveyed the site, head toward the river keeping the water to your left, and pick up Merrimack River Trail. At the end of the lawn, a path to the right leads to Rhododendron Dell, reportedly planted in 1903. Staying with Merrimack River Trail, walk beneath the pines and hemlocks growing along the steep riverbank. Linked to the Bay Circuit Trail, which begins at Plum Island and runs through Newbury's Old Town Hill. Merrimack River Trail spans the length of Maudslay and if plans pan out, the trail will eventually extend to Canada.

Continuing downhill, you soon come to a wooden bridge and commingled mountain laurels. Ahead a swath cut in the laurels affords a view of the river below. Three hundred years ago, looking from here you might have seen Penacook fishermen netting salmon and sturgeon; today recreational boaters fill the scene. On the other side of the clearing, the trail resumes its course under heavy branches of oak, hickory, and white pine. After encountering two sections of chain-link fence and a concrete dam, the path merges with a packed-earth trail. Climbing the banking, the route leads to a memorial bench.

Merrimack River Trail continues uninterrupted until it reaches Moseley's Flowering Pond, where it detours to a gravel road. From the road, descend left to a stone bridge and dam at the foot of the pond.

F. S. Moseley undertook several ambitious waterworks projects—one in 1906 to bring plumbing into his house, and others later to provide irrigation to lawns and gardens.

Midway through the estate, Merrimack River Trail reaches Laurel Hill. Watch for the great horned owls and pileated woodpeckers that nest here, and if winter is setting in, keep an eye out for bald eagles. In fact, this trail is closed from November 1 through March 31 to provide peace and protection to a number of these spectacular raptors, that retreat from Canada to this spot every year. Frederick's father, Edward, purchased much of Laurel Hill in 1860 to preserve the delicate habitat.

From the eagle's roosting grounds, stay with Merrimack River Trail until it reaches a broad fork. At this juncture, proceed left up a rocky slope to arrive at a large intersection.

Stay on the river until the trail arrives at an avenue of sugar maples ascending in a regal line to the top of Castle Hill. Back in the 1600s, a man named William Moulton settled these acres and earned a fortune mining silver along the river. In 1860, his descendant Henry Moulton acquired the hillside and built a gothic castle of wood on the highest point. In 1896, Charles Moseley gained possession of this parcel and in 1900 tore the castle down.

From the castle's footprint, follow the gravel road as it corkscrews around the other side of the hill. Arriving at the bottom, make a hairpin turn to take up a westward trail on the right. Look for engaging eyes staring through the woods from the dairy goat farm across the way.

The trail forks twice in quick succession; hike right at the first split and left at the second to travel downhill on a gravel carriage route under a canopy of hemlocks. Pass through the next junction to continue straight on this path, which is aptly named Cathedral Road. Stay on Cathedral Road through each four-way intersection and upon arriving at a fork, hike downhill to the left. Soon after this junction, the trail reaches yet another split; continue straight, and at the next fork bear left. Proceed straight on the wide carriage path. Before long you will see a sign that reads "parking," with an arrow pointing to a trail to the left. Resisting this direct route to the parking lot, bear right. In a moment, this road passes a narrow footpath running off into underbrush to the left. This, too, will take you back to the start. But, for the pleasure of crossing the eastern end of the Flowering Pond by way of a magnificent stone bridge, stay on the gravel carriage road. Referred to as Main Road, this route promptly reaches a T-intersection. Travel straight on to rejoin Pasture Trail and retrace your steps back to the parking lot.

WARD RESERVATION HIKE 21

IN BRIEF

Touring a 700-acre parcel of former farmland and forest, this hike begins with a hike up Holt Hill for a view of Boston then rounds Cat Swamp switching from footpaths to cart roads and back again to ascend Boston Hill then arc back to the Ward family's farmstead.

DESCRIPTION

Established in 1940, the Ward Reservation is a stunning example of the ongoing success of the landscape architect and conservationist Charles Eliot and his ambition to preserve New England's open space. Initiated by Mabel B. Ward's gift of 153 acres to the Trustees of Reservations, the reservation grew to 700 acres as private individuals made similar gifts. Over several decades, 40 separate parcels were united, preserved, and made available to the public for passive recreational use.

Look for the trailhead to the left of the kiosk and set out heading south toward the bog at Pine Hole Pond, crossing a grassy meadow next to a house on the left. Where the path approaches woods, a sign reads "X-country ski trail, follow orange markers." Hike left here to climb a steep hill overlooking the bog. After a steep ascent, the trail runs along the edge of a sloping apple orchard.

KEY AT-A-GLANCE INFORMATION

LENGTH: 4.7 miles

CONFIGURATION: Loop

DIFFICULTY: Easy to moderate

SCENERY: Farmland reverted to woods, centuries-old abandoned cart roads, solstice stones, and a rare quaking bog

EXPOSURE: Mostly shaded

TRAFFIC: Light

TRAIL SURFACE: Grass, packed earth, and an occasional boardwalk

HIKING TIME: 3–3.5 hours

SEASON: Year-round 8 a.m.–sunset

ACCESS: Free

MAPS: Available at the entrance

FACILITIES: None

SPECIAL COMMENTS: The Ward Reservation offers visitors great variety. For those with children or limited time, an interpretive trail along a 700-foot boardwalk through a fascinating quaking bog provides a satisfying shorter hike. Especially intrepid ramblers might consider linking from here to the Mary French Reservation and onward to the Harold Parker State Forest by way of the Bay Circuit Trail.

WHEELCHAIR TRAVERSABLE: No

DRIVING DISTANCE FROM BOSTON COMMON: 25 miles

Directions

From Boston take Storrow Drive east staying to the left; after 0.3 miles merge onto I-93 north. From I-93 north, exit onto MA 125 north and go 5 miles. Turn right onto Prospect Road and follow it 0.3 miles to the reservation entrance; there is a parking area on the right.

Ward Reservation Hike

UTM Zone (WGS84) 19T

Easting: 326825

Northing: 4723082

Latitude: 42° 38' 26"

Longitude: 71° 06' 44"

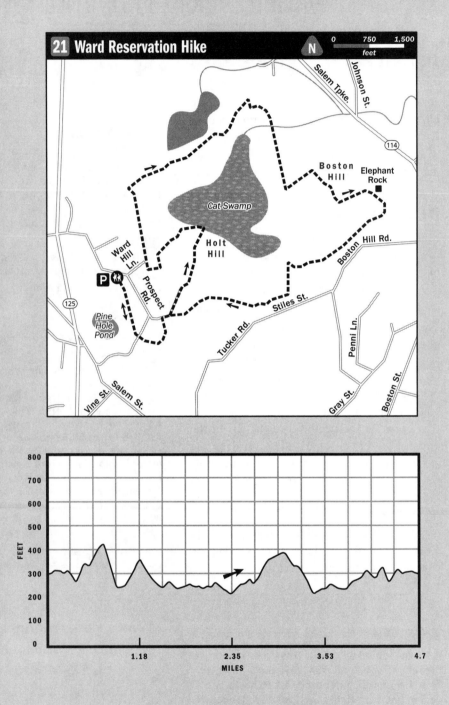

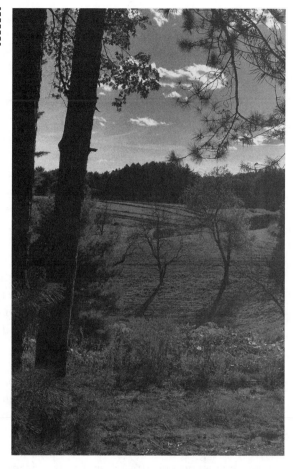

Fruit trees border hay fields at the foot of Holt Hill.

At the orchard's end, continue through a wide gap in a ramshackle stone wall and cross the gravel drive to a rounded hay-field spread before a clutch of houses. Bear left across the grassland to a valley on the hill's eastern side. Approaching the edge of the woods, two trailheads become visible; aim for the one farthest to the left and follow it on its meandering markerless course to another stone wall.

At the wall, a sign states that on the other side of the wall, the orange trail splits to the right and the Bay Circuit Trail continues straight on to the summit of Holt Hill. It's worth noting that the Bay Circuit Trail, in making its arc around Boston, is always identified by white trail markers; but on the Ward Reservation map, the Bay Circuit Trail is marked in green and is referred to as "the green trail."

From the stone wall, the Bay Circuit Trail bends northwest toward a farmhouse built on a verdant cleft in the hill. Reaching an elevation level with the homestead, the trail arrives at a three-way junction distinguished by an epic birch tree. Parallel stone walls run due east from the spot, with two trails traveling in their shadows. One of these, the Bay Circuit Trail, identified with green blazes, tracks the topmost wall briefly before veering north to girdle the hillside. Take this route as it curves through woods of monumental pines to approach Holt Hill, briefly winding eastward before taking the hill head-on. Though the well-trod path is easy to follow, the ascent is sudden and sharp.

Besides being a good test for the heart and lungs, Holt Hill's 420-foot elevation, with its bald southern face, boasts wonderful views of Boston and the Blue Hills. On June 17, 1775, settlers climbed to this vantage point to witness the raging fire in Charlestown set by British soldiers on orders of General Howe during the Battle of Bunker Hill.

Mabel Ward's solstice stones, arranged to mark the path of the sun on the longest and shortest days of the year—the summer and winter solstices—and at the spring and autumn equinoxes, also add interest.

From the solstice stones, hike 100 yards farther north to the imposing fire tower, then, following a stone wall on the right, locate a trail leading back into woods. On a sunny day, the transition from the heat and bright light of the hill-top back to the damp cool of shade cast by oaks and pines is jarring. That the trail plunges straight down the hill's dark northern face toward the mysterious Cat Swamp only heightens the contrast in mood.

Upon reaching the swamp, the connector trail forms a "T" with the San-born Trail. Turn left at this junction and continue along the base of Holt Hill, heading west. Gradually, the trail leaves the wetland to wind around the hill's more benign western slope and to reascend the peak.

Reemerging from the woods to find a paved access road to the hilltop reservoirs, turn right and following Bay Circuit Trail markers southeast a short distance to where this route joins a trail heading into the woods on the right. Change course here to follow a stone wall northeast. Along this approximately 0.3-mile section of sloping rocky terrain, the trail crosses the wet periphery of Cat Swamp. Past a boardwalk and after a brief climb, the trail reaches a three-way intersection.

Two trails bend off to the left. One is the Bay Circuit Trail; the other, making a tighter turn, is a 0.4-mile route back to the parking lot. To continue on the tour of the reservation, opt for the path to the right, Margaret's Trail.

Traveling northeast on level ground, Margaret's Trail parallels a wetland rife with beavers and vocal waterfowl. Upland rises beside it to the right. In autumn, the smell of apples wafts in the air, probably from orchards now overgrown by pine and sassafras. Turning away from the wetland, the trail arrives at a three-way junction. Take the path identified as "the shortcut to Chestnut Street" on the right, which serpentines to its promised destination.

Lined by two robust stone walls, Old Chestnut Street cuts a near-straight north–south line through former pastureland. Much of this ancient road, named for the tree that once flourished in this woodland, is still in active use beyond the reservation's borders, but the section within the property was abandoned in 1933. Access this still-impressive cart road by bearing right through a gap in the upper stone wall.

After crossing a stream, Old Chestnut Street meets the Sanborn Trail dropping in from the right off of Shrub Hill. Passing a valley on the left as it climbs the side of this hill, the cart road soon arrives at a crossroads. Leave Old Chestnut Street here, turning left onto Graham's Trail and hiking east toward Boston Hill. At the next split in the trail, which comes quickly on a rise, stay to the left on Graham's Trail. After climbing a bit farther to another junction, continue to the right, to continue your ascent. Laminated directions posted at junctions along here confuse more than they enlighten; so you are better off ignoring them

To proceed, stay on Graham's Trail, following it southeast. When Graham's Trail itself becomes vague, arrows point the way.

Curving around the top of Boston Hill, the trail passes a lovely vantage point above a meadow on the hill's western face. Have a look, then continue east alongside a stone wall and a wire fence to a second meadow on the hill's eastern side.

Lying several yards ahead amid goldenrod, the seed heads of grasses, and purple asters is the curious glacial erratic named Elephant Rock. Angular yet rounded, eyed through a squint, the boulder does resemble an adolescent elephant in the sun.

Take in the view looking south toward the City of Boston then hike down the hill, passing a service road, to a dense grove of birch saplings. Approaching the base of the hill edged by a stone wall, the trail meets another route merging from the right. An ancient birch, perhaps an original property marker, stands steadfast here in a corner formed by two stone walls. At this spot, the trail veers left to run along the outside of an abandoned walled-in avenue.

Ahead, the trail crosses a broad stream via a boardwalk and, after navigating a series of stone walls, climbs gently to connect with Old Chestnut Street. Bear left on this familiar avenue and continue several hundred yards to another trail, well marked with an arrow, branching off to the right.

Pass another path that splits northward, and if the sun is low, keep an eye out for deer attracted to a nearby spring. Climbing away from the wetland, the trail skirts private property. Shortly, where it splits again, arrows point the way. Somewhat sketchy now, yet sufficiently marked, the trail brushes past an enormous oak tree that, judging from planks nailed to it, doubles as a lookout.

A few feet farther, at a junction, a sign directs hikers right to the summit of Holt Hill and left to Prospect Road. Choosing the path to the left, ease southeast along the hillside that tapers downhill past a convergence of stone walls to join up with an old cart road. Striding up the last rise, imagine men clucking at teams of horses and oxen, cracking whips to urge them on to the homestead just beyond. Once back where the Bay Circuit Trail marches up Holt Hill, follow the trail left and retrace your steps to the parking lot.

22 INDIAN RIDGE LOOP

KEY AT-A-GLANCE INFORMATION

LENGTH: 2.93 miles
CONFIGURATION: Loop
DIFFICULTY: Easy to moderate
SCENERY: Woods, meadowland, pond, views from two tall eskers
EXPOSURE: Mostly shade
TRAFFIC: Moderate
TRAIL SURFACE: Gravel, packed earth, and some muddy areas
HIKING TIME: 1.5–2 hours
SEASON: Year-round sunrise–sunset
ACCESS: Free
MAPS: Andover Village Improvement Society (AVIS) guides can be purchased at the Andover town hall and from Moor & Mountain (3 Railroad Street, North Andover, [978] 475-3665). GPS coordinates and directions for the many Andover Bay Circuit Trail links can be found at www.baycircuit.org/section3.pdf.
FACILITIES: No
SPECIAL COMMENTS: Andover offers hikers a tremendous number of trails through hundreds of acres of conservation land. By accessing the 200-mile-long Bay Circuit Trail, short jaunts can easily be expanded into lengthy expeditions.
WHEELCHAIR TRAVERSABLE: No
DISTANCE FROM BOSTON COMMON: 24 miles

IN BRIEF

This hike links three properties conserved by AVIS. Starting in woods beside Andover's historic West Parish church, the hike crosses a meadow then negotiates a 50-foot-tall esker, dips to wetland, continues over a second esker, then loops around a large beaver pond to end feet from the start.

DESCRIPTION

Starting at Cutler Road, hike southeast several hundred yards to a large Andover Village Improvement Society (AVIS) sign indicating the trailhead on the left of Reservation Road, then continue northeast across a wooden footbridge several yards into woods brightened in summer by blossoming waist-high jewelweed.

After traveling along the level banking of a stream, the trail departs the damp shade of the woods to cross a meadow. In the near distance, the starch-white spire of the West Parish church stretches to the sky like the righteous boughs of goldenrod blending with the green below. Curving eastward over the domed field once grazed close by cows and now mowed by AVIS on a schedule that coordinates with bobolink nesting, the narrow trail parts clusters of milkweed and clover then returns to woods.

Indian Ridge Loop
UTM Zone (WGS84) 19T
Northing: 4724791
Easting: 322608
Latitude: N 42° 39' 19"
Longitude: W 71° 09' 52"

Directions ————————————➤

From Boston, take Storrow Drive east and merge onto I-93 north (Concord, NH) via the ramp on the left. At 21.1 miles, take Exit 43 to MA 133 east toward Andover. Bear right onto MA 133 and continue 0.8 miles. Turn right onto Cutler Road and follow it approximately 0.4 miles to the intersection at Reservation Road. Park beside the West Parish Garden Cemetery.

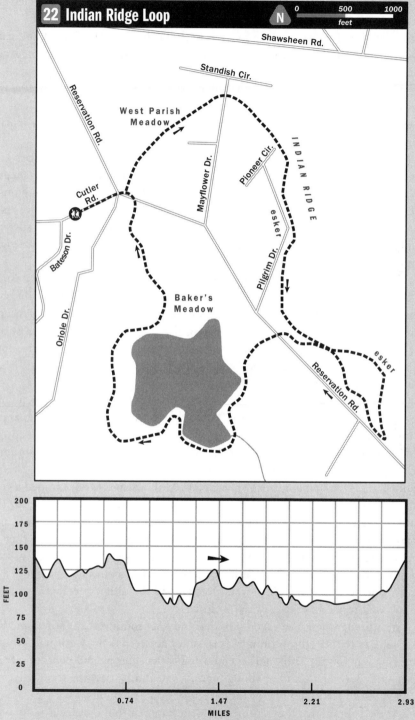

Wetland formed 10,000 to 12,000 years ago by the Wisconsin Glacier lies at the base of the field; here the trail continues across a lengthy span of boardwalk. A harbor for species such as high-bush blueberry, ferns, and skunk cabbage, this primordial morass sets the stage for the equally striking glacier work that lies ahead.

Conveyed to a gravelly crossroads on the far side of the boardwalk, the trail continues to the right heeding Bay Circuit Trail markers as they lead up an esker's slope of cascading glacial grit. Climbing higher and higher, the trail eventually reaches the height of the rooftops of neighboring houses.

As suburbs spread and tracts of land are leveled and filled by graders and bulldozers, it is easy to lose sight of the terrific geologic activity that shaped the New England landscape. However powerful and transformative the human impact on the land, this enormous mound, like 30-foot ship-crushing waves it matches in size, demonstrates the superior strength of nature. Formed of silt carried by meltwater beneath hundreds of feet of ice, this esker is a quiet but vivid reminder of the significance of climate conditions.

Passing well over the heads of the students and faculty of the school nestled on the esker's northwestern flank, the trail continues south, rising and dipping along the rocky ridge. Sheathed in the foliage of oaks, hickories, maples, and birches, the esker provides a well-camouflaged vantage point—a fact that wasn't lost on the generations of Algonquians and Penacook who hunted here until Chief Cutshamache of the Penacook sold the territory to white settlers for six pounds and a coat in the early 17th century.

Before King Philip's War in 1675–1676, relations between the Algonquians, the Penacook and the settlers of the Massachusetts Bay Colony were generally peaceful, if tenuously so. Practical knowledge the Penacook passed on to the settlers of Andover certainly helped keep many alive through the plantation's early years before farms were well established. Reciprocally, the Penacook and Algonquians, who had long been subjected to Mohawk aggression, gained a crucial ally in the English. Change was set in motion, however, in 1662, when the Wampanoag chief Massasoit's eldest son, Alexander (Philip's brother), was summoned at gunpoint to a meeting by the Plymouth Court and died soon after of what was suspected to be poisoning. The incident enraged the Wampanoag, who read the hostile actions of Plymouth's leaders as part of a power play intended to control and subdue them. This event precipitated the ultimate collapse of King Philip's well-tested tolerance of the whites.

At a point where the esker subsides and lists southwest, another, smaller esker joins in to the right, forming a deep valley between them. Continue straight following Bay Circuit Trail markers ignoring paths entering and departing from either side. Beyond a stand of young pines, a vale, and a rise, the trail arrives at an AVIS bench placed on one of Indian Ridge's highest points.

At the split on this downhill run, bear left onto a trail that leads to an oak-filled dell lying between wetland and the esker now tapering eastward. Crossing this floodplain, the trail soon arrives at a junction; bear left here and continue east on the Bay Circuit Trail. Bear left at the split that follows, then right at the next to mount another, smaller esker. At the top, a boulder dressed with a bronze plaque memorializes Andover conservationist Alice Buck, who in 1896 led a crusade to save Indian Ridge as permanent open space.

Arriving at the esker's southern end, the route dips back to lowland, turning sharply north upon reaching level ground (the Bay Circuit Trail continues south to join Reservation Road). White pines fill this glade with few hardwoods in sight as the trail gradually rises again on a gentle grade. Another fork comes quickly; here choose the left prong to hike on toward Indian Ridge.

Along this stretch, several superficial paths cut in from the left and right; disregard these and climb an esker tail to return to a triangular crossroads marked with the familiar white bars of the Bay Circuit Trail. Do not pick up the Bay Circuit Trail—instead, bear sharply left on a second esker tail to exit onto Reservation Road and continue to Baker's Meadow. Cross this quiet road with care, aiming for the brown-and-yellow AVIS sign posted on the other side.

Hiking west on the narrow footpath that leads to the shore of a pond, the realization dawns that Baker's Meadow is nothing of the kind. In fact it hasn't been a meadow since muskrat fur turned heads in the 1920s. Noting that there was more money to be made in fashion than in milk or hay, landowner Alexander Henderson built a dam and started a fur farm. Fortunately for all animals involved, the 1929 market crash brought it all to an end, and in 1958 the Henderson family was persuaded to sell their "meadow" to AVIS.

To navigate this part of the hike, follow white markers around the pond's periphery, being mindful that due to muskrat and beaver work, the pond's depth and therefore its contour is in constant flux. Between ducking under cherry boughs and lilting birches, cast a glance at the water to catch sight of animal life. Hiking through on a September afternoon, I spotted a family of three wild swans preening in the weedy shallows.

Beyond Henderson's dam, about 0.2 miles along, the trail bends due west to stay flush to the water's edge, encountering remnant stone walls as it goes. Crossing a small footbridge on the pond's far side, the route cuts across a wooded peninsula then weaves through a stone wall keeping close to the water. Nearing houses on Oriole Drive, the trail passes a path on the left then crosses another bridge as it swings back eastward.

Upland banking closes in to the left as the trail eventually winds north passing wetland extending from the pond. In time, the pond retreats from view as the trail enters the heavy shadows of woods and eases along the side of a sharply sloped hill. In spots where water percolates through underfoot, the boardwalk ensures dry crossing. Joining up close to a stone wall on its left, the trail soon makes a final climb to Reservation Road. To finish the hike, step from earth to pavement and bear left to retrace steps to the West Parish Garden Cemetery and parking on Cutler Road.

23 SKUG RIVER LOOP

KEY AT-A-GLANCE INFORMATION

LENGTH: 3.05 miles

CONFIGURATION: Out-and-back with loops

DIFFICULTY: Easy to moderate

SCENERY: Wetlands, farmland reverted back to woodland, the millrace of a centuries-old mill, and a 19th-century soapstone quarry

EXPOSURE: Mostly shade except for sun exposure along boardwalks

TRAFFIC: Light

TRAIL SURFACE: Clay dust, packed earth, boardwalk, and exposed rock

HIKING TIME: 2–2.5 hours

SEASON: Year-round sunrise–sunset

ACCESS: Free

MAPS: Available at the Groton town hall and from the town's Web site, www.townofgroton.org

FACILITIES: None

SPECIAL COMMENTS: This gem of a hike crosses land conserved by three distinct groups, the state, the Andover Conservation Commission, and the Andover Village Improvement Society, which, founded in 1894, is one of the oldest conservation groups in the country.

WHEELCHAIR TRAVERSABLE: No

DRIVING DISTANCE FROM BOSTON COMMON: 23 miles

IN BRIEF

Prior to the Civil War Andover was an enclave of strong antislavery sentiment. This hike passes near the home of William Jenkins, whose home was a stop on the Underground Railroad.

DESCRIPTION

The trailhead for the Mary French Reservation is marked on Korinthian Way with the modest square insignia of the Bay Circuit Trail. From this point, set out south on a narrow trail surfaced with clay dust. A kiosk posted by the Andover Conservation Commission greets hikers several yards in, where the initial incline touches bottom. Dedicated to a former town selectman who was both a nature lover and a hiking devotee, the Mary French Reservation is a recent addition to Andover's share of the 200-mile Bay Circuit Trail.

A moment later, the path rolls out from under tree cover to reach a wetland tucked in behind neighborhood houses. A dense buffer of shrubs and reeds permits little outside noise to penetrate. A lawnmower's tearing and grinding becomes almost zoological, its sound waves quickly decaying as they pass over the swamp.

Where water floods to meet the forest, a

Skug River Loop
UTM Zone (WGS84) 19T
Easting: 327749
Northing: 4721848
Latitude: N 42° 37' 47"
Longitude: W 71° 06' 03"

Directions

From Boston, take Storrow Drive East, then merge left onto I-93 north. Continue 16.5 miles to Exit 41. Drive 0.3 miles to where the road forks and bear right onto MA 125. At 4.5 miles, turn right onto Salem Street and continue straight onto Gray Road. At 0.4 miles, turn right onto Korinthian Way. Park at the dip just before Athena Circle.

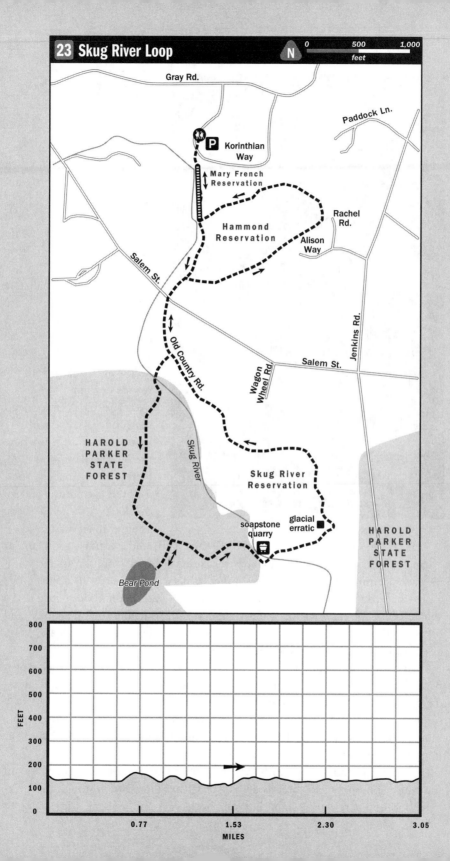

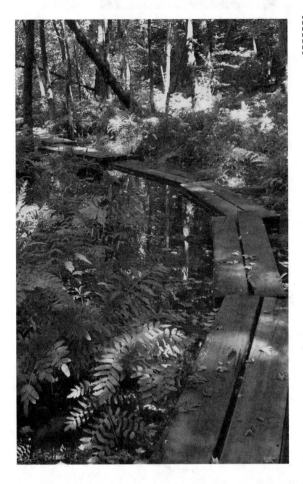

wooden deck built by kids from Andover's Youth Services and a school-based Youth at Risk program invites people to take a seat at a bench and while away an hour or two soaking up the sun or admiring dragonfly acrobatics. If not seduced by the palpable tranquility of the place (or plagued by bugs), step off the terrace onto the 1,000-foot boardwalk and follow as it zigzags into the woods beyond.

The Bay Circuit Trail reasserts itself with a marker on a pine tree where the boardwalk rejoins land. Here, in a shaded spot, a lovely sculptural bench overlooks a scene as poetic as any Monet masterpiece.

From the bench, resume the Bay Circuit Trail and continue south under a canopy of oak, beech, and hickory, brushing by fern fronds. Passing mammoth white pines the trail bends southeast, bisects a stone wall, and mounts an earthen causeway built by farmers to create a watering hole for cattle and a source of ice for their iceboxes. Bear right at the stooped grandfather oak, and hike along the top of the heap of stones. Wooden bridges fill gaps now and again as the causeway spans varying depths of bog.

Arriving shortly at the causeway's end, the trail continues southwest over packed earth navigating through and alongside lengths of lichen- and moss-dappled stone wall. Liberally marked with Bay Circuit Trail markers, the trail soon arrives at a junction. The path loops left here, but continue straight to cross mounds of submerged boulders and convex muddy spots often dimpled with the impressions of raccoon toes, to reach Salem Street.

Though seeming to abruptly vanish, the trail continues up the driveway of the house at number 315 directly across the street. The traffic through this quiet neighborhood is relatively light, but look both ways and, putting aside concerns about trespassing, hike up the drive. Once a public way, the route running over what feels like private property is Old Country Road. Reclaimed by the Bay Circuit Trail Committee, the path is once more open for public use.

The trail cuts back into woods just past a brown saltbox house. Reminiscent of the old cart road it once was, the trail starts off wide and clear with stone walls on either side. When it begins to lose ground to unruly shrubs and brambles. Forge on past a pile of brush to find a wide junction posted with AVIS and Bay Circuit Trail markers. Heed the AVIS arrow and bear right onto the Bridge Trail, which being a link in the Bay Circuit Trail, is also marked with white swatches.

Making a beeline west, the trail quickly reaches mud and a boardwalk leading over the soggy bank of Skug River to a bench. The view upriver on a certain September day revealed the lithe trunks of flame-red maples leaning over a basin overflowing after a summer of heavy rain. The river's name—"Skug"—is a phonetic spelling of the Nipmuc word for skunk.

Hiking along the opposite riverbank, making use of the stone-wall border to keep dry, you'll reach a split in the trail at the boundary of Harold Parker State Forest. Take this right and, for the time being, leave the river behind. An easy climb under pines on a southwest trajectory promptly ends at a "T" made by a second trail, running parallel to the river. Bear left onto this wide cart road edged by a stone wall and follow its even course southeast to where it crosses a path to Bear Pond. A quick trip for a look-see at this turn found neither bears nor much of a pond, just berry bushes and one pleased mockingbird.

From the intersection with Bear Pond, continue straight, hiking southeast. Ahead, beyond a slight rise and rocky pitch, the trail rejoins Skug River. At a junction defined by stone walls, the trail splits abruptly. One route veers sharply right and another pitches left through bushes. What lies beyond is William Jenkins's soapstone quarry and mill site. For a look at the site from atop massive stone walls built to control the water flow, take the left-hand path. Afterward, return to the junction and follow the path to the right farther downriver. Keep an eye out for the first left turn and follow a short winding path down a rocky slope to a bridge.

Built where the turbulent water spills into a quiet pool, the solid bridge provides a peaceful vantage point. Blocks of stone cut and discarded, or left for a pickup that never occurred, lie partially submerged in sudsy water. In the country's first centuries, the soft, easy-to-work stone was a popular material for tombstones and hand-warming blocks.

To the right, beyond a narrow channel, the river empties into a sprawling wetland. Once across the bridge, take a path to the right marked with the white of the Bay Circuit Trail. Starting up a rough slope, the path passes a large soapstone slab lying swamp-side. Look for messages scraped on its smooth face, and, if inspiration strikes, pick up a stone and log a new one. Running along a ridge above the wetland, the trail broadens to the width the carts that frequented the

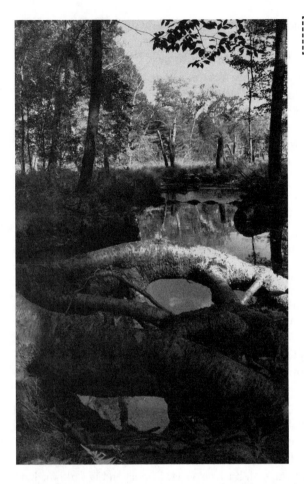

A bend in the Skug River provides a scenic spot to picnic.

place long ago to hauled out stone. Gnawed maple stumps poking through debris confirm suspicions that beavers have moved in and are imposing their ambitions on the swamp.

Leveling out as it aims east, the trail proceeds through sparse woods grown in on old pasture-land and converges with a stone wall opportunis-tically propped against a glacial erratic of astound-ing proportions. Here since the last Ice Age, the boulder that was once just another stone in a wall now popular with rock climbers. At least one bird has given the rock added purpose by building a nest in a southeastern crevice.

A road named for William Jenkins lies at the bottom of the hill to the northeast of the boulder. Aside from being an industrious man, Jenkins was an abolitionist and good friend of those who shared his sympathies, including William Lloyd Garrison, Frederick Douglass, and Harriet Beecher Stowe. Not only a meeting place for those who condemned slavery, Jenkins's house also served as a station on the Underground Railroad.

To reunite with the Bay Circuit Trail, circle the boulder counterclockwise and head off to the northwest. Progressing uphill amid glacial erratics lying about like unmelted hail, the trail nears a white house on the right. Pass this and the minor paths weaving in and out and continue straight through a junction marked with two white bars and a red marker.

Serpentining over land populated with oak, young pine, and the odd birch and beech, the red trail traces the edges of an obsolete pasture and eventually angles northwest to run back to the junction of Old County Road and the Bridge Trail. Having closed the loop, hike northwest back to Salem Street.

Returning to the Hammond Reservation, backtrack to where the trail

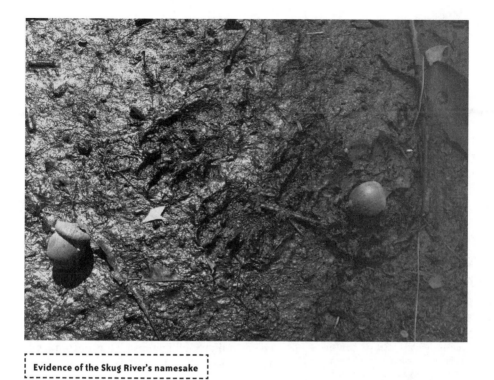

Evidence of the Skug River's namesake

splits and bear right. Traveling east, the trail traces the periphery of an all-but-impenetrable wetland, passing suburban homes shrouded by tree cover. Near where the boardwalk begins, the Bay Circuit Trail detours to the right. Let it go and continue north on the boardwalk, staying with the AVIS trail. Shortly, this trail turns downhill and, heading west, reaches the causeway bordering the Mary French Reservation. Hike along this curious mound of stone and, when you arrive at the grand oak in the junction, bear right and retrace the boardwalk back to the start.

NEARBY ATTRACTIONS

The Addison Gallery of American Art, located at Andover's Phillips Academy, 180 Main Street, (978) 749-4015, offers a chance to see exciting art in a peaceful setting. Created by Thomas Cochran in 1913 to promote art appreciation and learning, the gallery is part of Andover's Phillips Academy but is free to the public. The gallery is open Tuesday through Saturday, 10 a.m. to 5 p.m., and Sunday, 1 to 5 p.m.

24 GOLDSMITH WOODLANDS LOOP

KEY AT-A-GLANCE INFORMATION

LENGTH: 3.67 miles

CONFIGURATION: Loop

DIFFICULTY: Easy to moderate

SCENERY: Woods, wetlands, and a large pond

EXPOSURE: Mostly shaded

TRAFFIC: Light

TRAIL SURFACE: Packed earth, gravel, and boardwalk

HIKING TIME: 1–1.5 hours

SEASON: Year-round sunrise–sunset

ACCESS: Free

MAPS: Andover Village Improvement Society (AVIS) maps can be purchased at the Andover town hall and at Andover's sports outfitter, Moor & Mountain, at 3 Railroad Avenue, (978) 475-3665.

FACILITIES: None

SPECIAL COMMENTS: Though short in miles, Goldsmith Woodlands Loop is long in interest. Be sure to allow enough time for birding, botanizing, and, if the season is right, blueberry sampling.

WHEELCHAIR TRAVERSABLE: Zack's Way, which leads from the parking area to Foster's Pond, is rough but passable.

DRIVING DISTANCE FROM BOSTON COMMON: 22 miles

IN BRIEF

This hike explores the fabulously glaciated woodland landscape surrounding a large pond named for one of Andover's first settlers.

DESCRIPTION

In 1634 the Great and General Court of Massachusetts set in motion the establishment of an inland plantation northwest of the already burgeoning settlement of Boston. To encourage colonists to leave the comfort and security of the coast for the wild, wolf-ridden frontier, the court offered the first settlers three years of immunity from taxes, levies, and services—except military obligations. Thus encouraged, Andrew Foster and another 21 game individuals from Newbury and Ipswich ventured forth and, together by pooling resources that amounted to six pounds currency and a coat, they transacted a land deal with Chief Cutshamache of the Pennacook.

According to the evidence, Andrew Foster won the gamble for after amassing a sizable parcel of land—including the pond that now bears his name. He lived to the remarkable age of 106. His widow, Ann "Goody" Foster, fared not nearly so well. During the madness of the Witch Trials of 1692, she and her daughter Lacey were called before the

---

Goldsmith
Woodlands Loop

UTM Zone (WGS84) 19T

Easting: 325803

Northing: 4719767

Latitude: N 42° 36' 38"

Longitude: W 71° 07' 26"

Directions ⟶

From Boston, take Storrow Drive east and merge onto I-93 north via the ramp on the left toward Concord. At 16.5 miles, take Exit 41 to MA 125 toward Andover. Continue 0.3 miles and keep right at the fork to access MA 125. Drive 2.3 miles and take the MA 28 north ramp. Merge onto MA 28 and drive 0.3 miles. An AVIS sign marks the entrance to the parking area on the left.

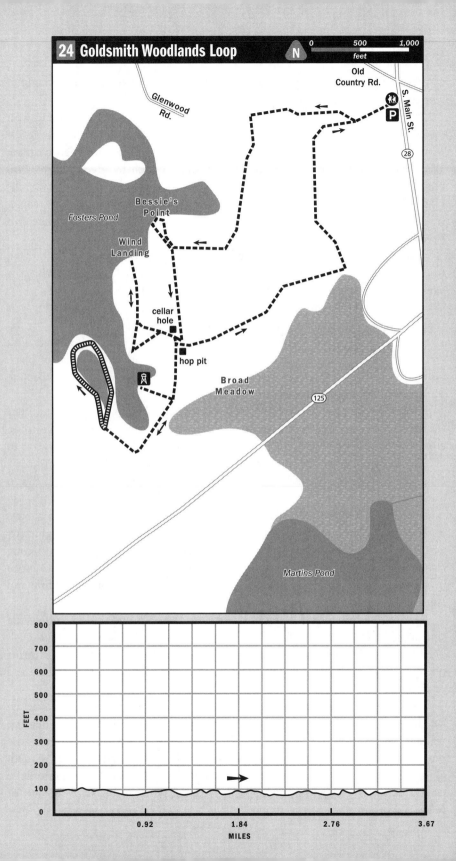

Old
Country Rd.

Glenwood
Rd.

S. Main St.

28

Bessie's
Point

Fosters Pond

Wind
Landing

cellar
hole

hop pit

Broad
Meadow

125

Martins Pond

0   500   1,000
feet

judges. Lacey survived, but Ann, who sacrificed herself to save her daughter, was condemned and died during her 21st week in jail.

From the trailhead at the far end of the parking area, set out hiking west on Zack's Way, a level path the width of a farm cart. Easing downhill alongside a brook past a kiosk and AVIS signs, this even, old-time service road nests on a banking beneath rock, sand, and gravel shoved high by glacial ice 10,000 to 12,000 years ago. Ahead, where Zack's Way swings left, bear right on the High Trail to ascend a great ridge rimming wetland to the north. Dark, steeple-straight pines varied with lissome birch veil the view of the gurgling waters of Frye's Brook far below.

Edged for a brief while by a slapdash or weatherworn stone wall, the trail traces the ridge west, passing an unmarked path to the left before leaving the stone wall and descending to a clearing on the shore of an old millpond.

Steer left, taking up the Pine Trail, which joins in off the hillside and travels south keeping within sight of Foster's Pond and its swampy border.

Rolling over gentle dips and swells through mixed woods accented with young aspen, the trail soon rises to a broad junction cut into a stand of black pine. Noting Zack's Way entering from the left and a new trail, make a beeline for the pond by heeding the sign for Bessie's Point.

Sloping downhill on a gentle grade, the path quickly dovetails with another (Meeting House Road) then carries on through an avenue of black pine to an elevated enclave rich with rhododendron and laurel planted a century or so ago. Landowner Bessie Goldsmith, kept house on this peaceful hummock in a rough-hewn cabin through World War II, the psychedelic 1960s, and the Nixon presidency.

Cast of a mold all her own, Bessie is said to have been more than a little possessive of her blueberries in picking season. Any trespasser she caught harvesting was met with a shotgun pointed at their bucket. Though indeed strong in her convictions, Bessie was not ungenerous—in 1974 she entrusted her entire property, blueberry bushes and all, to the Fund for Preservation of Wildlife and Natural Areas.

From the crest of the hillock where Bessie's cabin once stood, follow the trail as it tapers to a slender spit of moss-covered rocks sleeved in high-bush blueberries and honeysuckle. Water lies all around, rippling with life forms peculiar and spectacular—from polliwog and water strider to wood duck and painted turtle.

To continue the hike, reverse direction and ascend the steps to a bench beside Bessie's homesite; when ready, retreat on Meeting House Road. Bearing right at the junction encountered earlier, stay with the cart road as it leaves the pines behind and enters a wood of oak and maple to soon arrive at a crossroad. Here a sign alerts passersby to the former location of Zack's cottage on the right and, kitty-corner to it, his hop pit. Zack likely never met with the butt of Bessie's shotgun since Bessie employed him as a caretaker for the woods and as

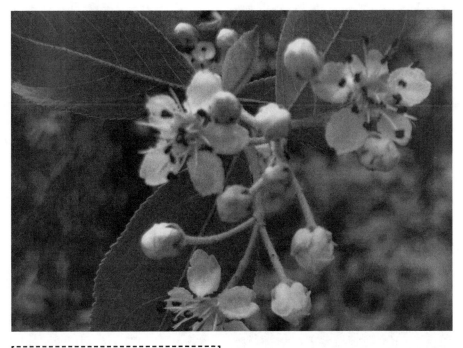

Red chokeberry (*Photinia pyrifolia*) in bloom

a seasonal handyman in the summer months when she rented out cottages to vacationers.

After surveying the cellar hole of the cottage where Zack once tucked into hearty meals and kicked up weary feet for a good night's sleep, follow the "new path" (Pond Road) west back toward Foster's Pond. After meeting with a path to the left, this rutted cart road bears north and rolls downhill rounding a shrub-hidden bend or two to meet the water's edge at Wind Landing. In spring, amid the raucous cackling of red-winged blackbirds and black-purple grackles, keep an eye out for blossoming lady's slippers.

To vary the route on the return trip, split to the right when the trail forks and hike along the pond's steep banking to loop back to Pond Road, heading east again.

On returning to Zack's house, turn right and follow Al's Trail south, first downhill then across a causeway between wetland and Foster's Pond. Don't be turned away by the chain—its purpose is to bar vehicles not hikers. Opposite a path that ventures up a steep rise pond-side, the trail travels past meadowland fringed by woods to the east. Once around a weedy cove settled by wood ducks, the trail ascends into a hemlock grove arcing high and wide of the water to follow an earthen finger to "Journey's End."

From the peninsula's narrow point, backtrack to a path branching to the left and follow its lead across a boardwalk to the tiny island of Point Judith. After

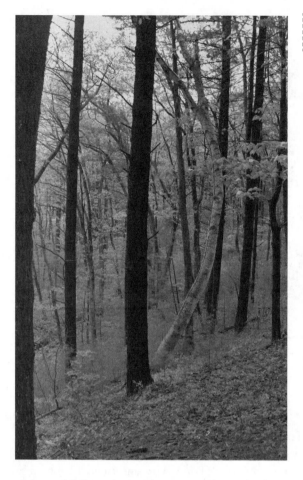

A supine birch and stately pine grow on an esker's slope.

some bird-watching or picnicking, follow the path as it crosses to another oblong island via boardwalk and loops back to the hemlock wood.

Aiming southeast now, retrace steps over Al's Trail past Birch Cove back to the junction at Zack's house— detouring to the left along the way for one more gander across the pond. Turning from the pond, pass Zack's hop pit and follow Pond Road (marked "New Trail") as it dives eastward. Continuing over and through great swells and swales, the trail swerves west at a brook then converges with the level plane of Zack's Way. At this triangular junction, bear right and follow the sandy cart road east back to the reservation's entrance and parking lot.

NEARBY ATTRACTIONS

Those interested in extending their stay in Andover might like to camp at the nearby Harold Parker State Forest. The park 91 campsites and, most importantly, hot showers. The campground is open from mid-April to mid-October. Trails in the 3,000-acre park connect with the Skug River hike (page 140) and the Bay Circuit Trail. The state forest is at 1951 Turnpike Street, Route 114, North Andover, (978) 686-3391.

WEIR HILL LOOP

IN BRIEF

Touring land that was once the estate of a 19th-century industrialist, this hike circles the base of a massive drumlin poised beside Lake Cochichewick then climbs along its axis to reach a scenic vista atop a second conjoined drumlin.

DESCRIPTION

From the information kiosk above Stevens Street, climb the grass-covered hill to a gap in a stone wall and ease into the cool shade of woods, heading northeast. Tracing the property's periphery along the base of Weir Hill, stay left at each of the next two intersections to take up the gently arcing Edgewood Farm Trail. Be alert for the next fork (it is less pronounced than the others), and bear left again to remain on this same trail as it descends to a streambed marked by skunk cabbage and mud the color of bittersweet-chocolate. A footbridge (and during wet season a few acrobatic leaps) provides dry conveyance to the upland opposite.

Ahead a trail entering from private property to the north interrupts Edgewater

KEY AT-A-GLANCE INFORMATION

LENGTH: 2.46 miles

CONFIGURATION: Loop

DIFFICULTY: Easy to moderate

SCENERY: Hills, woods, open fields, and views across Lake Cochichewick

EXPOSURE: Mostly shaded

TRAFFIC: Moderate

TRAIL SURFACE: Packed earth. Some sections can be muddy at times.

HIKING TIME: 1.5 hours

SEASON: Sunrise–sunset year-round

ACCESS: Free

MAPS: Available at the reservation while supplies last. Maps can also be printed from the trustees' Web site, www.thetrustees.org; select "Weir Hill" from the properties menu.

FACILITIES: None

SPECIAL COMMENTS: An ideal time to visit Weir Hill is an hour to an hour and a half before dusk to reach the hike's scenic vista in time for sunset.

WHEELCHAIR TRAVERSABLE: No

DRIVING DISTANCE FROM BOSTON COMMON: 28 miles

Directions

From Boston, take I-93 north to MA 125 north (Andover bypass) and go 7.3 miles. At the traffic lights, merge left onto MA 114 west. At the traffic lights opposite Merrimack College (on the left), turn right onto Andover Street (MA 125) and follow it 0.2 miles. Turn right at the traffic lights (still on Andover Street) and go 0.6 miles. Bear right at the fork and continue 0.2 miles to the intersection at Old North Andover Center. Go straight another 0.1 mile, then make a left onto Stevens Street. Continue 0.8 miles to the entrance on the right.

Weir Hill Loop

UTM Zone (WGS84) 19T

Easting: 307195

Northing: 4714344

Latitude: N 42° 33' 27"

Longitude: W 71° 20' 55"

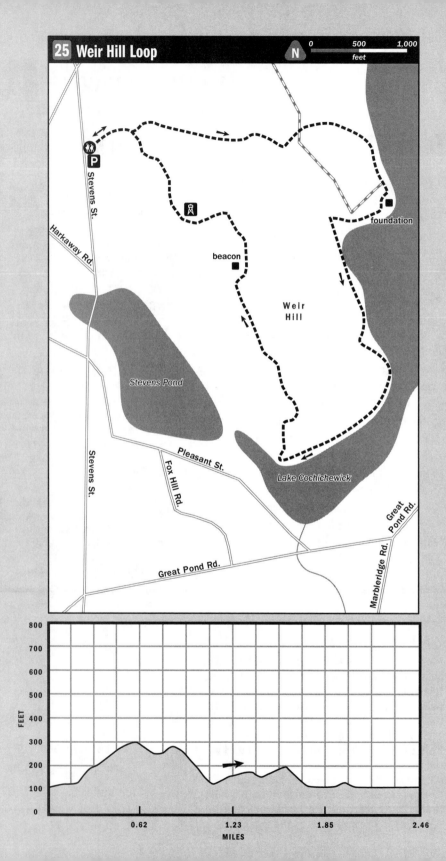

Farm Trail. Hike this wide path several yards south and bear left again where Edgewater Farm Trail continues on its eastward tack through a stand of young birch trees.

After being bisected one last time, Edgewood Farm Trail coasts downhill amid a blend of beech, pine, and birch to the shore of Lake Cochichewick. Even on windless days, vector currents of air propel ripples of surf to land. Again and again, breaking wavelets clink like glasses meeting in a perpetual champagne toast.

Bearing south a foot or two from the water, the root-tangled trail soon arrives at a sort of beach beside a stone foundation. Now little more than an abstract form that excites the imagination, this pit edged with granite marks where the clubhouse of the North Andover Country Club once stood. Back in the day, club members teed off on a golf course across the lake, and once the round was won—or lost—paddled to the clubhouse for cocktails, dinner, and dancing.

Leaving this site of many festive nights, continue along the lake on what now becomes Cochichewick Trail. Traipsing west around the base of the minor mound of glacial rubble that bumps shoulders with the more substantial Weir Hill drumlin, the trail crosses the watery gap between the two via a boardwalk. Then, like the many moccasins that wore it into being, the path trots south beneath the brilliant foliage of birch and hickory to where the tip of the great drumlin presses close to Lake Cochichewick's western bank.

It is likely that until Metacomet and allied tribes lost their war against colonial expansion, the Pennacook lived in seasonal if not permanent settlements here. Archaeologists digging in the area in 1968 uncovered a campsite near where the lake narrows as it bends west toward Stevens Pond. The setting offered all that the native people needed: shelter from northern winds, woods full of game, and proximity to the breeding grounds of bounteous alewives. The tribes set up woven traps fixed with wooden stakes just offshore to catch the coveted fish as they swam from brook to lake.

The presence of the Pennacook and their use of the land is evident in the name given the hill and—though far more subtly—in the natural history of the hillside. Before the arrival of white settlers, Native Americans altered the landscape almost as radically as did any farmer or timberman to come. To attract deer and facilitate hunting, the tribes practiced controlled burning, which had the immediate effect of clearing underbrush and promoting the growth of tender shoots and grasses—valuable fodder for grazing animals. Over the longer term, the burnings affected the profile of the woodland by promoting tree and shrub species that are resistant to fire.

Like the Native Americans, the farmers and mill operators who settled this area are gone, yet their mark on the landscape remains. Fragments of stone wall long ago stripped of their function haunt the woods, and geometric patches of successional species tell in whispers which tracts were once pasture and which

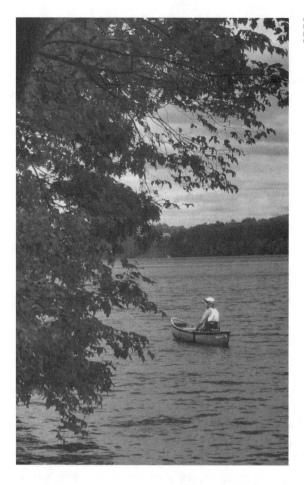

were timber lots. Many of the milldams are gone as well, but the effect of each persists in the character of the area's ecology.

A result of the property's complex land-use history is that ten distinct types of plant communities grow on Weir Hill. Besides an uncommon 60-acre oak and hickory forest, the hill harbors several rare protected species, including the white bog orchid (*Habenaria dilatata*), violet bush clover (*Lespedeza violacea*), and butternut tree (*Juglans nigra*).

At the tip of Weir Hill's blunt nose, Cochichewick Trail becomes Miller's Path. Remaining flush to the shore, the trail arches west, rising slightly to meet a path that emerges from woods below what appears to be former pastureland. Bear left to continue southwest along the foot of scruffy grassland dotted with scrub pine and oak. Improvised paths bleed off to the right now and again, but ignore these and the (unmarked) Weir Hill Trail and continue on level ground to where the lake curls north and a railroad trestle bridge comes into sight. Here take the next trail that bears north away from the water.

Looking something like a ski slope in summer pending a manicure by pruning crews, the southern face of Weir Hill—with its rangy blueberry bushes, ferns, and spotty oaks and pines—is a boon to bobolinks, goldfinches, bluebirds, and other songbirds dependent on open meadowlands.

The first stage of the ascent ends at a junction well up the hill. To climb higher along the drumlin's middle, bear left. Rising and sinking into and out of deep swales, the trail reaches a tilted T-intersection halfway up the hill. Turn left here and continue northwest on Scrub Oak Trail. Aptly named, this route winds between bristly oaks and graceful hickories on its approach to the hill's unpretentious summit.

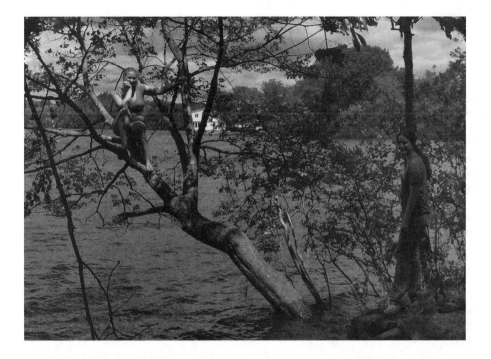

Just as the trail starts down the hill's western slope it meets a path entering from the right. Switch off here and head east briefly to pass an airport beacon erected amid trees at Weir Hill's highest point. On encountering Weir Hill Trail immediately ahead, bear left and follow it as it descends northward into a cleft formed by Weir Hill and its lesser twin.

Where depressions trap water and form vernal pools, another trail diverts left crossing a bog before mounting the eastern slope of the second hill. Take this mud- and rock-laced detour to reap the reward of a magnificent view looking west from a gorgeous hillside meadow. Those with foresight will plan to reach this picturesque summit in time to take in the light effects of the setting sun.

When ready, follow Stevens Trail as it descends along the hill's axis to Johnson Trail. Bear left at this last junction to return to the reservation's entrance on Stevens Street.

NEARBY ATTRACTIONS

If hiking Weir Hill sparks an interest in Native American history, consider paying a visit to the Robert S. Peabody Museum of Archaeology located at Philip's Andover Academy. This museum, one of the country's most important repositories of Native American archaeological collections, is located on the corner of Main Street and Philip's Street. The museum is open 8 a.m. to 5 p.m., and admission is free but by appointment only. To arrange a visit, call (978) 749-4490.

26 OLD TOWN HILL: Marsh and Farm Loop

KEY AT-A-GLANCE INFORMATION

LENGTH: 2.6 miles

CONFIGURATION: Loop

DIFFICULTY: Moderate

SCENERY: Salt marshes, woods, and hay fields, with a view of Plum Island from the hilltop

EXPOSURE: Mostly shaded

TRAFFIC: Light

TRAIL SURFACE: Mostly packed earth with grass sections and some gravel roads

HIKING TIME: 1.5 hours

SEASON: Year-round 8 a.m.–sunset

ACCESS: Free

MAPS: Posted at the entrance

FACILITIES: None

SPECIAL COMMENTS: If planning a hike here in the summertime, bring along a bathing suit, because at mid- to high tide on a hot day, a swim in the nearby creek is a pleasure you won't want to miss.

WHEELCHAIR TRAVERSABLE: No

DRIVING DISTANCE FROM BOSTON COMMON: 38 miles

Old Town Hill:
Marsh and Farm Loop

UTM Zone (WGS84) 19T

Easting: 348042

Northing: 4736893

Latitude: N 42° 46' 10"

Longitude: W 70° 51' 26"

IN BRIEF

Surveying salt marshes and Newbury's tallest hill, this hike explores a landscape that remains much as it was in the 1600s when a small group of colonists first settled the area.

DESCRIPTION

In 1633 a ship named the *Mary and John* hoisted sail and departed England's Thames River to deliver 71 passengers to new lives in the Massachusetts Bay Colony. Of these travelers, 2 were bound for Plymouth, 1 for Roxbury, 7 for Salem, 26 for Ipswich, 9 for Salisbury, 16 for undeclared destinations—and 9 for a new settlement they would call "Newbury." After wintering in Agawam (now Ipswich), Reverend Thomas Parker and eight others pushed farther north to rich land they found at the mouth of the Quascacunquen River.

Today a monument commemorating the settler's arrival sits on the Old Town village green. The monument is topped with a bronze replica of the *Mary and John* and bears the names of Newbury's first citizens. The one-room school they established stands across from the monument on the green's northern side. The meetinghouse they hastily built for a place to convene and worship was the 12th church of

Directions ⟶

From Boston, take Storrow Drive east and merge onto I-93 north via the ramp on the left and drive 1.8 miles, then take Exit 27, on the left, to head north on MA 1. Drive 0.4 miles, merge onto US 1 north, and go 13.9 miles. Merge onto I-95 north. From I-95, take Exit 54 and follow MA 133 east 4.5 miles. Turn left onto MA 1A north and drive 4.8 miles. Shortly after crossing Parker River, turn left onto Newman Road. The entrance and roadside parking for ten cars are approximately 0.5 miles ahead on the left.

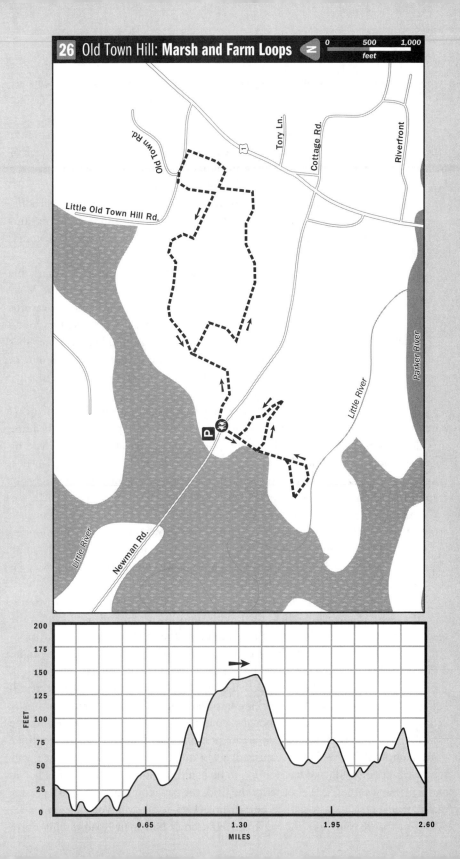

0   500   1,000
feet

Old Town Rd.

Tory Ln.

Cottage Rd.

Riverfront

Little Old Town Hill Rd.

Parker River

Little River

Little River

Newman Rd.

200
175
150
125
100
75
50
25
0

FEET

0.65   1.30   1.95   2.60

MILES

the Massachusetts Bay Colony. This rustic shelter and its several replacements are gone, but services continue at the Old Town Church, erected nearby in 1869. Since it opened in 1635, Newbury Congregational Church has had just 11 pastors.

Arriving with little but each other and the clothes they wore, this group of nine quickly set to work building homes and clearing land for farming. Fearing attack by malevolent beings, particularly American Indians and wolves, the settlers passed a law that no house could be built beyond a half mile from the meetinghouse.

The quality of life in Newbury proved good and the first farms productive, so the population quickly expanded. As families grew and new immigrants arrived, the settlement spread to what are now the towns of West Newbury, Bayfield, and Newburyport.

Much about the region has changed in the years since, but to a remarkable degree, much has stayed the same. Many descendants of those aboard the *Mary and John,* my family included, still live in the community. Thanks to various conservation organizations, the landscape has stayed largely as the setters found it. Farmers continue to harvest salt marsh hay on the vast and beautiful marshes that lie along the Quascacunquen River (renamed the Parker River in honor of Reverend Parker), and Old Town Hill, farmed for generations by the Bushee family, remains much as it was in horse and buggy days.

From the parking area on Newman Road, hike southwest on the wide packed-earth trail. Several hundred feet along you will pass a trail heading uphill to the left. Continue on descending the hill to arrive at a causeway leading between tracts of marshland. Looking west here, you will see the Little River, a tributary of the Parker River. To the northeast, you can scan acres and acres of fragrant wetland dominated by a salt-tolerant grass called spartina.

On the far side of the causeway, a path splits off to the right, but continue straight up a slight rise to reach a cedar and oak grove on an island surrounded by tidal-zone marshland. The narrow path winds as it leads to a lovely small "beach." If the day is hot and the tide high, pull off your shoes and jump in for the water is clean and the current gentle.

From this spot, the trail continues northwest along the edge of the woods, switching east to cross a hayfield thick with timothy, vetch, and patches of milkweed. At the end of the field the trail descends to the causeway crossed earlier.

Double back a short distance to the path running up a steep hill to the right. A climb up this banking leads to a wooden bench where you can relax and look out over a gorgeous view of the river below. From this spot, continue hiking east, paralleling a stone wall on the left. Ducking into the shade of hickory branches, bristly cedars, and scrappy black cherry boughs, continue until you come to a break in the wall marked with daylilies and an arrow pointing left. Heed the arrow and hike north alongside the hay field. As it is still a working field, you are likely to see huge shrink-wrapped bundles of hay waiting to be hauled off to feed the county's horses and remaining cattle. At the corner of the field, the path continues through a parting in the weeds, reenters woods then quickly links back to the trail you came in on.

To expand your hike to Old Town Hill, cross Newman Road aiming north

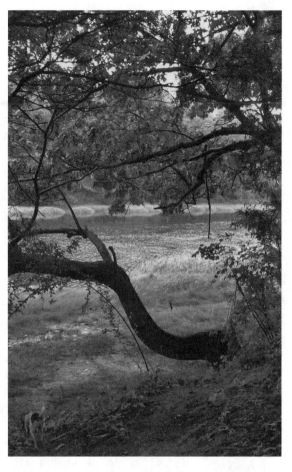

The clean water of the Parker River tempts fishermen and swimmers alike.

to find the trailhead marked by a white sign bearing a symbol of a hiker. Another sign posted nearby identifies this path as part of the Bay Circuit Trail. Traveling east through woods bordering Newman Road, the trail leads to an intersection near a pine grove planted in rows. Bear left to pick up a wide, packed-gravel trail. Swinging southwest as it gains elevation, this old wagon route leads to a pasture atop Old Town Hill. The Bushee family's herd once grazed on timothy and clover here, now the meadow is a butterfly haven choked with milkweed and Queen Anne's lace. Turning southeast to cross the hilltop, the mowed-grass path passes several old fruit trees holding out among the vigorous young Norway maples. The path reenters woods briefly before spilling out to a second field. From here, the township's highest point, you can see for miles on a clear day. Thick clouds or summer haze may hide Plum Island and the sea from view, but you'll know they are there by the fresh scent on the breeze.

To find the trail, walk east along the edge of the field 100 feet or so. Leaving the clearing, the path slants off to the right to retreat back into woods. Curving east, it then spills down a stony slope and arrives at a wide, open hay field at the foot of the hill. Loop around this tract of green, walking the periphery counterclockwise. When nearing where you began, look for the symbol of a backpacker on a white sign, and return to the woods, heading northwest.

As the trail bends this way and that, sections of boardwalk help keep your feet above water. After much twisting and turning, the trail arrives at a two-pronged fork. Pass the path that heads uphill under the pines and continue on the route bearing right. At the next split, stay to the left to rejoin the wagon road that scales Old Town Hill. Take up this route once more, hiking right to return to the intersection at the pine grove off Newman Road and head back to the parking area.

27 APPLETON FARMS: Grass Rides Loop

KEY AT-A-GLANCE INFORMATION

LENGTH: 2.6 miles

CONFIGURATION: Loop

DIFFICULTY: Easy

SCENERY: Forested wetlands, view across a giant pasture of a farm granted to the original owner by the King of England

EXPOSURE: Mostly shaded

TRAFFIC: Light

TRAIL SURFACE: Packed earth and grass

HIKING TIME: 2 hours

SEASON: Year-round 8 a.m.–sunset

ACCESS: Free

MAPS: Posted at the entrance

FACILITIES: None

SPECIAL COMMENTS: Now managed by the Trustees of Reservations, Appleton Farms still operates as a working farm, producing high-quality hay, milk, meat, and produce.

WHEELCHAIR TRAVERSABLE: No

DRIVING DISTANCE FROM BOSTON COMMON: 30 miles

IN BRIEF

Grass Rides Loop explores the northwestern acres of Appleton Farms, following an old steeplechase course and trails through forested wetlands.

DESCRIPTION

In 1638 Samuel Appleton was granted a 460-acre parcel of land spreading between the towns of Ipswich and Hamilton. Over the centuries nine generations expanded and maintained what grew to be a magnificent 1,000-acre farm. Today Samuel Appleton would be delighted to know that though the property has passed from Appleton hands to the protective care of the Trustees of Reservations, its life as a productive farm continues. A full-time farm manager oversees a meat and dairy program in addition to a commercial vegetable and haying operation.

Starting at the parking area, cross the field, following the avenue of maples to an entrance to the Grass Rides located beyond a bog at the edge of the woods. Enter through a break in a stone wall to access trails cleared generations ago for the purpose of equestrian sport. Head immediately to the left and follow the path along the edge of the woods to where it meets another gap in the wall. Turn

Appleton Farms:
Grass Rides Loop

UTM Zone (WGS84) 19T

Easting: 346737

Northing: 4723579

Latitude: N 42° 38' 58"

Longitude: W 70° 52' 10"

Directions ────────────────▶

From Boston, take MA 1 north to MA 128 north to Exit 20N and follow MA 1A north 4.5 miles. Turn left onto Cutler Road and follow it 2.2 miles. At the intersection with Highland Street, turn right. There is a parking area immediately on the right.

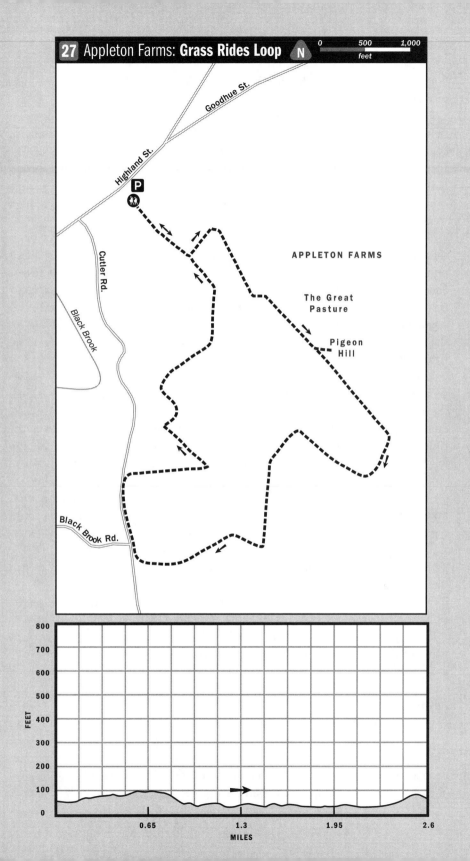

N

0   500   1,000
feet

Goodhue St.

Highland St.

P

APPLETON FARMS

The Great
Pasture

Cutler Rd.

Black Brook

Pigeon
Hill

Black Brook Rd.

800
700
600
500
400
300
200
100
0

FEET

0.65   1.3   1.95   2.6

MILES

left again and continue uphill just beyond the shadows of the hemlocks and oaks to your right.

Over your left shoulder you will see the soft contours of the wide-open field known as the Great Pasture. Where the climb levels off a well-placed bench invites you to stop and scan this fabulously vast field. At 133 acres it is the largest grassland in northeastern Massachusetts. Looking through bushes that grow along its edges, you might meet the warm gaze of a cow or, then again in the fading light of dusk, you might spot a triad of coyotes making a stealthy retreat.

Leave the bench and continue along the pasture. Follow the path as it winds through trees, descends, then climbs, to the peak of Pigeon Hill, the highest point in Appleton Farms. Break from the path here and walk out into the Great Pasture. In the center of the hill, you will see a large granite pinnacle. Salvaged from Gore Hall of Harvard University, the pinnacle was placed on the hill to commemorate Colonel Francis Randall Appleton Jr. (1885–1974). Looking to the southeast from Pigeon Hill, it is possible to see as far as Hog Island and Crane Beach.

Continue along the edge of the Great Pasture to where the path eases southwest downhill and turns northwest. A commuter rail line slices through the property between wetlands on the southern border of the Great Pasture. Spilling off the hill the trail widens as it meets another route joining in from the right. This broad, even track once served as a steeplechase course. Riders atop hot-blooded thoroughbreds once tore through this turn heading into the speed zone of the avenue ahead.

Before long, the trail arrives at a four-way intersection. At this juncture, take a sharp left and continue westward. The trail is raised through here, forming a causeway between wetland on either side. Soon the trail bends to the left as it passes a small meadow surrounded by woods. Resuming a straight course, the path takes you to a second pinnacle positioned at the center of a clearing shaped like the hub of a wheel with trails radiating in all directions.

Stay your course walking south beyond the pinnacle to the next trail on the right and proceed northwest. Unlike the avenues radiating from the pinnacle, this new trail has curves. Look for the occasional swamp oak among more plentiful beech and shagbark hickory trees. Shortly you will reach a stand of exotic evergreens planted in clean rows on the left and right. Directly ahead, look for a stone wall and, beyond it, a lightly traveled road. Turn right to parallel the wall on your left.

Following alongside wetland once more, you will pass a trail on the right, but continue straight. Soon you will notice a brown house on the left across the dirt road beside the Grass Rides Trail. Follow the trail as it arrives at a three-pronged fork and continue up a short rise. Just beyond the rise, the trail arrives at another elegant avenue of cultivated evergreens.

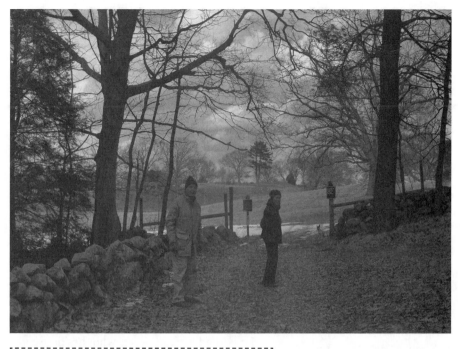

Two hikers pause before an entrance to the Great Pasture.

Heading east now, the trail takes you downhill briefly over soft footing. Passing through another intersection the trail continues straight and crosses wetland via a short causeway. Just beyond this, the trail joins one of the avenues that leads to the second pinnacle off to your right. Across the avenue lies a small meadow.

Turn left to head northeast. Evergreens stand on either side of the trail, with wetlands behind them. Upon reaching another grove of conifers, turn right to travel northwest. At the next intersection bear right to cross a narrow causeway. Beyond this continue straight heading northeast. Following a dip, the trail rises again and forms a "T" with another path. Cross here, bearing slightly left following the trail as it heads upward beneath a canopy of hemlocks. When the trail reaches the next junction, turn left to arrive back at the hike's starting point.

28 WILLOWDALE STATE FOREST:
Pine Swamp–Milldam Loop

KEY AT-A-GLANCE INFORMATION

LENGTH: 7.6 miles

CONFIGURATION: Loop

DIFFICULTY: Easy to moderate due to the length

SCENERY: Woods, kettle ponds, vernal pools, the Ipswich River, a fish ladder, and a 19th-century milldam

EXPOSURE: Mostly shaded

TRAFFIC: Moderate

TRAIL SURFACE: Mostly packed earth and gravel and potentially muddy areas

HIKING TIME: 3 hours

SEASON: Sunrise–sunset year-round

ACCESS: Free

MAPS: Available at www.mass.gov/dcr/parks/northeast/wild.htm

FACILITIES: None

SPECIAL COMMENTS: Deer ticks are common in these woods; be sure to check yourself and your clothes for hangers-on after hiking. Also note that hunting is allowed in November and December.

WHEELCHAIR TRAVERSABLE: Bradley Palmer State Park has wheelchair-friendly trails.

DRIVING DISTANCE FROM BOSTON COMMON: 31 miles

IN BRIEF

This hike explores the Pine Swamp of the popular Willowdale State Forest, taking a detour halfway through to travel along the Ipswich River to a scenic 19th-century milldam.

DESCRIPTION

Something about the Ipswich River and its rugged, placid, and fertile watershed attracts ambitious men with expansive appetites. Its first "owner" in recorded history was Chief Masconomo of the Agawam. The next was John Winthrop—son of Massachusetts's first governor. The last was Bradley Palmer, a Harvard-educated lawyer, who, besides representing Sinclair Oil in the Teapot Dome scandal, served President Wilson at the Versailles Peace Conference in the final days of World War I. Bradley Palmer's holdings were likely the smallest—just 10,000 acres spread over five towns. Perhaps the soul of Masconomo, who was said to have been a wise and generous man, still watches over the land. It's a curious notion but one that would explain what moved Bradley Palmer to donate all his vast acreage to the Commonwealth of Massachusetts well before his death in 1948.

From the parking area on the side of Linebrook Road, navigate the green steel

---

Willowdale State Forest

UTM Zone (WGS84) 19T

Easting: 344581

Northing: 4727597

Latitude: N 42° 41' 06"

Longitude: W 70° 53' 50"

Directions

From Boston, take Storrow Drive east toward I-93 north, then merge onto US 1 north toward the Tobin Bridge. Drive 15.1 miles and merge onto I-95 north. After 3.7 miles, take Exit 50 (toward Topsfield) to US 1 north. At 6.8 miles, turn right onto Linebrook Road, Ipswich. Continue about 1.3 miles. The parking area is on the right at the bottom of a hill before Marini's Farm Stand (259 Linebrook Road).

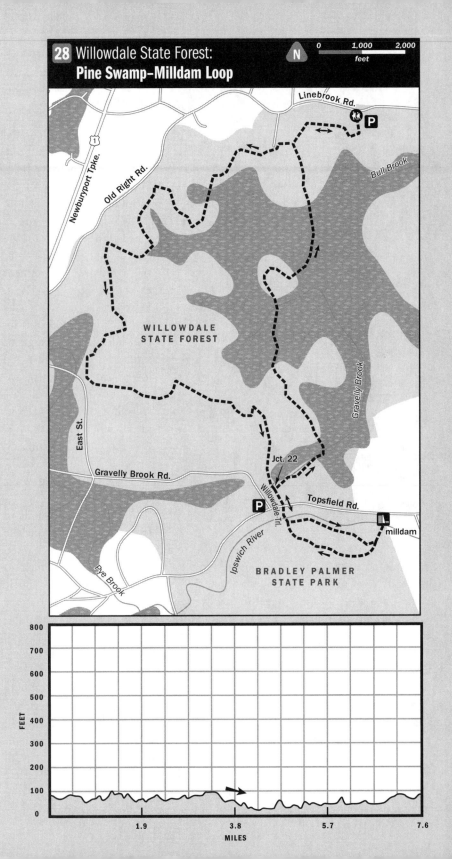

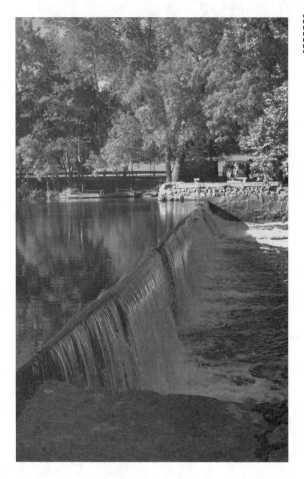

fence and hike south on the mowed path to the left of a cultivated strawberry field. Sloping to the edge of the farmland the trail divides in two as it reaches shade. Heed white markers for the Bay Circuit Trail and enter the woods via a prominent esker bridging wetland. Hardwoods, mostly oaks and hickories, nod in from the sides as the ridge of sand and gravel eases to lower ground. Except for the filtered sound of cars traveling on US 1 a couple of miles away, there is little to hear but buzzing insects, woodland birds, and the crunch of your own footsteps.

A stone wall plods in from the right, meeting the broad trail as it travels west, gently undulating to a triangular crossroads marked "24." Stay to the right, and continue hiking west to junction 25. Here, pick up a wide cart road heading southwest. Soon, the monotonous swish of the traffic vanishes into the pines. Sloping to more wetland, the woodland road flattens and narrows precipitously as it nears the next intersection (which may be number 26 but is unmarked). Choose the route to the left and continue southwest, passing a rough-and-tumble fragment of stone wall. Guided by parallel stone walls, the cart road passes through reforested farmland to reach junction 27.

Bearing right the trail begins climbing, swings west, and keeps climbing to arrive at another junction. Far out of numerical sequence, this intersection is marked 37. Here, the cart road exits to Old Right Road, which lies to the north. A less-used and narrower footpath splits off to the left. Take this route to continue south hiking over rounded hillocks straight through junction 38. Ahead, a wetland basin rife with pine lies at the foot of upland. At junction 39 leave the primary trail, blazed with small blue and red markers, and hike left, bearing closer to the wetland. Rapidly filling in with frilly white pine saplings and bushy ferns, this moist enclave of formerly cleared land is an ideal environment for deer. Guided by a brook the trail bends gradually northwest to reconnect with the trail from which it diverged earlier. At this unmarked juncture descend a slope heading southwest to a causeway spanning the brook's overflow.

Atop the opposite rise the trail arrives at junction 41. Continue straight to reunite with the Bay Circuit Trail as it comes rolling in from the east on another broad cart road at junction number 10. Picking up with this long-distance traveler, aim for its white markers posted across the way, and hike west through the next junction (11) to a large pond nested in bogland brush. Destined for Hood Pond in Boxford, the Bay Circuit Trail rounds the swamp and directs itself to the Topsfield–Ipswich town line.

Depart this trail at junction 12 and hike south a few hundred yards farther to a broad four-way intersection that is missing a marker (but is likely number 29), and hike left. Following a stone wall up and over a modest hill, the route travels along a broad avenue through uncluttered woods of beech and pine to arrive at junction 45. Continue straight (east) through this crossroads and the next, gradually curving north to reach junction 33. Bear right, away from Pine Swamp, to follow an expansive trail edged with sweet-smelling ferns over languorous contours to junction 35. Deviate from this southeastern trajectory briefly to hike north to a deep-woods version of Grand Central Station. At this junction (6), the Bay Circuit Trail sweeps in from the northeast, jackknifes, and continues on its 200-mile journey around Boston.

Quit the Bay Circuit Trail, turn right onto a cart road, and travel 0.4 miles to the western border of Willowdale at Topsfield Road. The trail continues across the road at Bradley Palmer State Park. Wait for a lull in traffic then cross to continue the hike. Several yards in, concealed by a curtain of hemlocks, a sturdy wooden bridge arches across the Ipswich River. Running 45 miles from its source in Wilmington to the Atlantic at Ipswich Bay, the Ipswich River today provides 350,000 people with drinking water. Wasting no time upon discovering this handsome river in 1638, John Winthrop shrewdly negotiated with Chief Masconomo to sell him the lands along it—together with exclusive fishing rights—in 1638. The price: 20 pounds sterling. Nearly four centuries later, Winthrop's Arbella Farm is still in the hands of the Winthrop family and remains largely intact.

On the far side of the river, by a Hamilton Conservation Commission sign, a trail diverges left. Turn here and follow blue paw-print trail blazes to trace the river's course eastward. Gouged and grated by glacial ice 10,000 years ago, the river lies like a black racer in the shade of a steep banking that looms from the south. Little but hemlocks grow along this heavily contoured edge made soft by their detritus. The only indication of the granite bedrock is the sand and grit lining the root-riddled trail.

On any given day, especially sunny ones, turtles line up nose-to-toe on fallen trees lying in the water. Night hunters, like raccoons, skunks, and fishers, keep well hidden during the day but leave plenty of evidence of their comings and goings. An occasional path splits off to climb away from the water, but stay with the blue trail on its riverside run to reach a dam built for a textile mill in the early 1800s. The mill turned out woolen blankets and stockings for half a century until an all-consuming fire put an end to the enterprise. Today, the mill site and old sluiceway stretching from the dam to Winthrop Street is held under the protective ownership of the Essex County Greenbelt Association.

While exploring the dam, have a close look at the fish ladder constructed beside it. From as early as April to sometime in June, daring alewives and herring, all but exhausted by their Atlantic exodus, leap from one step to the next, using all their might to reach still waters. Mature American eels migrating back to the Sargasso Sea use the ladder in autumn. Returning to ocean spawning grounds they leave equipped with newly formed fins and enlarged eyes—adaptations required for life at sea.

From the milldam hike away from the river on a path heading uphill past marker 10 to make a loop back to the park entrance. After a pulse-quickening climb the ground levels, and soon the trail arrives at junction 9. Take the wide grassy avenue to the right and continue southwest. As the route is both a hiking trail and a jumping lane for equestrians, don't be surprised to hear the beat of cantering horse hooves.

Follow this trail only a moment, then bear right onto a narrower path that ventures back into the woods. Light reflecting off the water jabs at the staid evergreens as the path passes high above the river. Odd strands of stone wall appear now and again as the path makes its way through the open understory to the trail that leads back to the bridge across the river.

Resuming the Willowdale Trail hiked earlier, retrace your steps to junction 22. Leave the cart road here and take up this narrower trail heading east. The outer reaches of the enormous Pine Swamp creep in from the left. Lifted above the wet by a natural and enhanced causeway, the trail runs on a plane through junction 32 and straight on to meet another cart road at junction 21. Turn left here to travel north across Gravelly Brook and the untamed wonderland of its floodplain.

Ahead, a fork presents an opportunity to venture from the cart road onto a less-traveled path. To feel closer to the woods and their inhabitants take this right. A few hundred yards ahead, the two paths meet again and the cart road continues on to junction 20. At this disorientating intersection, hike left and then straight ahead at the next split to reconvene with the Bay Circuit Trail, traveling north.

Managing to stay dry as it traverses swamp, the trail crosses a culvert here and there and winds past pools teeming with life. Frogs chirp as they leap out of the path where they have been sunning themselves or hunting insects. Bowing to the west and then east, navigating the swamp by misaligned hillocks, the wide, flat trail eventually straightens and climbs from the swamp. Ascending an

A great blue heron fishing near Bull Brook

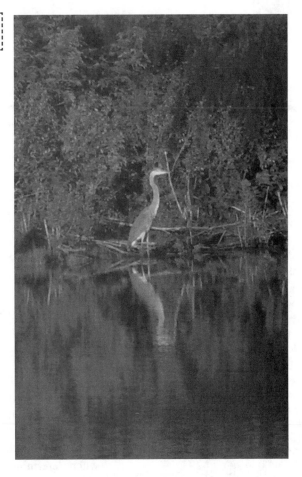

extended gravel slope, the trail passes several others diverging from it, and finally returns to junction 24. Having come full circle bear right and follow the familiar trail through the woods to Marini's strawberry field and Linebrook Road just beyond.

NEARBY ATTRACTIONS

After this long hike it is likely you will be ready for a bite to eat. If so, seek out The Clam Box restaurant close by at 246 High Street in Ipswich. Custom built in 1938 by Mr. Greanleaf to resemble an actual clam box, the eatery serves a full menu of fried freshly caught seafood. Their hours vary, so it is advisable to call before stopping by, (978) 356-9707.

Foote's Canoe Rentals, located opposite the milldam, has canoes to rent by the hour and by the day and will even organize overnight trips. Call for more information, (978) 356-9771; **www.footebrotherscanoes.com.**

29 | BALD HILL LOOP

KEY AT-A-GLANCE INFORMATION

LENGTH: 6.53 miles

CONFIGURATION: Loop

DIFFICULTY: Easy to moderate

SCENERY: Farmland reverted back to woodland, kettle ponds, vernal pools, a massive beaver dam, and the remains of an 18th-century farmstead

EXPOSURE: Mostly shade

TRAFFIC: Light

TRAIL SURFACE: Packed earth, loose gravel, mud, and flooded areas

HIKING TIME: 3 hours

SEASON: Open year-round sunrise–sunset

ACCESS: Free

MAPS: Available from the Boxford Trail Association/Boxford Open Land Trust; 7 Elm Street, P.O. Box 9,5 Boxford, MA 01921, (978) 887-7031, or the Boxford town hall; 7A Spofford Road, Boxford, MA 01931; open 8 a.m.–4:30 p.m. Monday–Thursday; (978) 887-6000

FACILITIES: None

SPECIAL COMMENTS: Sturdy water-resistant boots are recommended.

WHEELCHAIR TRAVERSABLE: No

DRIVING DISTANCE FROM BOSTON COMMON: 26 miles

IN BRIEF

This hike circles a great outwash plain of the Wisconsin Glacier and while scaling Bald Hill, passes through an 18th-century farmstead once owned by a veteran of the American Revolution.

DESCRIPTION

There is more to these quiet woods than first meets the eye. Sometime before or after the Wisconsin Glacier bulldozed through, volcanic forces convulsed at Crooked Pond. Drawn by abundant game, sheltering hills, and ponds rippling with fish, people of the Agawam tribe settled here. Colonial farmers came and went, and in the early 1900s the Diamond Match Company literally reduced much of the forest to matchsticks. In 1968 300 acres of the land nearly experienced the sad glory of becoming an antiballistic-missile radar site. A decade earlier Bald Hill survived its own close call when determined locals foiled a development plan. Over time, parcel-by-parcel, collaborative effort saved a total of 1,624 acres.

Start the hike directly behind the parking area on the wide cart road running west into a wooded landscape remeniscent of an unmade bed. At the first junction marked number 19, bear right to continue southwest.

Bald Hill Loop

UTM Zone (WGS84) 19T

Easting: 335780

Northing: 4723988

Latitude: N 42° 39' 04"

Longitude: W 71° 00' 12"

Directions

From Boston, take US 1 north toward Tobin Bridge/Revere. At 15.2 miles, merge onto I-95 north, and continue 6.3 miles to Exit 51. Take Endicott Road toward Topsfield/Middleton. Head west from the exit ramp 0.2 miles. Turn north onto Middleton Road and travel 2.4 miles to the pullout on the left located just beyond a small, white house.

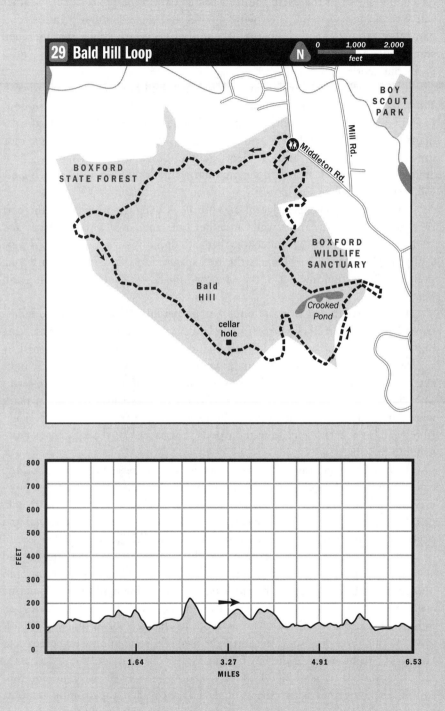

29 Bald Hill Loop

0   1,000   2,000
feet

N

BOY
SCOUT
PARK

BOXFORD
STATE FOREST

Middleton Rd.

Mill Rd.

BOXFORD
WILDLIFE
SANCTUARY

Bald
Hill

Crooked
Pond

cellar
hole

Ascending a fold in the earth the trail passes two kettle ponds, one on either side, as it bridges wetland. After winding over and between hillocks in the company of red squirrels and chipmunks, the trail meets up with a weather-loosened stone wall. At an unmarked junction beyond the wall, bear left to descend a rocky but gentle slope.

Upon reaching a clearing stay with the cart road as it undulates northwest. Though not identified by trail markers, the rutted cart road is easy to follow. Passing by more vernal pools and kettle ponds, where rare blue-spotted salamanders and their lungless four-toed brethren *Hemidactylium scutatum* hide under logs and leaves, the trail meets another stone wall then narrows as it arrives at junction 18. Bear left here and left again at the next split immediately following to continue south.

Proceeding along the edge of an enormous expanse of wetland, the cart road now bordered by stone walls on either side, rolls over waves of earth and stone. Ferns thrive in the understory beneath spindly oaks and vigorous pine saplings. Velveteen moss blankets the rocks underfoot. Coasting down a long slope to intersection number 8, the cart road meets with the Bay Circuit Trail. Bear left here.

Curving southwest along a floodplain, perpetually flooded thanks to industrious beavers, the trail clings to eroding land. Here roots pop from the banking like veins on the back of an old man's hand. A foot away, water darkened by shadow and oak tannins glistens under bristly bush twigs. The trail then climbs away from the wet and travels along a slope of rocky silt, known in glacial terms as a "kame terrace." At the crest of this rise two logs laid a foot apart mark where another path splinters off to Middleton. As the trail continues beside a stone wall on a level stretch, and the woods thin, it feels as though there's more room to breathe.

Gaining momentum as it passes a hemlock grove beside a vernal pool, the trail descends and quickly devolves into muddy chaos. A human's chaos, however, is a beaver's order. Immediately to the left a dam constructed of maple, oak, birch, and any other fellable tree stacked on a 20- to 30-foot diagonal and packed with mud, holds back a sheet of water as flat and heavy as rolled steel.

Characteristic of construction sites, the dam has obstructed traffic and altered the pathway. On a bank opposite the mire, the trail climbs back onto upland beneath the boughs of hemlock trees. Continuing uphill in this quieting evergreen wood, the trail comes to a tree marked with two white dashes, an indication that the Bay Circuit Trail is about to change course. Junction 8A follows. At this three-way split, hike straight through, staying on what appears to be one of two branches of the Bay Circuit Trail.

The western slope of Bald Hill lies ahead. Composed of rock, silt, and topsoil squeezed together as two sheets of glacial ice collided, the drumlin amounts to a farmer's dream since the deep loam supported by layers of rock and gravel is fertile ground with excellent drainage. Beginning in the 18th century, the

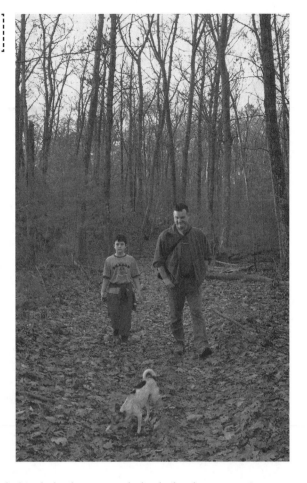

Bald Hill is popular but never crowded.

Gould family took owner-ship of 50 acres of the hill's southern slope. In 1784, the land passed into the hands of the Russell fam-ily, who in turn sold it— 71 years later—to Ebenezer Hooper, a ship captain from Marblehead who, it seems, had had enough of sea faring.

Tracing the hillside between parallel stone walls, the old cart road leads up a gravel slope to a turn indicated by marker number 10, and beyond a pasture. Swing left at the turn to climb northwest to the site of the Hooper fam-ily farmhouse. Though the house is gone, the founda-tion and remnants of the garden remain. Vinca vines still climb the garden steps behind the house, and rhododendrons continue to flower each spring. Across the way is a small meadow where the family cow once grazed. Two or three hundred yards farther up the rugged slope, the trail reaches a mowed field atop Bald Hill.

From the 247-foot peak, follow the track as it bends southeast and descends back into oak woods. At junction 12 bear left and continue northeast. As the trail descends farther water seems to percolate from all sides. And as condi-tions get wetter more species of ferns appear, along with birches. Sweet pep-perbush (*Clethra alnifolia*) and spicebush (*Lindera benzoin*) give the air a spicy twang. Spicebush wakes the woods in the crisp days of March and April with its greenish-yellow blossoms, and later its leaves nourish the caterpillars of swal-lowtail butterflies. Late-summer blossoms of white alder or pepperbush attract hummingbirds and honeybees.

Ahead, where a vast pond becomes visible through brush, the trail arrives at junction 13A. Leave the cart road here and bear right onto a lightly etched path heading southeast along the edge of Crooked Pond. Aiming for higher ground,

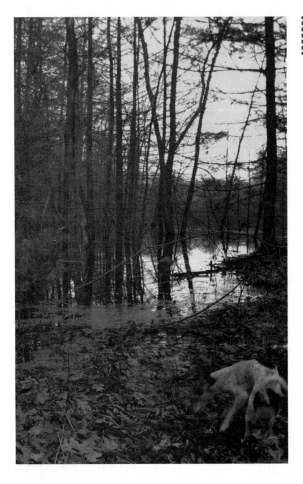

the trail ducks under hemlock cover on the pond's eastern side, veering wide of the wetland. In the dark woods bereft of underbrush, it can be difficult to be sure of the way. Ignore the arrow pointing uphill to the right and instead continue straight, hiking northeast.

Easing downhill then up again in great sine-wave undulations, the trail meets with several stone walls. On the north side of Crooked Pond, the trail rushes downhill over a streambed. Markers disappear for a spell, but the north-pointing route is easy to follow. By now the pond is starkly visible on the left constrained by upland immediately to the right. From this point on, the true route is anyone's guess—though before beavers got busy, it probably cut a trajectory farther west across land now covered by water. In any case, use the water as a guide until a marker for Bay Circuit Trail materializes near a stone wall close to the pond. A few feet farther on, there is a blue marker and then a sign posted by the Boxford Wildlife Sanctuary asserting the rights of the beaver. At this junction, bear left to follow Bay Circuit Trail markers as they lead northwest.

Still hugging the expanding pond, the trail aims west then arcs northward to higher ground. At the fork ahead, stay to the right with Bay Circuit Trail to climb away from the pond. After scaling the rocky side of another basin, the trail slips back down to wetland, then, negotiating sloping deposits of sand and gravel, arrives at junction 23. At this split, bear left, staying on Bay Circuit Trail. Junction 22 is just beyond a wet patch crossed by wooden planks; turn right here to continue northeast. Where it approaches a stone wall, the trail bends resolutely east. Ignore an arrow pointing north and stay with the trail until it reaches junction 20A, soon after. Bear left and continue to the fork marked number 20.

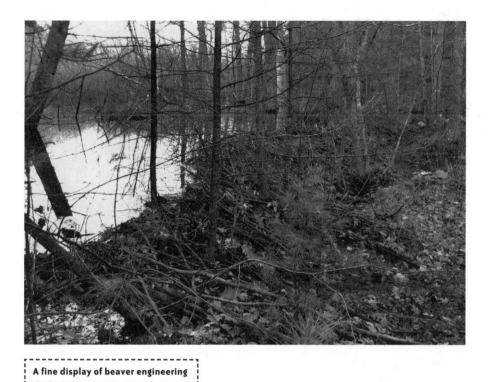

A fine display of beaver engineering

At this split, turn right and follow the trail north to junction 19. At this final fork, bear right once more to return to the parking lot.

NEARBY ATTRACTIONS

If the timing is right, consider coordinating your hike with a stop at the county fair. The Topsfield Fair is held every year from the last week in September through the first week in October and is open daily 10 a.m. to 10 p.m. To reach the fairgrounds from Boxford, take I-95 south to Exit 53 (MA 97). Follow MA 97 south to US 1, then follow US 1 south to the sign on the left. In addition to the fair, the fairground hosts other events year-round. Visit the Web site, **www .topsfieldfair.org** to view the schedule.

30 WINNEKENNI PARK:
Lake, Forest, and Castle Hike

KEY AT-A-GLANCE INFORMATION

LENGTH: 5.6 miles

CONFIGURATION: Out-and-back with two loops

DIFFICULTY: Easy

SCENERY: Two lakes, woods, and a restored castle built of stone

EXPOSURE: Mostly shaded except for sun-exposed stretches along the banks of Kenoza Lake and on the grounds of Winnekenni Castle.

TRAFFIC: Light to moderate

TRAIL SURFACE: Packed earth

HIKING TIME: 3 hours

SEASON: Year-round sunrise–sunset

ACCESS: Free

MAPS: Posted at the parking area; also available at www.ci.haverhill. ma.us/departments/econ/ conservation/trails

FACILITIES: None

SPECIAL COMMENTS: Winnekenni Castle hosts many special events, including Haunted Halloween Nights in October.

WHEELCHAIR TRAVERSABLE: The 2.5-mile Dudley Porter Trail that borders three quarters of Kenoza Lake is wheelchair-friendly.

DRIVING DISTANCE FROM BOSTON COMMON: 38 miles

IN BRIEF

After first surveying the magnificent expanse of Kenoza Lake from a carriage road and footpaths, this hike climbs to a 19th-century castle built of fieldstone.

DESCRIPTION

As the 17th century waned, so, too, did the Pennacook people, who from time immemorial had lived in villages along the Merrimack River from New Hampshire to Massachusetts. Nearly extinguished by disease and war with the Penobscot, Micmac, Mohawk, Dutch, French, and English by 1726, what was left of the tribe amounted to one village of five men living just north of Haverhill near Concord, New Hampshire.

Fear and hatred for Indians had long since dissipated when, in 1861, the chemist and agronomist Dr. James R. Nichols purchased the former Darling Farm and gave it the name "Winnekenni," the Pennacook word for "very beautiful."

Two years earlier, the poet, Quaker, and Haverhill native John Greenleaf Whittier had renamed Great Pond, beside the farm, "Kenoza Lake," meaning "lake of the pickerel" in the same Indian tongue. According to Katherine M. Abbott, author of *Old Paths*

Winnekenni Park: Lake, Forest, and Castle Hike

UTM Zone (WGS84) 19T

Easting: 330786

Northing: 4739673

Latitude: N 42° 47' 27"

Longitude: W 71° 04' 08"

Directions ———————————————→

From Boston, take I-93 north 22.4 miles to I-495 north. From I-495 north take Exit 52 to MA 110 west (toward Haverhill). Turn left onto MA 110. Winnekenni Park is 1.1 miles ahead on the left.

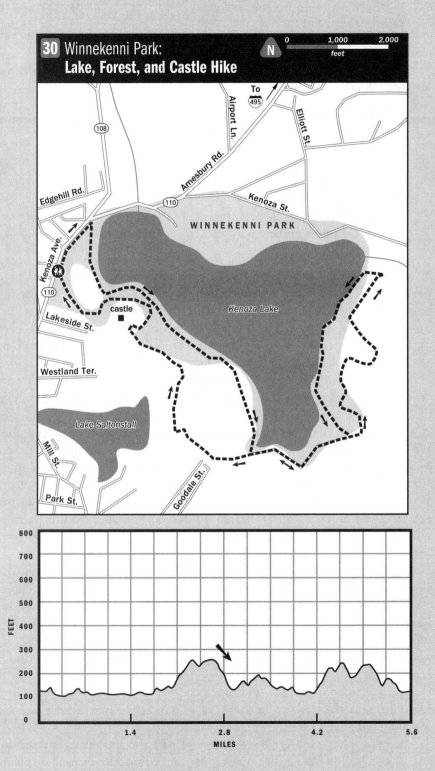

and Legends of New England, Whittier considered himself a friend of the Pennacook and never carried a weapon.

Likely then, John Greenleaf Whittier was sincere in his sentiments when in his poem "Kenoza," he wrote:

> . . . Lake of Pickerel! Let no more
> The echoes answer back "Great Pond,"
> But sweet Kenoza, from thy shore
> And watching hill beyond.
> And Indian ghosts, if such there be,
> Who ply unseen their shadowy lines
> Call back the dear old name to thee,
> As with the voices of the pine."

As told by Donald Freeman in *The Story of Winnekenni,* after a decade of summering at his Haverhill farm, Dr. Nichols traveled to England and was thunderstruck by the country's great cathedrals and castles of stone. Inspired, he returned determined to build a castle at Winnekenni of granite excavated from his hillside. Dedicated to helping farmers improve their lot, Dr. Nichols was quoted at the time as saying, "We desire to prove to farmers and others in a practical way the value of boulders and rocks as building materials."

When finished two years later, Nichols's summer castle boasted a Grecian drawing room, a Pompeian-style dining room, and a Roman-tiled, black walnut–finished library, as well as a kitchen, sleeping room, storeroom, and laundry, all on the first floor. Above, atop a sprawling stairway, there were nine bedrooms and a "bathing room." Climbing even higher by means of corner towers, one could access the roof that, back when the landscape was cleared for farming, afforded views of Mount Monadnock, Mount Agamenticus, and the ocean.

In 1885, after 24 years of summering at Winnekenni Castle and conducting experiments with chemical fertilizers on the farm, the elderly doctor sold the castle and a parcel of land to his cousin. A decade later, the City of Haverhill acquired the property and made Winnekenni its first public park.

Begin the hike heading north toward MA 110 on the path that runs wide along the bank of the Basin of Kenoza Lake. Shortly after passing a children's play area, the path cuts close to the road and dips into a wooded corridor. Emerging on the other side, stay right, and continue south on a wide packed-earth path that leads between Kenoza Lake and the basin. Straight ahead, the woods end at a dam bridging the waters; cross here to arrive at the Dudley Porter Trail.

Turn left at this junction and proceed eastward on the old carriage trail, edged by beech trees. In the short days of autumn, the leaves turn vivid shades of yellow and gold.

Keeping a fairly level grade, the carriage path rounds wide bends as it follows Kenoza's bank. About 0.25 miles along, lanky rhododendrons loom among

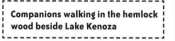
Companions walking in the hemlock wood beside Lake Kenoza

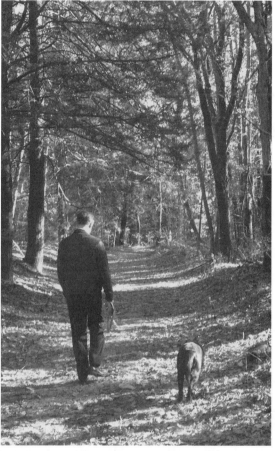

the beech and oak, adding a tone of sobriety to the rousing colors. Ahead, on the right, the path approaches a monument erected in memory of the trail's namesake, Dudley Porter, who died in 1906. Generous to passersby and to Porter himself, the monument is designed as an elegant, granite, watering trough, with benches on either side. Missing is the fox-head drinking fountain that once decorated the center plaque.

Across the lake to the north, you will see an alluring forest of hemlock. Almost entirely devoid of deciduous species, these woods are at once forbidding and alluring, like those of fairy tales. Ahead, the trail arrives at a broad junction equipped with a bench, a sign pointing east to the Castle Trail, and a map board (missing a map as of this writing). Make a detour here for a quick trip to the castle, or hike on, staying with the Dudley Porter Trail, which winds around the eastern tip of the lake, forms a causeway, then crosses wetland as it heads north.

Passing an old upland meadow laced with weathered barbed wire, the trail turns away from the lake and ascends into woods. Once the water is out of sight, the trail arrives at a two-way split. Hike up the hill to find the ruins of a small gazebo or cabin poised on the edge of the path. Stop to have a look from this vantage point, then follow the road into the hill's hemlock-shaded recesses.

Following the pronounced contours of the land surrounding the lake, the trail bends this way and that as it gains elevation. Finally, the path levels on a lofty plateau. Here, the trail's left side falls away to a steep banking open to all but sunlight. Nothing but a few ferns and velvety silence fill the void beneath the hemlocks.

Passing a thin path that leads to a dome-shaped field beyond woods to the

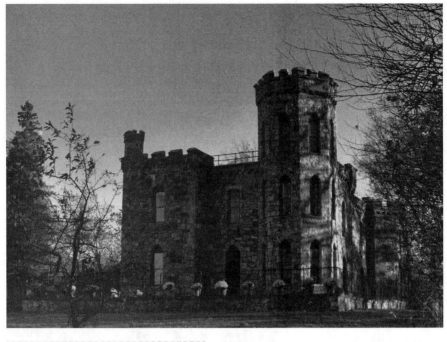

Winnekenni Castle overlooks Lake Kenoza.

right, the trail weaves from the east to the west then north as it descends back to Lake Kenoza. After sloping to the water in an arc to the left, the trail levels at a junction. Pick up the Shore Trail, running southwest, to double-back to Winnekenni Hill.

A far cry from the civilized carriage road of the Dudley Porter Trail, this path seems to have been cut by goat hooves. Roots, rocks, and occasional muddy spots force attention to your feet until chattering red squirrels and rafts of ducks gliding on the silvery lake quickly snatch it away again.

On the left, just past a birch with three trunks, the trail climbs away from the lake to meet the Dudley Porter Trail at an intersection passed earlier. Turn right here and retrace your steps to the causeway. After crossing between the lake and the wetland to the left, look for a narrow trail marked with red diverging from the carriage road. Take up this stony path and follow it southwest to another split. Stay with the red trail here, and continue uphill to a second junction. This time, choose the path to the right, changing course to follow a loose stone wall running horizontal to the hill. The path is clear from use but otherwise poorly marked. However, where the direction gets sketchy, a light-blue arrow painted on a tree points the way. From the arrow on, light-blue dots appear with sufficient frequency.

At the next fork, bear left and hike downhill. Continuing in this direction leads to a sister lake of Lake Kenoza, Lake Saltonstall. Soon, though, the path forks again. This time, take the trail to the right and continue uphill on an old

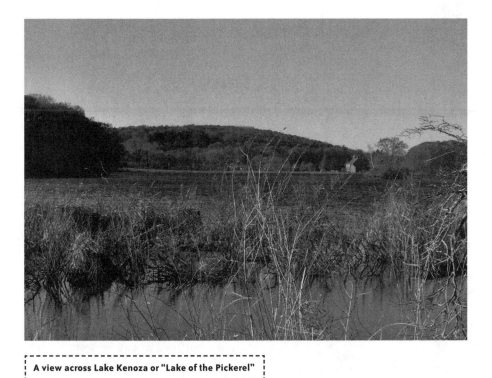

A view across Lake Kenoza or "Lake of the Pickerel"

road surfaced with fractured asphalt disguised by moss and grass. At the top of the hill, on the left, you will spot the stone and brick foundation of a building and, a few feet higher on the hill, a second foundation with a crumbling tower. Offspring of trees cut centuries ago have returned the Darling Farm meadows to dense woods obliterating this home's once-magnificent view of the lakes below. Facing Lake Kenoza, find a path to the left of the homesite and follow it on its northwest course down the hill. Soon after it winds north to face the water, this path meets a crossroad. Turn left here and continue several yards farther to join a carriage road to Winnekenni Castle. Since this road makes a rear approach, the first structures you see are outbuildings; the castle stands beyond these, overlooking Lake Kenoza. After taking in the castle and the bronze elk—frozen in a open-mouthed bellow—arranged on the lawn before it, find the head of the Castle Trail on the edge of the woods to the right of the paved drive and descend toward Lake Kenoza. Meeting the Dudley Porter Trail, turn left and hike to the trail's end at the paved entrance to the park.

31 BEAVER BROOK HIKE

IN BRIEF

Located just over the Massachusetts/New Hampshire border, the Beaver Brook Preserve presents a landscape where beaver abound and loons or even a wandering moose wouldn't come as a big surprise.

DESCRIPTION

Like many conservation projects, the 2,000-acre Beaver Brook Preserve exists because a small group of individuals with a passion for the environment got an idea and acted on it. It all began in the early 1960s when two cousins, Hollis Nichols, a Boston mutual fund manager with a powerful love of nature and the outdoors, and Jeff Smith, a farmer, forester, horticulturalist, and already active conservationist, put their heads together and founded the Beaver Brook Association. The first donated parcel was 17 acres surrounding a house Nichols had built for his mother. Nichols possessed the resources and financial expertise to get the

KEY AT-A-GLANCE INFORMATION

LENGTH: 5.69 miles

CONFIGURATION: Loop

DIFFICULTY: Easy to moderate

SCENERY: Forested wetlands, beaver ponds, and views of sustainable forestry in action

EXPOSURE: Mostly shaded

TRAFFIC: Light

TRAIL SURFACE: Packed earth, wooden footbridges, and some rugged, rocky areas

HIKING TIME: 2.5–3 hours

SEASON: Year-round sunrise–sunset

ACCESS: Free

MAPS: Available online at www .beaverbrook.org/bbtmaps.htm, and at the Beaver Brook Association's office at 117 Ridge Road, Hollis, NH, open Monday–Friday, 9 a.m.–5 p.m., and Sunday, 10:30 a.m.–3:30 p.m.; closed Saturday.

FACILITIES: None

SPECIAL COMMENTS: The Beaver Brook Association manages a cabin facility that accommodates up to 22 people—two bunkhouses, a cookhouse, a well house, a campfire circle, and a primitive latrine.

WHEELCHAIR TRAVERSABLE: No

DRIVING DISTANCE FROM BOSTON COMMON: 50 miles

Beaver Brook Hike

UTM Zone (WGS84) 19T

Easting: 285404

Northing: 4734547

Latitude: N 42° 44' 01"

Longitude: W 71° 37' 17"

Directions

From Boston take Storrow Drive east to I-93 north. After 5.4 miles, merge onto I-95 south/ MA 128 south via Exit 37B toward Waltham. Take the US 3 north/Middlesex Turnpike Exit 32B-A. Merge onto US 3 north via Exit 32A toward Lowell/Nashua, NH, and continue 27.1 miles. Take the Broad Street Exit 6 toward Hollis, driving 0.2 miles. Bear left to take the MA 130 west ramp toward Hollis/Brookline, driving 0.1 mile, and turn left onto Broad Street/ NH 130. Pass through one roundabout and continue 5.4 miles. Turn right onto Ash Street/ NH 130. Continue to follow NH 130 to the sign for the Beaver Brook parking lot on the right (note that you will first pass another Beaver Brook parking lot on the left).

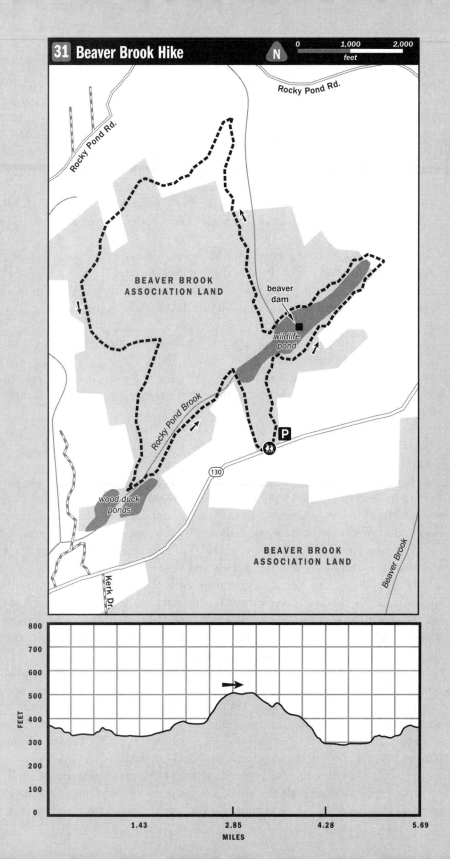

31 Beaver Brook Hike

N

0   1,000   2,000
feet

Rocky Pond Rd.

Rocky Pond Rd.

BEAVER BROOK
ASSOCIATION LAND

beaver
dam

wildlife
pond

Rocky Pond Brook

P

130

wood duck
ponds

BEAVER BROOK
ASSOCIATION LAND

Beaver Brook

Kerk Dr.

800
700
600
500
400
300
200
100
0

FEET

1.43   2.85   4.28   5.69

MILES

project off and running, and Hollis native Jeff Smith, who had been a town select-man and member of the conservation commission, knew the community and its eligible property.

Today Beaver Brook is composed of 90 separate parcels located in the Merrimack River watershed, most of which lie in the town of Hollis; an additional 200 acres lie in neighboring Milford. Invested in more than conserving land and protecting wildlife, the Beaver Brook Association runs a model sustainable farm, educational programs for children, public festivals, and horticultural classes. All told, the overarching goal is to demonstrate how forestry, recreation, and wildlife can thrive side by side.

From the notice board located in the right corner of the parking lot, hike north on Wildlife Pond Trail. Passing through woods along a stone wall. Starting out wide and level, the path soon reaches a junction, where it splits in two. Take the path on the right to join Wildlife Pond Trail; marked with yellow diamonds.

Becoming narrower, the trail dips and bends over soft ground riddled with roots to reach the southwestern end of Wildlife Pond. Turning eastward, briefly leaving the bank, the trail returns to the water's edge, and what first appears to be a modest pond is revealed to be something more. Greatly elongated, this magnificent pond stretches on and on.

Five hundred feet ahead, Wildlife Pond Loop Trail is bisected by Old City Trail, which runs to the northwest. Crossing Route 130, this trail links the northern and southern halves of Beaver Brook.

Rising from the water just past this junction is a Taj Mahal of beaver lodges. Beyond this tooth-wrought architecture, the trail leads to a bench arranged on a mossy nub of turf. Stop here to scan the watery landscape for a moose, a flashy wood duck, or a heron standing in shallows like a frozen shaft of lightning.

Winding onward Wildlife Pond Loop Trail encounters a path to the right and a small footbridge. Mountain laurels add elegance, and the plump fruit of well-irrigated high-bush blueberries incite greed as the pond reaches northward. Close by, too, is another beaver lodge similar in size to the first. Finally, rounding the slender tip of the pond, the trail turns and traces the opposite bank to its western end. Yellow-flowered lily pads grow densely on this murkier side, and flycatchers swoop from drowned trees to chase damselflies.

Short of completing the loop around the pond, the trail veers away from the wetland into a hemlock wood. A few yards farther, after a stone wall interrupts the trail, the path rejoins Old City Trail. Turn right toward upland here to hike along a wide logging road. Climbing on a slight grade between stone walls, the dirt road cuts through a forest thinned over time of its choicest lumber. White pine and hemlock dominate with hardwoods poking through here and there.

At about 0.3 miles, the trail comes to what a posted notice identifies as a full-scale prototype for a portable skidder bridge. As the notice explains such bridges promote sustainable timber extraction by protecting rivers and streams from wear

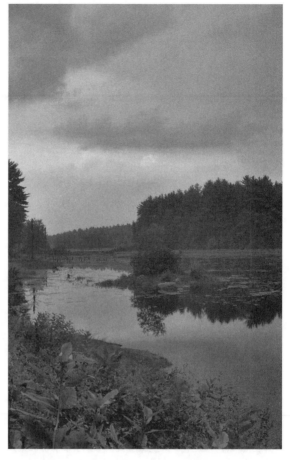

A stormy sky reflected on the waters of Wildlife Pond

and tear and from contamination caused by eroded soil and other waste.

Passing the skidder bridge, the blue-marked Old City Trail proceeds along a sliver of land between the wetland bordering Rocky Pond Brook to the right and rugged upland to the left. Leafy mountain laurel thrives on both sides and hemlocks tilt at odd angles, tightly grasping the granite ledge which creeps to the swamp.

Not far along this dramatic passageway, Old City Trail passes Rocky Ridge Trail, which cuts to the left. If a shorter, steeper hike has more appeal than a longer but less strenuous one, head west here; otherwise, continue north on Old City Trail. Soon crossing a wooden bridge, this trail runs along the brook. Basswood trees, maples, and aspen do a good job of hiding the action in this wetland, but through breaks in the foliage you might catch a glimpse of a resident kingfisher squawking in the high branches or diving for trout fingerlings.

Where the trail begins to sweep northwest, a notice alerts visitors that in August 2005 acreage on both sides of the trail was given to the Beaver Brook Association by Debra Worcester Hildreth in memory of her father, John Worcester. A century ago, the Worcester Brother's Mill located upriver off Rocky Pond Road, fueled its business with timber cut from this forest. Old City Trail continues north to the millpond and the site of the Worcester Brother's milling operation.

At a junction farther on, take Rocky Pond Trail to visit the nearby mill, or turn left onto Tupelo Trail. Immediately crossing a bridge, this trail heads southwest, narrowing as it ascends a moderate grade, and passes plentiful mountain laurel.

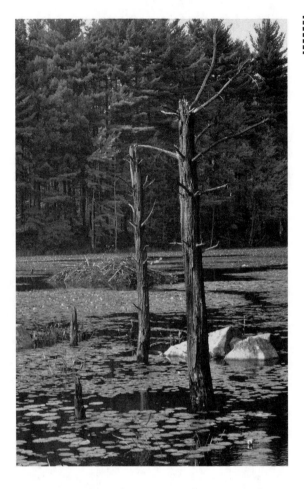

One of Beaver Brook's easy-to-spot beaver lodges

Nearing the top of the hill, the trail skirts a tract where the effects of logging are more obvious. Fueled by increased sunlight, grasses and shrubs have gotten the upper hand, to the benefit of deer and songbirds. A chestnut oak or two grow where the trail crosses a logging road and levels off. The commercially desirable tupelo trees, for which the trail is named, were undoubtedly heavily logged.

Making its way downhill between stone walls, the trail passes above Heron Pond and, moments later, opens to a wide triangular intersection amid pine and oak. Continue straight, heading southwest. As I hiked on a September afternoon, the lemony smell of witch hazel drifted on the breeze as rain clouds rolled in.

Behind the hill in a choice resting spot, a throng of granite chunks sits just off the trail like weary bystanders. Hereafter, the incline shifts decidedly downhill. Winding eastward, the trail soon arrives at another intersection. Take Mary Farley Trail on the left for a shortcut back to Wildlife Pond, or follow my lead and bear right onto Wood Duck Pond Trail.

Marked with blue, this wide path tapers unhurried to wetland. In autumn amanitas shaped like goblets, and honey mushrooms feeding on eroded life poke out from the dark humus. After passing a glade on the left, the trail dips then rolls steadily downhill past young beeches.

Settling onto level ground in view of the twin Wood Duck Ponds, the trail makes a "T" upon meeting Jeff Smith Trail. Marked with yellow, this new trail emerges from between the ponds to the right and heads abruptly eastward. Whatever the season, the pond detour on Jeff Smith Trail is highly recommended.

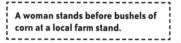

A woman stands before bushels of corn at a local farm stand.

Having been coaxed back to life by Beaver Brook Association volunteers, the Wood Duck Ponds are always beautiful—even in the smudgy gray light of an impending storm. In dim light, the red blossoms of cardinal flowers (*Lobelia cardinalis*) growing here spark like flares. Like Old City Trail, Jeff Smith Trail connects the north and south sides of Beaver Brook. A half-mile or so past the Wood Duck Ponds, this trail crosses Route 130. But to complete the loop back to the parking lot, return to the intersection at the end of Wood Duck Trail and follow Jeff Smith Trail northeast.

Weaving between rocks, roots, and trees in a valley at the foot of the hill, the trail follows a brook connecting Wood Duck Pond to Wildlife Pond. Coarse granite rubble makes for uneven footing, while moist conditions bring orbs of pure quartz to a mysterious glow. After passing through a stone wall and over a footbridge, the trail breaks from the woods and arrives at a junction at the head of Wildlife Pond. Turn right here to cross a constructed causeway and, once on the southern side follow Dam Road back to the parking lot.

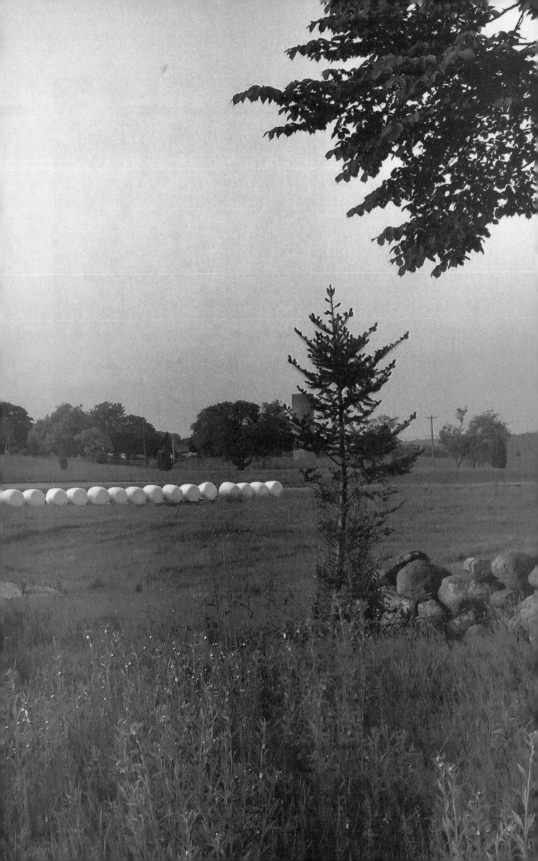

SOUTH OF BOSTON

32 BLUE HILLS: Hemenway Hill Loop

i KEY AT-A-GLANCE INFORMATION

LENGTH: 3.9 miles

CONFIGURATION: Loop

DIFFICULTY: Moderate

SCENERY: Woods, ponds, streams, wetlands, and hills

EXPOSURE: Mostly shaded

TRAFFIC: Peaceful, though popular with horseback riders, mountain bikers, runners, cross-country skiers, and leisurely hikers

TRAIL SURFACE: Soil and stone, rough in places from erosion

HIKING TIME: 1.5 hours

SEASON: Year-round sunrise–8 p.m.

ACCESS: Free

MAPS: $2 at the Blue Hills Reservation Ranger Station near the trailhead

FACILITIES: Restrooms located at the ranger station.

SPECIAL COMMENTS: Trail may be wet in the spring and any time after heavy precipitation

WHEELCHAIR TRAVERSABLE: No

DRIVING DISTANCE FROM BOSTON COMMON: 9 miles

IN BRIEF

Located just outside Boston's southern border, the vast 7,000-acre Blue Hills Reservation offers a glimpse of the past and a sense of the land before the birth of Boston.

DESCRIPTION

The Blue Hills Reservation exists thanks in large part to landscape architect Charles Eliot, who campaigned hard for its creation in the late 1800s. A progressive visionary, Eliot knew that, "for crowded populations to live in health and happiness, they must have space for air, for light, for exercise, for rest, and for the enjoyment of that peaceful beauty of nature."

A refuge for deer, birds, amphibians, and a few footloose coyotes well versed in urban living, the Blue Hills—quite literally a stone's throw from Mattapan's hair-braiding parlors and ethnic eateries—is a soothing green ripple in time and place. Its woods of hemlock, beech, and oak spreading over hills of granite quiet the far-reaching sounds of the city and subdue them with birdsong and trickling streams. Old stone walls, like gray lines of slowed motion, divide the trees, casting the last shadows of Milton's farms.

Directions ———————————————→

From the junction of I-93 south and US 1 south, travel 11.4 miles on I-93 to the Ponkapoag Trail, Exit 3. Drive 0.1 mile toward Houghton's Pond. Turn right onto Blue Hill River Road and drive 0.4 miles, then turn right onto Hillside Street. Continue 0.7 miles until you see the sign for the Blue Hills Reservation Headquarters. Parking is available on the other side of Hillside Street facing a gray barn. The trailhead is at the top of the drive beside the reservation's headquarters.

Blue Hills:
Hemenway Hill Loop

UTM Zone (WGS84) 19T

Easting: 327278

Northing: 4675709

Latitude: N 40° 12' 52"

Longitude: W 71° 05' 33"

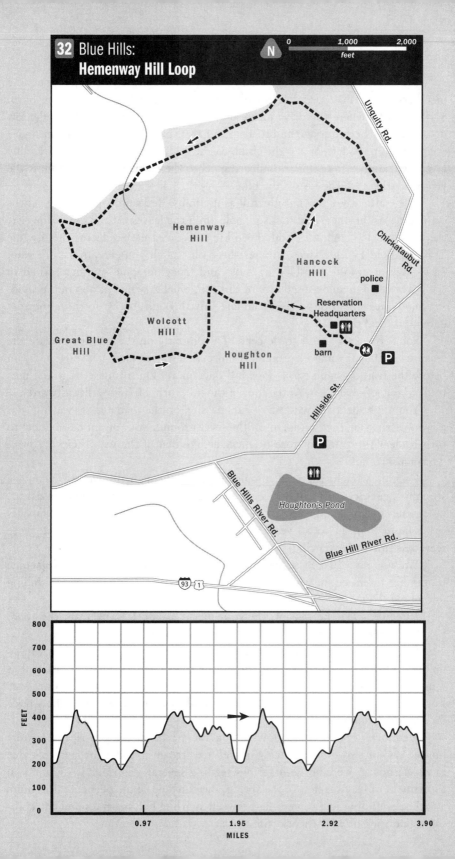

N

0   1,000   2,000
feet

Unquity Rd.

Chickataubut Rd.

Hemenway
Hill

Hancock
Hill

police

Reservation
Headquarters

Wolcott
Hill

Great Blue
Hill

Houghton
Hill

barn

P

Hillside St.

P

Houghton's Pond

Blue Hills River Rd.

Blue Hill River Rd.

93 1

800

700

600

500

400

FEET

300

200

100

0

0.97   1.95   2.92   3.90

MILES

Before beginning the hike, or on your return, stop to say hello to the equine members of the Boston police force turned out in paddocks behind the barn. Start the hike where the drive meets the woods just above the barn to the left of the office. Before long the broad gravel trail picks up with a stream and a boggy basin to its left. When the climb eases, this trail joins another marked by a yellow triangle. Take this trail, bearing off to the right. From here, follow the yellow markers for the rest of the hike.

The trail cleaves through the hill as it climbs. Red squirrels hustling acorns or fending off brothers and foes squabble amid the leaves. At the top of the rise, the trail surface smoothes and the hiking becomes easier. Here, the Skyline Trail, marked by blue signs, crosses the path. Catch your breath as you walk past crags of granite humbled by moss and tenacious pine saplings rooted in their crevices. On an exposed face of this hill, blueberry bushes abound, providing many pies worth of berries from late July through August to those intrepid enough to find them.

Soon, the trail begins to descend. Though easy on the legs, here again the feet are kept busy by uneven ground. A short causeway elevates you above a stream before the trail dips and turns downhill once more. On this descent, you'll pass trails to the left and right. At the foot of the hill, turn left and walk eastward.

You might hear the whoosh of cars passing on the road a short way off, but as you catch your rhythm again on the level ground, your attention is likely to turn to deer footprints or forest delicacies like hen of the wood (*Grifola frondosa*) mushrooms.

On this stretch, the trail undulates gently through the woods keeping a straight trajectory. You will notice an assortment of oak species, pine, sassafras, mockernut hickory, and a few birch and beech. Only the occasional tree appears to be more than 25 to 50 years old. The generation of trees preceding these served as timber for fencing, boat hulls, and houses.

Walking on, you'll encounter a slight downhill. A short way ahead, you come to another intersection, where an opening in the trees reveals a stream spilling into pools.

After crossing the stream, the trail meets a path leading from the road. Bear left, staying on the yellow trail. Vernal pools providing sanctuary to salamanders and hunting grounds for raccoons lie to the right, with hemlock-filled upland to the left. At the next junction, look for a sign for trail 1135 as well as a marker for the green trail. The yellow and green trails join and become one. Looking to the right, you can see a stone wall meandering through the woods on a parallel course

Hemlocks cast dark shadows along the trail, shielding a sleeping great horned owl or two. An interlacing of well-fed streams trickles through this area most seasons. A wetland with springs feeding several small ponds supports an assortment of frog species. In the spring, the chirping of the peepers raises quite a racket, sounding like something between swirling ball bearings and the chilling soundtrack of a Hitchcock film.

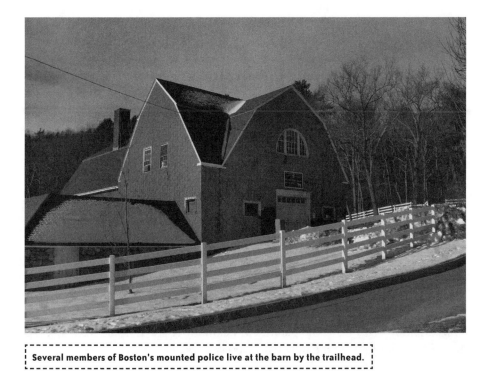

Several members of Boston's mounted police live at the barn by the trailhead.

As the trail continues, look to the right to see a red barn on private property abutting the Blue Hills Reservation. Behind the barn, a small meadow spreads to meet the woods beside the yellow trail. Though once common, fields such as this are now scarce and more vital than ever to bobolinks, bluebirds, and swallows.

You soon arrive at a point where the trail runs into a gravel road. Turning right here, markers confirm that the yellow trail and the green trail are still joined, even as they follow this road. Keep an eye out on the left for the point at which the yellow and the green trails turn back into the woods. The trail veers left sharply, climbing into upland. At the fork, bear left. A small hill stretches your legs as the trail winds upward. Chicken of the woods mushrooms (*Laetiporus sulphureus*) have been found in this general spot on ailing hardwood trees.

Keeping your eyes on the trail, you may see turkey footprints among the ubiquitous deer tracks. Turkeys have become common again in the region, and wherever there is an abundance of acorns, there is likely to be evidence of these magnificent birds.

After leveling, the trail descends again and arrives at a picturesque pond. A perfect kettle hole collared by a granite-studded ridge, this pond serves as a reminder of the glacial erosion that shaped the landscape in another age.

A trail cuts back into the woods on the pond's left. The yellow trail, however, continues along the near side of the pond, heading right. The trail jogs up an incline then quickly back down a gravelly pitch. Through a thicket to the left, you can just make out another pond that all but roars with bullfrog song in the summer.

A sign for the blue trail marks the yellow trail's departure to the right up a steep rocky slope. On the yellow trail, wetlands hug one side while, on the other, the land drops into a deep basin. The trail bends left away from a trail heading right. At the intersection with a trail marked "1120," markers indicate that the green and the yellow trails are still conjoined. Head uphill again to an opening where the green and the yellow trails meet the same gravel road you initially set out on.

Resume hiking on the gravel road, walking downhill. This, the final section, leads back to the trailhead. For more information about the Blue Hills, pay a visit to the reservation's headquarters, housed in the gray-shingled house on the hill to the right. A bulletin board on the porch outside presents a calendar of upcoming events, trail condition updates, and nature news. Visitors are invited to help themselves to maps for a contribution of $2.

NEARBY ATTRACTIONS

Farther down Hillside Street on the left is Houghton's Pond. This recreation area offers swimming, fishing, and picnicking. Restrooms, picnic tables, and barbecue grills are provided free to the public. Also close by is the Trailside Museum, the Blue Hills Ski Area, and the Blue Hills Observatory and Science Center.

BLUE HILLS: Skyline Trail **33**

IN BRIEF

Covering 7,000 acres, the Blue Hills Reservation boasts 125 miles of trails over terrain varying from granite-hewn hillsides to placid forest sheltering vernal pools and kettle ponds teeming with life. This hike follows the reservation's single-longest trail which stretches from the town of Dedham to Quincy, the birthplace of both John Adams and his son John Quincy Adams.

DESCRIPTION

From the parking lot set out hiking south toward Houghton's Pond following a path surfaced with clay. Straight ahead you will see a playground and visitor center to the left. Bear left as the path bends southeast coasting downhill beside the sandy beach that draws cheerful crowds in the summertime. Beyond a bog on the left and a boathouse with public restrooms on the right, the path eases away from the pond and into the shade of woods. Just after a green trail marker on a tree to the left, look for a narrow dirt trail bearing away from the pond and take this brief path north to link with a paved service road. Continue north following this road as it winds eastward and merges with the Bugbee Trail which enters

KEY AT-A-GLANCE INFORMATION

LENGTH: 13 miles

CONFIGURATION: Loop

DIFFICULTY: Strenuous

SCENERY: Views from the peaks of the Blue Hills, woods, wetlands, several large ponds, and a good deal of wildlife

EXPOSURE: Mostly shaded, with sunny lookouts

TRAFFIC: Medium

TRAIL SURFACE: Variable, packed earth, very rocky in places

HIKING TIME: Allow a full day

SEASON: Year-round sunrise–sunset

ACCESS: Free

MAPS: Available at the Blue Hills Reservation Headquarters on Hillside Street in Milton

FACILITIES: Restrooms and picnic tables can be found at the Blue Hills Reservation Headquarters and Houghton's Pond.

SPECIAL COMMENTS: To enjoy this hike to its fullest plan to setout early, and if the day is hot bring along a bathing suit to be ready for a celebratory swim in Houghton's Pond upon reaching to end.

WHEELCHAIR TRAVERSABLE: No

DRIVING DISTANCE TO BOSTON COMMON: 15 miles

Directions

From Charles Street on Boston Common, drive north to Storrow Drive East. From Storrow Drive merge onto I-93 South. Continue 13 miles on I-93 South to Exit 3, the Ponkapoag Trail, toward Houghton's Pond. At 0.1 mile turn right onto Blue Hill River Road; continue 0.4 miles and turn right onto Hillside Street. The parking lot for Houghton's Pond is 0.7 miles ahead on the right.

Blue Hills:
Skyline Trail
UTM Zone (WGS84) 19T
Easting: 326699
Northing: 4675121
Latitude: N 42° 12' 32"
Longitude: W 71° 05' 58"

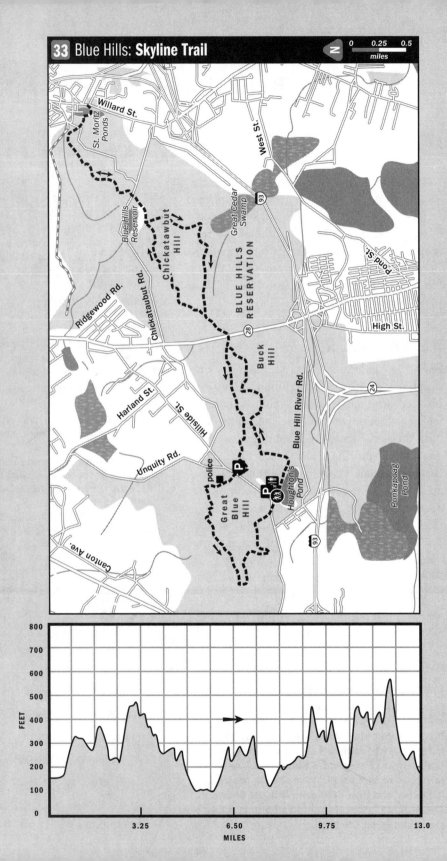

from the west. Hiking east on a steep incline, you soon arrive at a broad turn-around where park maintenance has piled sand and campfire ash. Here aim left to find a wooden post marking Massachuseuck Trail, a route that ascends sharply uphill quickly leaving the road behind. This point marks your first encounter with the rocky slopes of the Blue Hills. In May, plentiful white, bell-shaped flowers on low bushes foretell the blueberry harvest two months off.

Pass junction 2094, traveling east to reach wetland. Here Massachuseuck Trail traipses along the wooded rim of an overgrown pond. Dense underbrush conceals shallow waters teeming with amphibians. Varieties of hickory and oak mix with beech and evergreens in the uplands.

Abruptly the trail leaves the wetlands and makes its way up the side of Buck Hill. Stay with the Indian highway's eastward course about 0.5 miles longer to reach Skyline Trail, marked with blue. Descend the stone-riddled banking to the base of the hill, where MA 28 cuts a swath through the reservation.

The Massachuseuck and Skyline trails pick up again directly across this two-lane road. The two trails travel north together parallel to the road before diverging. Where they split, switch to Skyline Trail. From the intersection at 3042, follow the blue markers to begin your ascent of Chickatawbut Hill. It is a strenuous 517-foot climb to the peak. Because of the cascade of chipped granite, horseback riders and sensible mountain bikers leave this section of trail to hikers with nimble feet and good boots.

Upon reaching the top, the trail eases as it navigates between the peaks of two lesser hills, Kitchamakin and Nahanton, situated beside Chickatawbut. Short of the summit is a sunken plateau where the hills meet. Here you will find a monstrous boulder resplendent with fern fronds.

For a brief respite from the physically demanding Skyline Trail, follow yellow trail markers west to Chickatawbut Tower. Otherwise, forge on to the ridge of Nahanton Hill.

Skyline Trail drops steeply down the eastern face of Nahanton to the foot of Wampatuck Hill. Across Wampatuck Road, Skyline Trail rolls boldly on, leading you over tumbling granite rubble to the peak. Coming down the hill's northern side, you soon arrive at an old granite quarry, now a deep pool fed by trickling springs. The Bunker Hill Monument in Boston's Charlestown neighborhood, commemorating the battle said to be the bloodiest of the American Revolution, was built from stone cut from Quincy's quarries.

After Wampatuck Hill, the path levels and the onslaught of rock lets up. The last elevation on this, the eastern side of the Blue Hills, is Rattlesnake Hill. Far less imposing than the peaks you have crossed, this hill is milder than its name suggests. However, on our Memorial Day weekend hike, my partner and I were told of several snake sightings. The black rat snake, though endangered, seems to be fairly common here. Timber rattlesnakes are known to live in the Blue Hills but are rare and reclusive.

From Rattlesnake Hill, Skyline Trail continues about 0.5 miles to arrive at

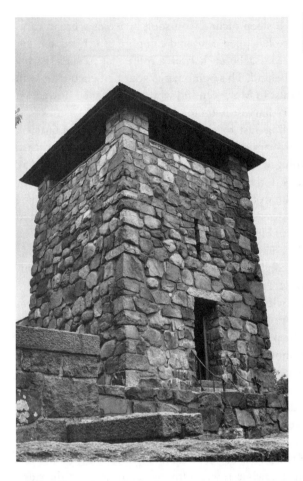

Saint Moritz Ponds. Cross Wampatuck Road and head southeast down a wide, sandy path to the twin ponds rife with pond lilies. After cutting between the two, the trail curves southward up a hemlock-shaded banking. Continue a short distance farther to arrive at the trail's end in the peaceful neighborhood of Quincy. Straight ahead, you will see Shea Skating Rink. Around the corner, hidden from view, is an active riding stable.

Though a sleepy bedroom community now, West Quincy was famous for its Saint Moritz Winter Carnival held annually from 1929 through the mid 1940s. Tens of thousands of people came to the area to see skiers launch themselves from a 400-foot jump on a nearby hill and to watch Olympic skaters carving the ice at Saint Moritz Ponds.

Resuming your hike from Saint Moritz Ponds, take Skyline Trail back over Rattlesnake and Wampatuck Hills. Ascending Nahanton, look for intersection 3144. Turn left off Skyline Trail here and hike south into Squamaug Notch. Foliage envelops you as you descend this less-frequented route. Bear right at intersection 3143 to join Curve Path, marked with red. Soon the trail turns sharply right at 3130 and becomes Bouncing Brook Path. Skirting the bases of Nahanton, Kitchamakin, and Chickatawbut hills, this route runs westward 1 mile to meet Skyline Trail at junction 3042.

Retrace your steps across MA 28 and follow the blue markers up the rugged face of Buck Hill. From this open peak at the midway point of Skyline Trail, look south to see Ponkapoag Pond. The twittering in the shrubs you hear is likely to be that of the rufous-sided towhees that nest here.

Stretching westward, Skyline Trail leads you down a steep drop to a peaceful tree-shaded plateau then drops to a root- and boulder-riddled pitch in a lowland hollow.

Look for blue markers to lead you out of the quagmire to the side of Tucker Hill. You will need ready arms and legs to climb this next section. But it is a quick trip to the top, and soon you reach a clear view west to Great Blue Hill.

Wind your way downhill again, crossing the green trail before merging with Bugbee Path at junction 2054. Turn right and take this paved road a short distance to Hillside Street. Make your way across to the Blue Hills Reservation Headquarters next to the state police station and the gray barn. A gateway beside the shingled headquarters marks the trailhead. Enter here and make an immediate right to start back on Skyline Trail. Zigzagging first up Hancock Hill then on to Hemmenway Hill, listen for the warning snorts of startled deer.

Coming off Hemmenway Hill, you will cross the green trail. Enjoy level ground for the few yards that lead you to the foot of Great Blue Hill, then begin your ascent of this, the final and highest peak. Granite steps laid by the Civilian Conservation Corps in the 1930s make the arduous climb a smidgen easier.

Press on, up another steep rise, then lift your eyes to the stone monolith directly ahead. Named Eliot Tower, it honors the landscape architect Charles Eliot.

Have a look from the tower and a celebratory snack and, when ready, walk south toward the weather observatory to find junction 1066. From here, pick up Skyline Trail's southern branch and head east back downhill along a stream. At junction 1094, leave Skyline Trail and take up Wildcat Notch Path, running off to the right.

Far less traveled than Skyline Trail, this path of packed leaves and earth descends gradually. At junction 1093, turn left to travel east on Half Way Path to cross two hillocks split by a stream. Pass straight through junction 1110 to reach Coon Hollow Path a bit farther on. Take this next right and walk along the deep hollow toward the road.

Cross Hillside Street on a diagonal to find the yellow trail on the west side of Houghton's Pond. Follow this trail east keeping the pond to your right to return to the parking lot.

NEARBY ATTRACTIONS

Once you have discovered the Blue Hills, you'll want to return again and again. For rock climbers and history buffs, one irresistible draw is the Quincy granite quarries accessible by car, public transportation, or hiking trail just over 0.5 miles from Saint Moritz Ponds in Quincy. The "Father of the Granite Industry," Solomon Willard, chose the site as the source of stone for Charlestown's Bunker Hill Monument in 1825. In short time Willard's innovative building techniques made Quincy granite a much-coveted construction material and thus launched America's granite quarrying industry. The last blocks of granite were cut from Quincy's

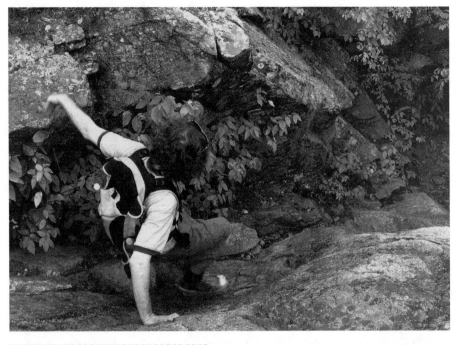

Sections of the trail are quite challenging.

quarries in 1963. Now linked to the Blue Hills Reservation, the quarries are open to the public for climbing and various programs run by the Department of Conservation and Recreation year-round. To reach the quarries on foot, follow Wampatuck Road northeast from Saint Moritz Ponds about 0.12 miles to Quarry Foot Path diverting to the left. At trail marker 4238, continue straight, crossing Ricciuti Drive to a paved access road which leads to the quarries. If traveling by Boston's "T," take the Red Line to Quincy Center, then MBTA bus #215 to Copeland and Willard Streets. Turn left on Willard, cross under the Expressway, and take the first right onto Ricciuti Drive. Quarries are just ahead on the right.

If traveling by car, take I-93 south to Furnace Brook Parkway (Exit 8). Follow signs to Willard Street and cross under I-93. Take the first right onto Ricciuti Drive at Mr. Tux. Quarries are just ahead on the right.

WILSON MOUNTAIN HIKE

IN BRIEF

Tall enough to fit its name, yet accessible to hikers of all abilities, Wilson Mountain is minutes away from the center of Boston's neighbor, Dedham. Following a trail that loops around the mountain's base then climbs to its rocky peak, you will enjoy peaceful woods, gurgling streams, and a meadow that at the height of summer is resplendent with wildflowers and butterflies.

DESCRIPTION

In 1995 an out-of-town developer visited Wilson Mountain and conjured a plan to grade its ruts, backhoe out its boulders, and, once it was bare, "improve it" with a shopping mall. The scope of the development meant zoning would need to be considered, reconsidered, and possibly changed. A special town meeting was therefore scheduled to give the townspeople a chance to voice their thoughts and vote yea or nay, not only for the acres of asphalt, linoleum, and accompanying goods, but for the last sizable tract of open space in Dedham. The vote was unanimous, and Wilson Mountain's 216 acres were saved.

Head uphill from the parking lot, following the wide gravel-topped path into woods. Keep to the right, passing another path bearing

KEY AT-A-GLANCE INFORMATION

LENGTH: 3.47 miles

CONFIGURATION: Loop

DIFFICULTY: Easy to moderate

SCENERY: Woods, spring-fed wetlands, and a meadow sown with wildflower species especially attractive to butterflies

EXPOSURE: Mostly shaded

TRAFFIC: Moderate to heavy

TRAIL SURFACE: Packed earth topped by loose gravel, some rock face

HIKING TIME: 1–2 hours

SEASON: Year-round sunrise–sunset

ACCESS: Free

MAPS: Posted at entrance

FACILITIES: None

SPECIAL COMMENTS: A good hike for families

WHEELCHAIR TRAVERSABLE: No

DRIVING DISTANCE FROM BOSTON COMMON: 19 miles

Directions

From Boston take I-90 west 9.4 miles to I-95 south via Exit 15. From I-95 south take Exit 17 to reach MA 135. Continue on MA 135 toward Dedham. The parking lot is 0.5 miles ahead on the right.

Wilson Mountain Hike
UTM Zone (WGS84) 19T
Easting: 318737
Northing: 4680850
Latitude: N 42° 15' 32"
Longitude: W 71° 11' 52"

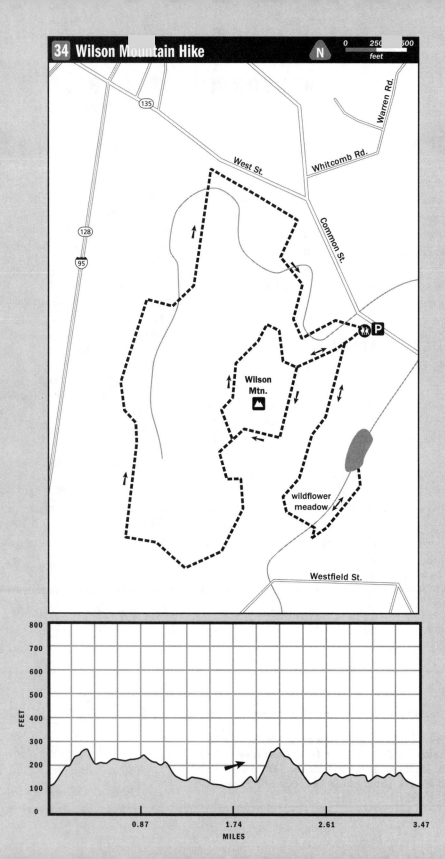

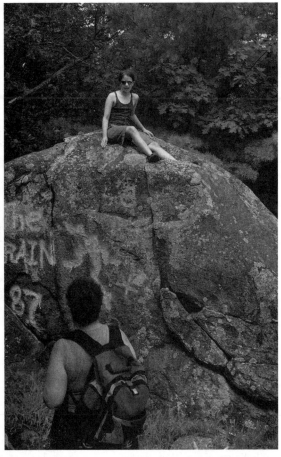

left. Within a few hundred yards, this path, identified by green blazes, forms a "V" with the red and green trail. A tree beside it bears the number 21. To escape city sounds and feel peaceful pines close by, take the narrow red and green trail. Traveling southwest over exposed roots and angular rocks spit up by the hill, and what looks like the forehead of an earth-enshrined granite giant, the trail reaches a high point.

From here, hiking becomes less strenuous. Less rocky, the path is now made of packed earth, mottled with patches of sand, the remains of pulverized boulders. After passing through a stone wall, perhaps built by Mr. Wilson for his family's cows, the trail rounds a bend and climbs to intersection 24. Here the red trail hikes up and to the right, and the green trail goes left easing downhill. On this slope cooled by shade cast by pines, hemlocks, ashes, and basswood trees, the acoustics amplify the whoosh of cars slicing through air on a nearby road.

At the next intersection, the trail is, disconcertingly, marked 18. Bear left to stay on the green trail. For a pleasant, virtually rock-free stretch, the trail travels south up a slight grade. Then, closing in on the reservation's boundary, it contracts in width and doubles back to head northeast, descending past knotted swamp oak and spry sassafras. This sheltered eastern side of the hill harbors mountain laurel and woodland wildflowers, including lady's slippers (*Cypripedium acaule*). Easy to miss, this endangered member of the orchid family can live for 100 years but may flower only 10 to 20 times in its lifetime. Because of its rarity, identifying the plant's twin oval leaves spread flat against the ground (to optimize photosynthesis), gives nearly the same thrill as spotting the single purple-pink blossom of the orchid in bloom.

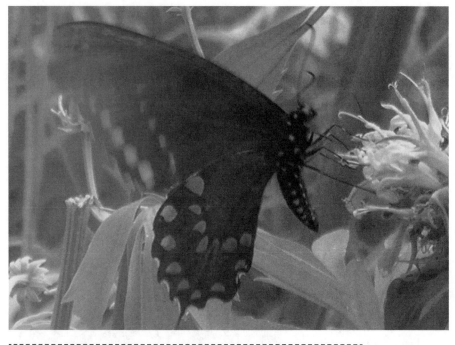

A monarch butterfly alights on a bergamot blossom at the wildflower meadow.

Several unmarked paths split off from the green trail as it sweeps uphill again over pine needle–fed humus, which, besides being easy on the feet, is the basis of life for myriad forest creatures ranging in form and appeal from the lady's slipper to American robins (thrushes misnamed by colonists who missed their British robins) to mushrooms (some deadly, some delicious). Stay on course with the green trail at both intersections 16 and 17, and at a split beyond, cross planks bridging a modest stream. In summer, the leaves of lindens and basswood trees fan the air above the trickling water. Nearby a fractured stone wall, looking tired and disorientated, traipses through this tract, which in farming days was pasture land.

Heading north past abutting residential property, the trail crosses more wetland. Rough slabs of wood provide dry footing over pooled tea-colored water. Granite-hewn upland casts shadow from the right. Pitching downhill, the green trail passes junction 15, veering away to cross a stream. Dazzling in the heat of a summer day, dragonflies and fluttering butterflies stir the vaporous atmosphere. Weaving north then west, up then down between hill and mire, the trail expands and flattens as it nears a road.

Insulated from the road and its light-but-steady traffic by a thick buffer of woods, the trail winds alongside it to a rock formation looking like the spine of a monster arching out of the earth. The trail then aims southwest, eases downhill, and frees itself from the road. Leveling at wetland once more, the trail meets an enormous boulder at the center of a clearing. Carried here by creeping ice thousands of years ago, the granite monolith is pinned in place by sassafras trees deeply rooted on opposing sides.

Wetland, perhaps born of glacial meltwater, picks up again beyond the boulder. An inviting pool to the left tempts passersby and dares jaded city slickers to give up inhibitions and at least dip their feet. Passing between the water and upland crag, the trail meanders southeast. Quiet that includes squawking blue jays and chirping chickadees takes over. Here, the city seems a thousand miles away. Dipping downhill over smooth ground, the trail arrives at junction 11. Sidetrack onto the right-hand path for an alternate route to the peak; otherwise, stick with the green trail to quickly reach the parking lot.

For those wanting more, steer right of the parking lot to take up the red and green trail once again. This time, bear right at junction 21 to take the red trail up Wilson Mountain's western slope. Featuring jagged ledges, cliffs, and plenty of mammoth glacial erratics, this route is a dramatic counterpoint to the green trail. A massive mound of granite marks Wilson Mountain's highest point, and, though it offers very little in terms of a view, it makes a perfect throne for anyone naming themselves " King of the Mountain." From this great rock, follow the red trail as it serpentines around the peak, rising and falling with hillocks and hollows to eventually arrive at junction 24, where it reunites with the red and green trail. Bear left here and hike back downhill.

If you still balk at returning to your car, there is yet another diversion to consider. Where the red and green trail filters toward the parking lot, a second trail veers off to the right. Climbing a gentle incline, this route leads to a hidden meadow passing a collapsed cabin with an intact chimney along the way. Attractive to deer looking for fodder in the drab winter months, this round acre or so is a fantastic butterfly garden bursting with blossoming bee balm, aster, Queen Anne's lace, and terrifically tall coneflower in the summer months.

When ready, follow the path of trodden grass southwest across the meadow back into woods. At the three-way junction you reach moments later, take the left-most trail and follow a stream on its northeast course to a pond below. Look for basking turtles, frogs, or a blue heron, and then turn heel and hike back to the parking lot.

NEARBY ATTRACTIONS

To round out the day before or after hiking, you can catch a movie at the Dedham Community Theater, established in 1927 and located in the town center (580 High Street, Dedham; [781] 326-0409). Besides showing the best in cinema, the theater houses the Museum of Bad Art. Unlike most movie houses, the concessions stand serves beer, wine, and hot chocolate in addition to sodas, candy, and popcorn.

35 NOON HILL LOOP
(with Charles River extension)

KEY AT-A-GLANCE INFORMATION

LENGTH: 4.6 miles

CONFIGURATION: Loops around Noon Hill and Holt Pond, with an extension to an overlook on the bank of the Charles River

DIFFICULTY: Easy

SCENERY: Views include forest wetlands, the Charles River, Holt Pond, and a panoramic overlook from the top of Noon Hill

EXPOSURE: Mostly shaded

TRAFFIC: Moderate

TRAIL SURFACE: Packed earth with some areas of gravel

HIKING TIME: 3 hours

SEASON: Year-round sunrise–sunset

ACCESS: Free

MAPS: Available at the trailhead or online at www.thetrustees.org

FACILITIES: Picnic tables

SPECIAL COMMENTS: Noon Hill is a link in Bay Circuit Trail; the latter connects green space in 43 towns in Eastern Massachusetts, from Newburyport to Kingston Bay.

WHEELCHAIR TRAVERSABLE: No

DRIVING DISTANCE FROM BOSTON COMMON: 23 miles

Noon Hill Loop (with Charles River extension)

UTM Zone (WGS84) 19T

Easting: 308509

Northing: 4670683

Latitude: N 42° 09' 54"

Longitude: W 71° 19' 05"

IN BRIEF

This secluded reservation provides 204 acres of peaceful hiking, with trails suitable for horseback riding, mountain biking, and cross-country skiing. Miles from the busy Charles River esplanade in downtown Boston, this location provides an opportunity to experience the river in its natural state.

DESCRIPTION

In 1676, a thousand warring Wompanoag tore through these parts, setting fire to 32 houses, 2 mills, and a slew of barns. Having lost patience with the English settlers, Wompanoag chief Metacomet, known by the English settlers as King Philip, instructed his man Monaco to eliminate them. The Wompanoag had succeeded in destroying a village called Mendon farther south—Medfield was next in line.

Furious fighting continued throughout the region all the way to the border of Connecticut for the rest of the year. King Philip came close to achieving his goal, once the Narragansett tribe joined his effort. But by making preemptive strikes, the English held

---

Directions ⟶

From Boston take Storrow Drive east to I-93 south. Take Exit 1 to I-95 south 7.3 miles. At Exit 9 merge onto US 1 south. Turn right onto Old Post Road and soon after turn slight left onto Common Street. After 1.8 miles Common Street becomes Elm Street. Stay straight to go onto Elm Street/MA 27 and continue to follow MA 27 for 2.6 miles. At the intersection of MA 27 and MA 109, take MA 109 west for 0.1 mile, then take an immediate left onto Causeway Street. Follow 1.3 miles and turn left onto Noon Hill Road. Entrance and small parking area is 0.2 miles ahead on the right.

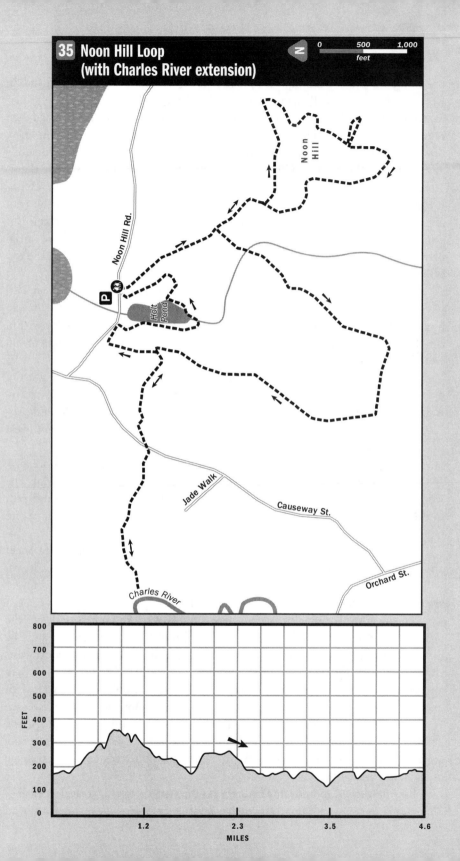

35 Noon Hill Loop
(with Charles River extension)

N

0   500   1,000
feet

Noon Hill

Noon Hill Rd.

P

Holt Pond

Jade Walk

Causeway St.

Orchard St.

Charles River

on. Come spring, the bloody conflict was put to an end when a Praying Indian working as a guide for Benjamin Church shot King Philip dead.

From the parking area, set off uphill, heading southeast. Pass the sunken remains of an old foundation, continuing straight on as the path tapers back downhill and enters the woods. The trail passes through a mix of hardwoods and evergreens before reaching a sign, bearing the number 1 and, shortly thereafter, a second marked with the number 2. Here you have the choice of following a fork to the left on a new trail, or continuing straight with the trail identified as a part of the Bay Circuit Trail. The day of my hike, the clamor of gunshots to the east made up my mind—I stayed the course, despite my initial plan to take the route to the left, which offers a slightly longer ascent to the top of Noon Hill.

Like most of the land of Massachusetts, the wooded acres of Noon Hill were open pasture enclosed for generations by stone walls. The oak, beech, birch, and hemlock have grown in over the last century. Because they lay within the floodplain of the nearby Stop River, the pasture and cultivated tracts of old were likely highly productive.

An intersection ahead offers a path to the right, but continue straight on, up what is the start of Noon Hill. Not much farther along, the trail splits again. Rather than following the path marked with yellow, keep to the right and proceed slightly downhill. From here, the trail, still level and wide, winds southwest in easy curves through the woods.

Arriving at marker 5, turn off and climb southeast on a slender, more rugged path through a grove of young white pines. In the first week of May, the woods are bright with half-sprung leaves in vivid shades of green—and red, in the case of some oaks and maples. Low-bush blueberries sport dainty white blossoms.

After winding around a ledge of granite, the trail noses north to meet another trail. Hike to the right, rounding the curve of the hill. Up ahead, you will come to a sign directing hikers away from a section of trail which is under restoration. Follow the blue markers to take the detour marked 8A.

This new trail gradually ascends over a track of packed pine needles to the peak of Noon Hill at 370 feet. Explore the hilltop's nooks and crannies as the view opens and the trail becomes obscure momentarily then continue southwest, traveling downhill to reach an intersection with a trail marked 7. Turn left here and ascend southeast a short distance to a scenic overlook. Ahead a mass of exposed granite serves as balcony seating for viewing Boston's skyline. Retrace your steps from the overlook back to marker 7 and continue downhill. At the next intersection, number 6, turn right to head northwest. A burbling spring makes for a wet zone, but for the most part the trail provides easy, dry passage as it winds through wetland.

Pass marker 5 and continue northeast on a piece of trail traveled earlier. Beyond marker 4, where the trail reaches another intersection, turn left to head

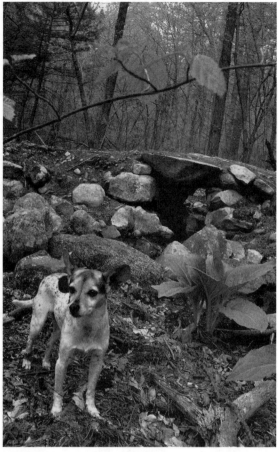

Luminous skunk cabbage brightens the trail in spring.

southwest. You will come to a granite boulder off to the side, and, farther on, to a bridge across a rushing stream. The trail along this part makes many twists and turns and becoming narrower by degrees. Well away from any houses or roads, the woods are peaceful here, the loudest noisemakers being blue jays. Fortunately, since there are few markers, the path is clear and easy to follow. However due to a newly fallen tree I briefly lost my way.

A seemingly forgotten small gray shack sits off the trail to the left, where the trail eases to the northwest. Continuing on, pass through a gap in a stone wall and walk down a long avenue between two stone walls. Keep an eye out for forget-me-nots and less-friendly poison ivy growing along the edge of the grassy way. Looking over the stone wall to the right, you might notice elm trees that have miraculously survived disease and clear-cutting.

Stay with the trail, heading northeast. Passing a trail on the left, you will shortly come to a dirt driveway. Cross here and continue on through more woods to a junction. Turn left and left again at the next split, marked 12 then follow this new path as it twists and turns westward. Beyond a small wooden bridge and another stone wall, the path bisects Causeway Street and arrives at marker 14.

Aim for the well-concealed river on this wide pine needle–strewn path by bearing left at the next two forks. As the land begins to slope to the Charles River, you will see marker 17 posted on a tree. By now you will be able to see the Charles River through the tangle of trees and shrubs growing along its banks. The path ends at a gorgeous spot beside a massive oak.

When you are ready to leave this idyllic scene, follow the trail back to the junction at marker 12. From here, take the path heading left. This less-used

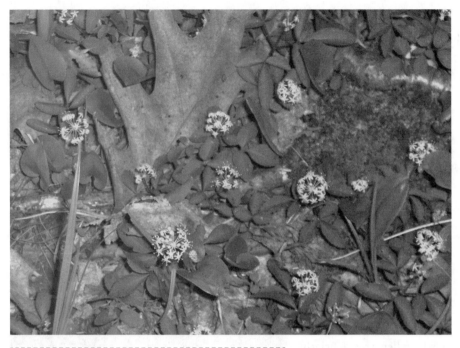

In spring rare wildflowers reveal themselves in the leaf litter.

route leads through a grove of young pines to Noon Hill Street. Emerging from the woods, turn right and walk briefly on the pavement to Holt Pond. On spotting a path alongside the road, reenter the woods following the path over a footbridge, then head right to circle the pond.

Holt Pond was formed in 1764 when the nearby Sawmill Brook was dammed to provide power for a mill. In the next century, the woods surrounding the pond were cleared and fenced for pasture. Today nature has reclaimed the land, and instead of a working mill or a dairy herd, you are likely to see herons and egrets fishing in its shallows.

Once you're around the southeastern bend of the pond, a second trail branches off to climb a banking to the right. Take this turn and follow the path uphill to a boulder. Press on through bushes concealing the path to find a more pronounced trail. To make your way back to the parking area, hike left, then left again at a wide junction.

NOANET WOODLANDS HIKE

IN BRIEF

This hike traverses undulating woodlands named for Noanet, a chief of the Natick tribe who was well-known among Dover's first white settlers. Circling the ravine carved by Noanet Brook, the trail diverts to the reservation's highest point, Noanet Peak, then passes near the site of a 19th-century mill.

DESCRIPTION

Like all the towns settled soon after New England's founding, Dover is rich in history. And although the acres within the Noanet Reservation were first farmed by colonial settlers a good many years ago—in 1720—the area has an even longer history. In fact, archaeologists from Harvard's Peabody Museum of Archaeology and Ethnology discovered that ancestors of the region's Powissett tribe quarried felsite for arrowheads from nearby sites around 3000 BC, around the time Egyptian pharoahs were building the pyramids!

Much of the credit for discovering and preserving Dover's history goes to Amelia Peabody, who, in 1923, purchased the first of what, in the course of 60 years, grew to be a nearly 800-acre estate. Born wealthy as the

KEY AT-A-GLANCE INFORMATION

LENGTH: 5.11 miles

CONFIGURATION: Loop

DIFFICULTY: Easy to moderate

SCENERY: Woods, ponds, a view of Boston from Noanet Peak, and the site of a mill built in the early 19th century on Noanet Brook

EXPOSURE: Mostly shaded

TRAFFIC: Moderate

TRAIL SURFACE: Packed earth with some more-rugged areas of loose gravel and exposed rock

HIKING TIME: 2.5–3 hours

SEASON: Year-round sunrise–sunset

ACCESS: Free

MAPS: Available while supplies last at the trailhead; can be printed from the Trustees of Reservations Web site www.thetrustees.org.

FACILITIES: Restrooms open seasonally

SPECIAL COMMENTS: The Noanet Woodlands is dog friendly, but dogs are not allowed in the parking lot at Caryl Park or in Caryl Park itself.

WHEELCHAIR TRAVERSABLE: No

DRIVING DISTANCE TO BOSTON COMMON: 21 miles

Directions

From Boston take I-90 west to Exit 15, I-95/MA 128 toward Waltham/Dedham, and merge onto I-95 south/MA 128 toward South Shore/Cape Cod. After 6.8 miles take Exit 17 to MA 135 toward Needham/Wellesley. Turn left onto MA 135/West Street. Continue 0.6 miles then turn left onto South Street. After 1.8 miles, South Street becomes Willow Street. Turn right onto Dedham Street and continue 0.3 miles to Caryl Park.

Noanet Woodlands Hike
UTM Zone (WGS84) 19T
Easting: 312811
Northing: 4679843
Latitude: N 42° 14' 54"
Longitude: W 71° 16' 09"

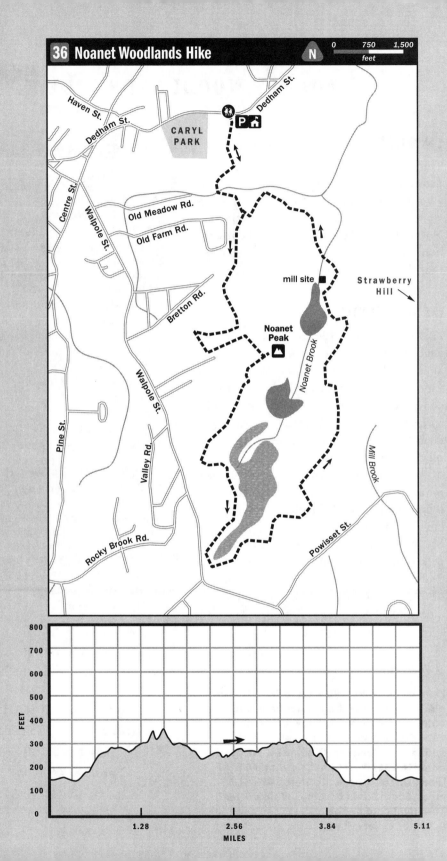

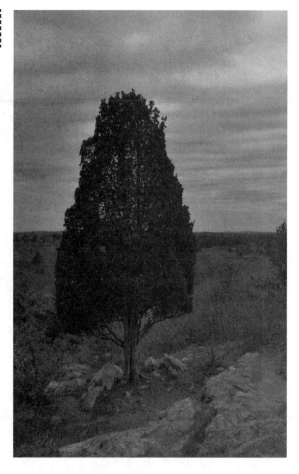

From the peak of Noanet Hill you can see for miles.

only child of the invest-
ment banker Frank E.
Peabody of the investment
house Kidder and Peabody,
Amelia chose to forgo the
life of a wife and mother
and instead devoted her
energies to her passions:
philanthropy, sculpture,
thoroughbred horse breed-
ing, sustainable agriculture,
and land conservation.

Rather than use her
money to insulate her-
self, Peabody used it to
reach out to the world
and to lend support where
needed. An ardent horse-
woman and member of the
Norfolk Hunt Club, she
maintained miles of bridle
trails not only for her own
enjoyment but also for that
of the entire hunt club.
Uncommonly appreciative of the history beneath her feet, Peabody hired the
archaeologist Roland Robbins, who had excavated the Saugus Iron Works, to
investigate the Dover Union Iron Mill site on Noanet Brook. For many years,
Peabody served as the chair of the Arts and Skills Service of the American Red
Cross. Upon her death in 1984 at age 94, Amelia Peabody left nearly her entire
estate to charity.

The hike begins at the trailhead to the right of the ranger's station at Caryl
Park, near the former home of Reverend Benjamin Caryl at 107 Dedham Street.
The region's first minister, Caryl built the house around 1777. To reach the
Caryl Trail (marked with yellow), follow this short clay path southeast to its end
at a dirt road. Bear right at this junction and proceed on this winding road past
a composting site on the right and an unmarked path on the left. Beyond a sign
reading "to Noanet Woods," the trail bends southwest to cross a stream. Several
yards farther, it encounters a junction marked number 2 and then reaches junction 3, where it meets the Larrabee Trail (red) and Peabody Trail (blue). For a
quick hike to the mill site, choose the Peabody Trail; otherwise, continue south
on the Caryl Trail to take a full tour of the reservation.

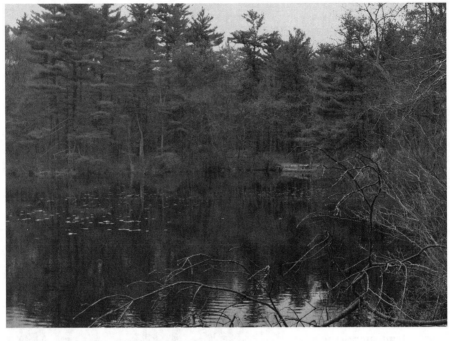

The mill pond is shrouded by woods.

For 0.25 miles, the wide woodchip trail has a suburban feel to it as it skirts the backyards of houses built on a cul-de-sac outside the reservation. But as it sways southeast beyond the houses, distractions from outside fall away. Beech trees become more numerous among robust red pines and wispy white pine saplings.

At junction 6, the Caryl Trail shoots westward and soon thereafter jack-knifes to head southeast to reach junction 7 as if following the scent of a fox pursued by Amelia Peabody and the rest of the Norfolk Hunt Club. From this turn, the Caryl Trail straightens, allowing for a full gallop to junction 9, over-shooting Noanet Peak. A fast pace is well and good for horse and hound, but hikers wanting a view over these lands should leave the Caryl Trail at junction 8 and bear left to head to upland. At the next junction, turn right and climb southeast to reach the pinnacle of Noanet Hill. Tree-covered except for an outcrop of granite, the hilltop provides a perfect view of Boston's skyline, which, in spring, appears to be floating on a sea of budding treetops brightened here and there by the rosy blush of blooming cherries.

To resume the Caryl Trail, locate a path several feet downhill from the peak marked with a white square, and follow it southwest over roots and stones to the base of the hill where the Caryl Trail sweeps by. Join this bridle trail and continue on level ground through junction 9, traveling southwest on an easy downhill slope. At junction 10, the Caryl Trail crosses the blunt swath of a gas line. Having reached the reservation's boundary, the trail swings southeast at junction 11. In May blooming violets, wild cherries, and blueberry bushes, far outdo the distraction of neighboring houses.

After pitching down a rocky slope, the trail steadies on the shoulder of a hill overlooking wetland. Upon leaving a burly oak stand, the character of the woods changes abruptly from deciduous to primarily evergreen. The sudden appearance of a well-built stone wall explains the transition— since the acres contained within it were once cleared pastureland.

Once around the tip of the wetland, the Caryl Trail traces the reservation's southern border, running parallel to the fencing of a private farm. To briefly break away from the border, bear left at junction 16 to hike on glacial debris mounded around the swamp. Beyond a horse jump, the path bends east, passing through a clearing shaded by looming red pines. Follow this deeply recessed path as it meanders through woods then climbs sharply to meet another traveling along a ridge. Bear right here to return to the Caryl Trail.

Traveling northeast a short distance farther alongside a horse farm, the Caryl Trail swings north onto a cart road entering from the right marked number 17. Several hundred yards ahead, this cart road becomes the Peabody Trail (blue) at marker 18. To follow the course of the Noanet Brook and the millrace, choose this route. Otherwise, at junction 18, bear right onto the Larrabee Trail (red) to complete a wide circumnavigation.

The Larrabee Trail is named for Thomas Larrabee, a well-loved citizen of Dover, who, after enlisting to fight in the Revolution was assigned to the guard company responsible for protecting General George Washington. He both fought in the battle of Ticonderoga and was one of the troops with Washington when, at Christmas 1776, the general crossed the Delaware River in a raging blizzard to attack the Hessians at Trenton, New Jersey. When at last free to attend to domestic life, Larrabee settled in Dover and built a homestead on Strawberry Hill. He was said to be a large man both in body and character, and local lore has it he drank many pints at William's Tavern, where he entertained patrons with colorful stories from his fighting days.

For 0.4 miles, the Larrabee Trail arcs gently northwest across upland. This section of easy walking over glacial grit offers several opportunities to visit neighboring conservation land. To add a loop around Larrabee's Strawberry Hill or an excursion to the Hale Reservation, travel east at junctions 22 or 25.

After bearing directly west at junction 22, the Larrabee Trail descends to meet the end of an esker then, veering north once more, climbs the finger of sand and gravel and continues along its narrow top. Junction 25 may or may not be marked (as of this writing it was not), but it is distinguished by being located at the northern end of the esker, where a path feeds in from the right near a confluence of stone walls. Strawberry Hill is named for the abundant wild strawberries growing on its slopes. If it is June and thoughts of the tart fruit compel you to set out to find them, bear right here; otherwise, stay with the Larrabee Trail as it switches westward toward Noanet Brook.

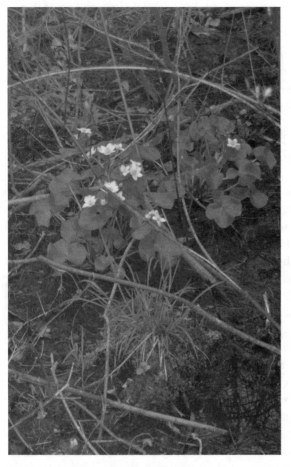

Marsh marigolds bloom from April to June.

Drawing near the brook, the trail meets another route rising from the left. From this vantage point at the bottom of a steep banking, you can see a pool that was shaped by the mill that once operated upstream. Follow paths to the left to explore the pond and mill site. When ready to continue, bear east at junction 27 on the Larrabee Trail. Around a bend sits a massive glacial erratic; being almost perfectly flat on top, it looks like a giant slice of cake or cube of cheese.

Departing from the stranded boulder, the trail veers sharply west to parallel a stone wall, then crosses Noanet Brook where it flows at a trickle. Several feet farther, a trail to the mill site branches off to the left. Continuing north, the trail leads to a wide, open clearing with a much-used horse jump in the middle, a smattering of imposing pines, and a second great boulder perched at the far side.

Cross on a diagonal, keeping the haunting boulder to the left, and follow red markers back into the woods. Stay with the Larrabee Trail as it aims northwest, then, bending like an elbow at marker 33, bears southwest traveling uphill to junction 3, where the yellow, red, and blue trails converge. Back at the Caryl Trail, bear right and follow it north to the parking lot.

NEARBY ATTRACTIONS

The Dolphin Seafood Restaurant is just 5 miles away at 12 Washington Street in downtown Natick, (508) 655-0669. This eatery is open seven days a week for lunch and dinner. From Caryl Park, follow Dedham Street west to Park Avenue and bear right onto Haven Street. After 1.2 miles, turn right onto Main Street and left onto Pleasant Street, which becomes Union Street. After 1.5 miles, turn left onto East Central Street (MA 135), and at 0.2 miles, turn right onto Washington Street.

BORDERLAND STATE PARK:
Pond and Quarry Hike **37**

IN BRIEF

The Pond and Quarry Hike is a great escape from the cheerful throng of visitors to Borderland State Park.

DESCRIPTION

Borderland State Park was, until 1971, the estate of Blanche and Oakes Ames, one of the most prominent and intriguing couples in New England history. Oakes Ames, revered as a foremost expert on orchids and a celebrated professor of botany at Harvard University, was the son of Oakes Ames of Crédit Mobilier infamy. The artist, inventor, and suffragette Blanche Ames, a graduate of Smith College, was the daughter of Brigadier General Adelbert Ames, the provisional governor of Mississippi under Abraham Lincoln. In his bid for a second term, Lincoln asked Ames to be his running mate; however, the general turned him down. The 20-room granite mansion Oakes and Blanche built has been preserved. Oakes's two-story research library remains intact, as does Blanche's studio, located on the third floor.

The Pond and Quarry Hike provides a varied tour of Borderland's northern reaches.

Directions ➝

From Boston, take I-93/US 1 south toward I-95/Dedham, then merge onto I-95 south (Exit 1) toward Providence, Rhode Island. Travel 5.3 miles to Coney Street (Exit 10) and head toward Sharon/Walpole. Stay on Coney Street 1.6 miles before turning onto Norwood Street. Turn left onto Upland Road/MA 27. Continue on Upland 0.5 miles to Post Office Square. Drive 0.1 mile and turn right onto Pond Street. At the roundabout, take the first exit onto Massapoag Avenue. The entrance to Borderland State Park is 3.8 miles ahead.

KEY AT-A-GLANCE INFORMATION

LENGTH: 6.18 miles

CONFIGURATION: Loop

DIFFICULTY: Moderate

SCENERY: Woods, ponds, streams, granite boulders, and granite mansion

EXPOSURE: Primarily shaded, with exposed lookouts

TRAFFIC: Light, except for the first 0.25 miles

TRAIL SURFACE: Variable, including a gravel multiuse path, soft level ground, rocky footing, and wooden bridges spanning streams

HIKING TIME: 3 hours

SEASON: Year-round 8 a.m.–sunset

ACCESS: Parking $2

MAPS: Available at the visitor center

FACILITIES: A visitor center with restrooms; many picnic tables

SPECIAL COMMENTS: Besides offering miles of hiking, Borderland State Park welcomes anglers, horseback riders, and Frisbee golfers. For a schedule of mansion tours and special events, visit www.friendsof borderland.org. Tour tickets cost $3.

WHEELCHAIR TRAVERSABLE: No, The recommended route for wheelchair users is the "Pond Walk" trail which circles Leach Pond.

DRIVING DISTANCE TO BOSTON COMMON: 27 miles

Borderland State Park:
Pond and Quarry Hike

UTM Zone (WGS84) 19T

Easting: 320918

Northing: 4658963

Latitude: N 42° 03' 45"

Longitude: W 71° 09' 52"

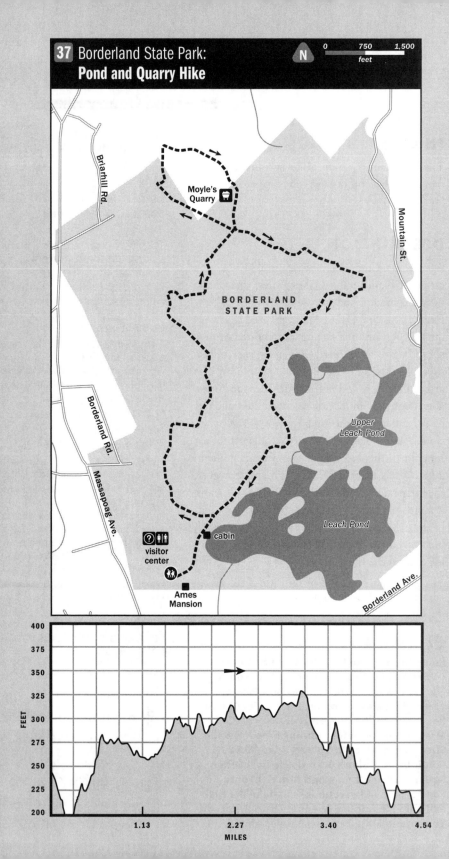

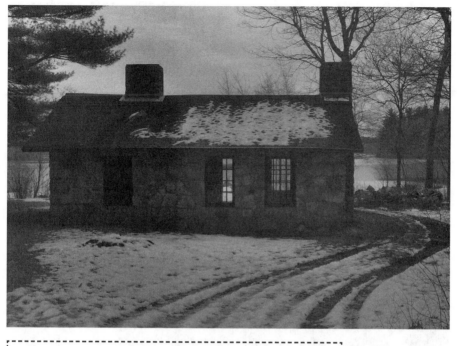

In winter a fire is kept burning in a hearth at the cabin beside Leach Pond.

The trailhead lies not far from the edge of the parking lot, just beyond the visitor center. Begin walking on the gravel road, bearing left. This path turns through woods briefly before arriving at the stone cabin on Leach Pond. After pausing at the cabin to admire a fisherman's catch or the fire in the hearth within, continue on the gravel road. Just ahead on the left, you will see a sign for the West Side Trail. Take this trail, leaving the pond behind.

The West Side Trail is entirely different from the gravel path. This narrow trail climbs gradually into dense woods littered with huge orbs of granite looking like golf balls lost on the edge of Hercules' driving range. In winter, snow and ice accentuate the contours of the boulders in stark contrast to the slender trunks of the hardwood trees swaying amongst them. Too rugged for strollers, fainthearted joggers, or equines—the West Side Trail leaves crowds and commotion behind.

A few minutes along the route, the trail forks where it meets the French Trail. The West Side Trail veers westward, but follow the French Trail east instead. Ahead the trail threads through a dramatic garden of stone then arrives at a massive boulder. As I passed, a boy brandishing a plastic sword paced atop it, telling his mother the laws of the forest.

The trail winds and weaves enough to be tricky to follow at times. Keep an eye out for painted blue rectangular markers on rocks and trees to stay on track. At the next intersection, where the French Trail meets the Northwest

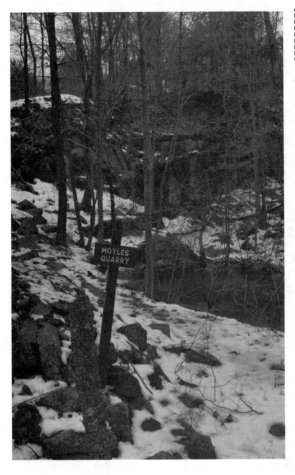

Moyles Quarry is closed for for quarrying, but there's still plenty of granite to be had.

Trail, stay left to switch to the Northwest Trail. The terrain remains stony and undulating as you head northward, passing numerous vernal pools and ponds. At streams and perpetually wet spots, well-laid wooden planks enable hikers to pass without getting their feet wet. Moss thrives in this well-watered world, and otherwise-austere stone is softened in cloaks of green. Through the woods to the left, you can see a pond surrounded by dense underbrush. In January, silent deer leave bold impressions in the snow and mud; come March, red-winged blackbirds liven the place with flashes of red and wild chattering.

Here the trail levels and briefly broadens as it passes an imposing wall of stone before reaching an intersection with the Ridge Trail. Leave the Northwest Trail at this point and bear right. Immediately ahead, you will see a great pile of granite. On the day I passed, a man, a girl, and two goats stood on its peak gazing down at me.

The Ridge Trail continues, passing scores of pools on either side. The footing remains rocky and rough but level except where the trail encounters the occasional monstrous boulder. On several sections of the hike, the trail cuts through gaps in stone walls, reminders of the farmland these acres were when Blanche and Oakes acquired them. You might notice at this point that the trail markers you were following earlier are no longer blue but white, designating the Ridge Trail.

Eventually, after weaving through grassy forage land, the trail leads to a crossroads where the Ridge Trail meets the Quarry Loop Trail. To pay a visit to the Moyles's Quarry on this circuit, you can go clockwise or counterclockwise.

If you prefer counterclockwise, take the path straight ahead; otherwise, bear left, heading northwest. Almost immediately, you will cross a wet bog via a small bridge. A bit farther along, the trail passes though a grove of young white pines which provide sweet relief to the drab gray trunks of inelegant swamp oak common in these woods.

Where the Quarry Loop Trail reaches its northern tip, a sign points left to "an emergency exit to private homes." Continue right, staying on Quarry Trail. Heading east, and soon southeast, the trail leads past a steep-faced granite monolith. Weathered holes drilled into it tell of the hard labor of the quarry-men who years ago cut blocks from the wall of stone. Rounding a bend, the now narrow trail opens to the site of the Moyles's Quarry. Today the quarry looks something like a stage. The cavity left by excavators is ringed by a wall of granite that provides a grand acoustic backdrop. Shortly after the quarry, the trail passes the tail end of the Morse Loop Trail. Stay right to complete the Quarry Loop Trail. Arriving back where the loop began, bear left to rejoin the Ridge Trail, heading east.

Ahead is the startling find of a vehicle abandoned many storms and sun-scorching summers ago. Reduced to flaking rust, the auto's style and vintage is any hiker's guess. On this stretch of trail, you will pass by dense underbrush. Lucky hikers making the trek in July and August might discover blueberries. Not long after meeting the Friend's Trail, the Ridge Trail jogs abruptly to the right. Be on the lookout for this turn; although not well marked, this elbow is a part of the Ridge Trail. From here, the trail winds south, heading downhill much of the way. After passing more boulders and crossing a wooden bridge, look for a pond through the woods to the left and, finally, a sign confirming that you are on the upper Granite Hills Trail. At the end of another long boardwalk, the trail eases to the right.

After crossing more wetland and climbing uphill, the trail reaches a fork. To the right is the Split Rock Trail, however, take the Granite Hills Trail, which continues left. Before long, this meandering trail breaks from tangled thickets to reconvene with the more civilized gravel path that hugs the banks of Leach Pond. To head back to the visitor center and parking lot, follow this road to the right. The sight of water rushing over the lip of a dam that divides Leach Pond may cause you to divert left at the split ahead. Once you have had a look, return to the gravel road and follow it westward to the visitor center.

NEARBY ATTRACTIONS

If it is strawberry, blueberry, or apple season, don't miss a chance to stop at Ward's Berry Farm, at 614 South Main Street in Sharon, just 6.34 miles up the road from Borderland. Besides offering seasonal pesticide-free produce grown on its 150 acres, Ward's has friendly farm animals, a sandbox for kids, and gourmet delights for sale year-round.

38 WHITNEY AND THAYER WOODS HIKE
(with Wompatuck State Park)

KEY AT-A-GLANCE INFORMATION

LENGTH: 6.12 miles
CONFIGURATION: Loop
DIFFICULTY: Easy to moderate
SCENERY: Woods, ponds, vernal pools, enormous glacial erratics, and garden with reflecting pool
EXPOSURE: Mostly shaded
TRAFFIC: Light to moderate
TRAIL SURFACE: Packed earth
HIKING TIME: 2.5–3 hours
SEASON: Year-round sunrise–sunset
ACCESS: Admission is free, but the trustees welcome donations.
MAPS: Available at a kiosk near trailhead and at www.thetrustees.org
FACILITIES: None
SPECIAL COMMENTS: The Whitney and Thayer Woods property combined with Trustees of Reservations–owned Turkey Hill and Wier River Farm covers 824 acres. Wompatuck State Park, another neighbor of the Whitney and Thayer Woods, adds another 3,500 acres. In addition, Wompatuck offers 262 campsites.
WHEELCHAIR TRAVERSABLE: The many carriage roads that weave through this property are traversable by wheelchair; however, several paths included in this hike are not.
DRIVING DISTANCE FROM BOSTON COMMON: 13 miles

IN BRIEF

Hiking miles of groomed carriage roads and rugged footpaths through hemlock and holly groves, visitors will take in such spectacles as a magnificent woodland garden and a glacier-made granite rooster.

DESCRIPTION

From the parking lot, set out hiking southwest on Howe's Road, the carriage path located at the head of the lot. Serpentining down a gentle grade, this road cuts an elegant route through woods, passing vernal pools on either side. After a few long, leg-loosening strides, the world outside, with its gas stations and convenience stores, fades as another replaces it—a place created by Wampanoags, early settlers struggling for a foothold, a handful of well-heeled folks, a down-and-outer or two, and the U.S. government.

The dense woods have grown in since New England's agriculture went bust at the end of the 19th century. A hiker here—say, in 1815—would have found barely a tree in sight. By then, woolly-backed sheep and stiff-gated goats had replaced the hardwoods and conifers that had previously sheltered grouse, deer, and other game coveted by Native Americans.

Whitney and Thayer
Woods Hike

UTM Zone (WGS84) 19T
Easting: 349479
Northing: 4677415
Latitude: N 42° 14' 04"
Longitude: W 70° 49' 27"

Directions ⟶

From Boston, take I-93 to MA 3 (Cape Cod). From MA 3, take Exit 14 to MA 228 north. Continue 6.5 miles through Hingham. Turn right onto MA 3A east and follow it 2 miles to the entrance and the parking lot on the right.

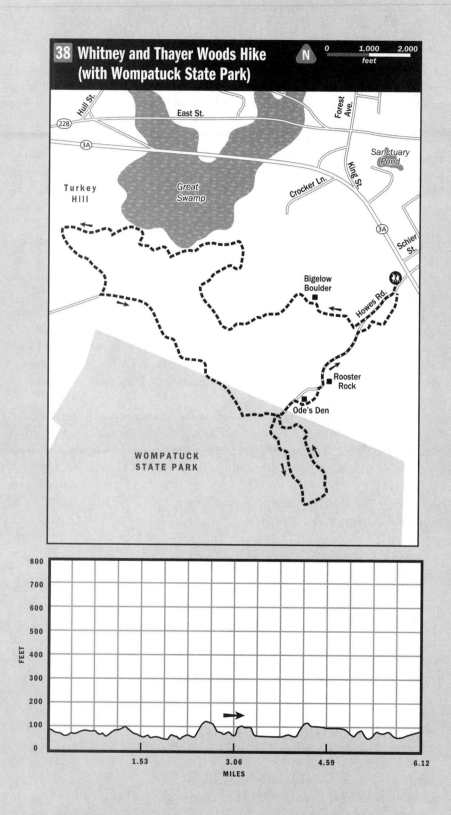

An unmarked trail or two diverts left and right, but stay with Howe's Road until it reaches a junction marked "2." Here, turn right to leave the manicured carriage road for a less-tamed footpath traveling westward over roots and granite rubble between two stone walls, one edging wetland, the other tracing a line across upland.

Ahead, the enormous boulder looking as odd as a goose egg laid on a frozen lake, is Bigelow Boulder, named after Reverend E. Victor Bigelow, the author of the first volume of the *Narrative History of Cohasset*. It was Henry M. Whitney, the owner of much of these 824 acres in the first half of the 20th century, who reshaped the stagnating farmland into a grand estate. A lover of horses and equestrian sport, Whitney had the bridle paths cut and carriage roads laid out and carved to enable him and his guests to enjoy his land and its natural wonders from the saddle or the seat of a smart buggy. As president of the West End Street Railway, Whitney presided over the development of the Boston rail system that is now known as the MBTA.

In 1889 Whitney's enterprise employed 9,000 draft horses and was growing by leaps and bounds, so much so that Boston's four-legged population seemed to be outpacing that of humans. But Whitney jumped aboard the technological wave and converted the light-rail to electrical power. Almost overnight, the horses were retired from streetcar duty. Faced with so many jobless equines, Whitney may have reassigned a flashy chestnut or two to the Bigelow Boulder route.

Bigelow Boulder sits at junction 3, where the footpath crosses Boulder Lane. To continue, pass to the left of the granite monolith, staying with the footpath as it travels northwest back into woods. Small white squares mark the way. Heading downhill at first, the path winds through young beeches and pines, passing an occasional spindly holly. Now and again it parts one of the many stone walls built after 1670, when the surveyor Joshua Fisher cleaved the land into mile-long 25-foot-wide strips to facilitate land trading among Cohasset's first settlers.

After crossing wetland via a sturdy 20- to 30-foot-long boardwalk, the trail bows south at a stream and rambles back uphill. Rocks with fleshy lichen ears loiter off to the side as if listening for gossip.

Breaching from the woods at junction 6, the trail continues across Boulder Lane. For the sake of variation, bear right and hike west on the carriage road.

Following a downward slope to a swampy brook, the route winds its way back uphill to meet Whitney Road. For a shortened loop, hike left; otherwise, continue northwest on this road packed hard by clopping hooves (and the trustees' maintenance personnel) and colored orange by a steady rain of pine needles.

At junction 8, leave the predictable footing of the carriage road for the root, rock, and water hazards of a wooded path to the right. Starting off with a steep but brief climb, the trail reaches a pinnacle then zigzags erratically on a northeastern course, mostly downhill, to a well sitting in a clearing.

At marker 12, the trail crosses Adelade Road, which stretches east toward Scituate Hill. Beyond this intersection the trail arcs westward, shedding hardwoods and hollies for hemlocks as it touches the outer reaches of Great Swamp. The area

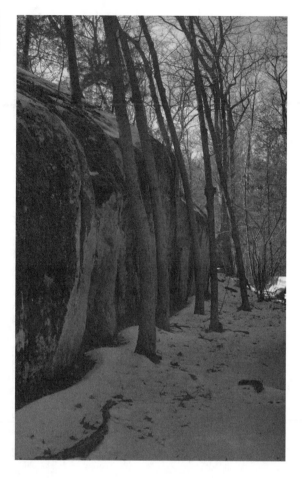

Trees contort around a massive boulder

is gorgeous in winter—when snow sparkles on low-hanging hemlock boughs, and in spring—when fists of skunk cabbage push through the last of the frost, and red-winged blackbirds wake the place with their raspy song and the shock of red against black. And the scene is stunning in fall—when maples and birch give up their green for riotous reds and cracking yellows. But for sinister mosquitoes, gnats, and deer flies, the swamp's loveliness peaks in summer when with their incessant buzzing and biting, they mask the beauty for all other beings. Arriving at the footpath's end at marker 13, hikers happy to be back on flat ground can continue to the right, on Turkey Hill Lane. But for a more adventurous trek, cross the carriage road and resume the footpath that leads back uphill into woods. Climbing the heap of glacial debris, the path shimmies past a boulder—crumbling like a last piece of layer cake sitting among crumbs—to reach an overlook at junction 14. After surveying the view and maybe settling in for a picnic, continue westward on the path to the right.

Follow white markers as the trail slopes back down to level ground and bears right at a broad, vaguely marked junction. Around a bend, the trail crosses a glade walled in by a great wedge of rock greened by ferns and moss. Lithe trees growing close to the mass bend from it like waves peeling away from an ocean liner.

Twisting its way north, the trail soon crosses paths with an abandoned railroad track that is being converted into a hiking trail. As of this writing, the project is nearing completion. In any case, stay with the footpath as it bisects the former rail line and continues into the American holly grove opposite.

Aiming west toward Turkey Hill, the trail continues to follow white markers. After winding through muddy lowland often imprinted with deer hoofprints, the trail gradually steepens as it gains traction beneath red pines on the eastern slope

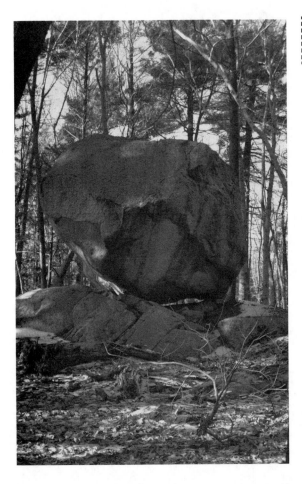

The Wisconsin Glacier carried the Burbank Boulder to where it sits today.

of Turkey Hill. Ahead, where the plane levels and the trees thin out, the trail meets One Way Lane.

At this junction (16), bear left and follow the cart road southeast down a gentle grade. The gangly woods, made up of early successional species, hints that this hilltop offered an open vista in the last century. Meadowlarks (*Sturnella magna*) and bobolinks (*Dolichonyx oryzivorus*) flitted about the hay fields then; today, pine siskins (*Carduelis pinus*) singing in the upper stories add variation to the throaty chirps of chickadees.

Reaching James Hill Lane at junction 17, hike left to descend to a glacier-scoured valley cradling the defunct rail line. Follow the lane across the valley and up and over the lofty drumlin beyond. At junction 18, at the base of the hill, steer right to leave the carriage lanes for the Milliken Memorial Path, a path Arthur Milliken cleared and made magnificent with densely planted azaleas, rhododendrons, mountain laurels, and other showy shrubs to honor his wife, Mabel Minott Milliken, who died in 1927.

After tunneling through an herbaceous corridor, the path spreads wide as it bridges wetland and ascends to another evocative boulder—this one looking like a loaf of bread with a slice tilting off the end. Behind it are more glacial erratics, clustered together in a picturesque spot equipped with a bench.

Farther southeast is a sculpted pool nested between the path and a curtain of granite embellished with velvety moss and extravagant fern fronds. It's futile to try to hurry through. Adopt "island time" and spend a moment or two drinking in the beauty from the well-hidden bench to the left of the pool.

Traveling between Brass Kettle Brook and the edge of upland, the path soon arrives at its end, at junction 19. Here Howes Road, bearing left, offers a neat link back to the parking lot. To add a circular jaunt through Wompatuck

State Park's nature study area, bear right.

In 1941 when World War II was intensifying, wishing to build a naval ammunition depot, the U.S. government took a third of the Trustees' Whitney Woods property, including these acres, by eminent domain. Twenty-five years later, in more-secure times, the government released the land, and the acreage was joined with that of Wompatuck.

The trail leads up a gravely slope, past a marker that reads NS7 to a map kiosk inside the state park's border. From this post, follow the hardscrabble trail to placid hemlock woods above. Stay left at marker NS6 to continue south to junction NS5. Here, the path to the right leads to Doane Street, the former property line of Whitney Woods.

Turn left and left again at each junction that follows, to complete the loop begun at the kiosk. Mounded and soft, the wooded landscape resembles a hastily made bed. Though disturbed by natural forces and axes many times, it is now remarkably quiet. About midway along this stretch, the trail passes the Burbank Boulder, another glacier-age vagrant biding its time.

Upon reaching the kiosk, reenter the Whitney and Thayer Reservation and take up Howes Road at junction 19. Elevated to evade seasonal flooding, the carriage road crosses Brass Kettle Brook, then taking a northeast tack, meets Bancroft Trail at junction 20. To visit two more points of interest, switch tracks and bear right. A handful of twists and turns away, the path reaches a castlelike rock cave. Made homeless in 1830, Theodore "Ode" Pritchard found the shelter to his liking and moved in. The accommodations were temporary, but the name "Ode's Den" stuck for good.

White markers lead right into and through Ode's grandly humble abode, heading through a rock garden rendered by clumsy fingers of ice. Every now and again amid the topographical chaos, a stone wall marches by.

As the trail swings northwest on the edge of a valley, it passes a massive rock configuration painted with the letter "R" to identify it as Rooster Rock. Catch it at the right angle in the right light, and it is the spitting image of a rooster sporting a fancy comb.

A few yards farther, the trail reconvenes with Howes Road at junction 21. Bear right to proceed northeast. Arriving at an orange chain gateway moments beyond junction 22, rather than ending, the route continues past a private home. Talk softly to the barking dog tied outside and continue on to junction 2. Here, leave the carriage road once more and hike the Bancroft Trail back to the parking lot.

NEARBY ATTRACTIONS

Seventy-five acre Weir River Farm, owned and managed by the Trustees of Reservations, boasts hay fields, managed woodlands, a stable and barn, and, best of all, friendly livestock. Access the farm via MA 228 in Hingham. From MA 228, turn right onto Levitt Street, continue 0.6 miles, and bear left onto Turkey Hill Lane. Follow it to the end.

39 DESTRUCTION BROOK HIKE

KEY AT-A-GLANCE INFORMATION

LENGTH: 4.07 miles

CONFIGURATION: Two linked loops

DIFFICULTY: Easy

SCENERY: Millworks first built in 1690; holly woods and abandoned farm established in 1853, American beech and Atlantic white cedar

EXPOSURE: Mostly shade

TRAFFIC: Light to moderate

TRAIL SURFACE: Packed earth

HIKING TIME: 2.5–3 hours

SEASON: Year-round sunrise–sunset

ACCESS: Free

MAPS: Available at kiosk by the trailhead and online at www.dnrt .org/pdfs/dbwmap1.jpg

FACILITIES: None

SPECIAL COMMENTS: Destruction Brook is one of 40 reservations of the Dartmouth Natural Resources Trust, which, to date, has helped preserve 4,000 acres.

WHEELCHAIR TRAVERSABLE: The red and yellow trails both offer access to wheelchair users.

DRIVING DISTANCE FROM BOSTON COMMON: 59 miles

Destruction Brook Hike

UTM Zone (WGS84) 19T

Easting: 331956

Northing: 4605110

Latitude: N 41° 34' 48"

Longitude: W 71° 00' 57"

IN BRIEF

Located upstream from Dartmouth's historic Russell Mills, this hike takes you on a tour of land preserved much as it was in the 1600s when the area was first settled.

DESCRIPTION

From the off-street parking, head southwest on the broad trail marked by the Dartmouth Natural Resource Trust (DNRT) sign. A hundred yards or so in from the road, the trail leads to a kiosk displaying a map of the property and DNRT news and information. Continue from here along the yellow trail to reach a three-way intersection. At this junction, turn left to hike east along the yellow trail, paralleling Fisher Road through woodland composed of pine, oak, and maple.

Ahead where the yellow trail meets the blue trail, bear left to hike southeast behind houses on Fisher Road. Then, turning away from backyards, follow blue trail markers to the uneven terrain of a weathered esker. At the next split, bear right switching back to the yellow trail to retreat to deeper woods.

Directions ⟶

From Boston, take I-93 south 12 miles, then take Exit 4 on the left to merge onto MA 24 south toward Brockton. Drive 38.1 miles to Exit 4 to merge left onto I-95 east toward New Bedford. Continue 4.6 miles and take Exit 11 toward US 6/Dartmouth to merge onto Reed Road. Take Reed Road 2 miles and turn left onto Beeden Road. Continue 0.7 miles and turn right onto Old County Road. After 0.1 mile, turn left onto Fisher Road. Look for a wooden Dartmouth Natural Resource Trust sign for Destruction Brook Woods on the right. Park just off Fisher Road, adjacent to the sign.

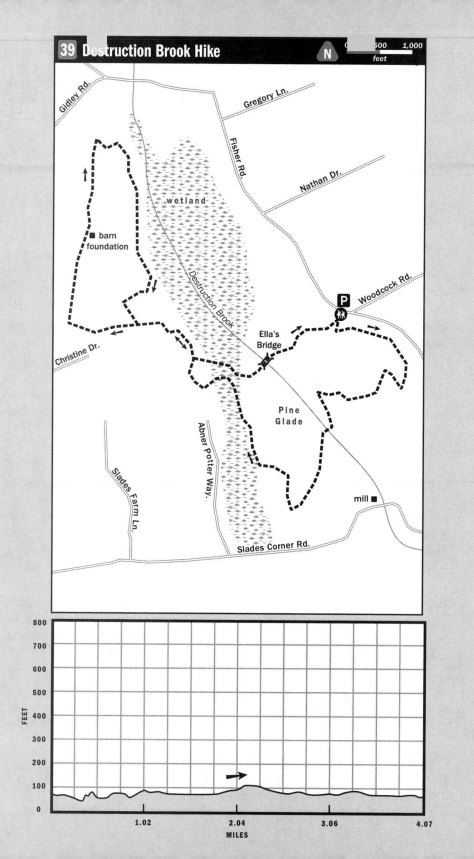

Becoming narrower as it runs under a canopy of trees, the trail dips and climbs then merges with another trail. Continue following yellow markers. At a somewhat baffling intersection follow the path to make an about-face and head north. Continue downhill off the ridge to reach another junction. Stay to the left to hike southwest on the wide yellow trail over level ground. Undulating westward the trail passes a stream and scattered birches. Bear left again at the next fork to follow the yellow trail as it swings to the south. Snaking onward through the landscape the trail soon leads to a bench on a banking overlooking Destruction Brook and remnants of the millworks first established here around 1690.

From this spot, descend the banking and turn left onto the red trail which traces the flow of the brook. Shortly, this route joins the yellow trail, and the two continue as one. Passing a gate to the left, the trail curves south and crosses a wide bridge. On the opposite bank, the trails separate; stay with the red trail and continue hiking south. Although the coast is nowhere in sight, the dead-level ground dusted with silver sand bespeaks the land's position just a hair above waves coursing to the seashore nearby.

Ahead, the trail eases westward to pass a white house sitting among pines on the left. Just beyond this, the trail reaches another intersection. The path to the left leads to alternative parking for the reservation, and a path straight ahead leads to an open meadow. Steer away from these and stay with the red trail, bearing right. A moment later, a red arrow at knee level redirects the trail left, back on a westward course.

Here knobby American holly trees (*Ilex opaca*) punctuate the woods otherwise dominated by red oak and white pine. If you are hiking through in mid-autumn, when the female hollies are bearing berries, watch for goldfinches and cedar waxwings. Ahead, the land to the left dips to a valley, while on the right it remains even with the trail, which now eases northward. At the next two forks, stay to the left on what remains of the red trail, which is scarcely marked through here.

Dipping beside wetland on the left, the trail swings on several points of the compass but continues generally northward. Holly trees grow more thickly along this avenue, mixing with maples, beech, and omnipresent oak and pine. At one point, the trail passes a magnificent beech tree growing flush to an equally magnificent oak. Equivalent in height and girth, they make an odd pair.

Weaving through wetland, the red trail eventually aims northwest to meet the green trail. This junction is marked both with the letter "D" on a stone and a sign that reads "Start of Green Loop." Leave the pine-thick red trail here and continue northwest down a slight grade on the green trail. Thick woods and a stone wall lie to the right.

A few hundred yards ahead, where the trail forms a "T," turn left and continue west toward a house neighboring private property. Where the trail forks a few feet farther on, bear right to hike north tracking a stone wall built back in the mid-1800s, when a farm was established on the 90 acres encircled by the green loop.

The wetlands surrounding
Destruction Brook harbor a great
diversity of species.

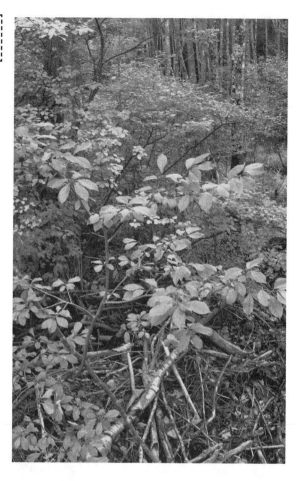

Along this section of former cart road, boughs of giant hickory trees arch overhead. Bittersweet clings to many of the trees like cobwebs on the furnishings of a deserted mansion. Though nearly retaken by nature, the place has not yet fully given up its former self. Like mud-caked draft animals eager for work, the root-jostled wall and ancient fruit trees humbled by sucker growth and competition from pines appear to long for the return of their master. It's been many years since this land was a working farm, but the spirits of those who shaped this place hold on. Midway down the path on the right is a foundation for what was once a great barn. All but the deep rows of stone it sat upon are gone.

Beyond the barnyard, the path leads across a stream that feeds into wetland to the east. Take a moment here to notice how the stone wall paralleling the path was artfully engineered to bridge the flowing water.

A short distance farther, the path reaches a point where the DNRT reservation ends. The land beyond this border is also protected and open for public use. In any case, the green trail continues ahead, emerging from the woods briefly as it passes privately owned land lying to the west. Watch to the east for a path leading into a thicket of pines to an intriguing cemetery where several of those who lived on this land in its most productive days are buried.

Trust the trail as it forges northward; the way is clear though momentarily bereft of markers. Coming to the end of the avenue draped voluminously with vines, the trail arrives at a junction. "No trespassing" signs rule out the paths to the left and center, leaving two paths to the right. Of these, choose the soft right and hike southeast down a pitch. A sandpit lies ahead on the left and, in it, the

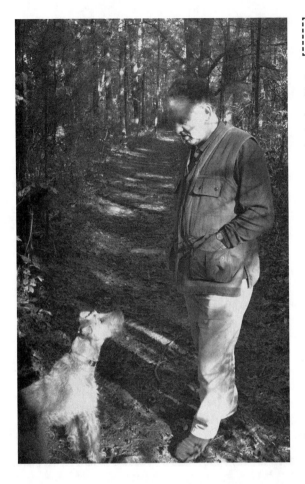

carcass of a sedan pinned between two pine saplings. As if spooked, the trail cuts sharply away from this wreck and runs into woods of cedar and holly.

Looping around the eastern side of the wetland, the trail splits briefly upon reaching an esker. For the sake of the view, bear left to ascend the 30- to 50-foot skeletal mound of glacial debris. A century ago, cows lulled in a pasture below; today little stirs but red squirrels and crows.

As the esker subsides, the land on the right falls away to a deep glade. Having the hushed feel of a room just made empty by a crowd, this natural basin held grazing cows. Scrappy trees have grown in over time, but none look as though they will ever achieve the height and girth of the tremendous oak that stands at the center. Known as the Pasture Oak, this tree may have been rooted here since King Philip's father, Massasoit, sold this territory to Pilgrim colonists intent on moving beyond Plymouth. If not, it was certainly here in 1773 when colonists disguised as Mohawks heaved 342 chests of tea into Boston Harbor from the *Dartmouth,* a ship built by Joseph Rotch, a native of these parts.

From this old meadow, the barely marked green trail continues southeast through swales and over bumps until, bending westward, it returns to the start of the loop. To complete the hike, return to the junction where the green and red trails meet and bear left onto the red trail, heading east. Running wide and flat through wetland thick with maples, this trail is easy to follow. Plentiful red markers guide the way to Ella's Bridge lying just ahead at Destruction Brook.

Upon crossing to the opposite bank, quit the red trail and pick up the yellow trail once more, and continue straight ahead. Weaving through woods draped with curtains of bittersweet, the trail soon reaches a vibrant pine grove. Look for

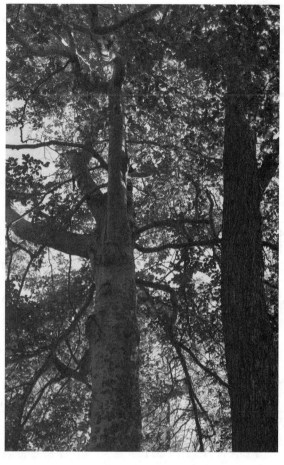

Beech and oak grow side by side.

where the trail splits left to return to the start at Fisher Road.

NEARBY ATTRACTIONS

Another place worth visiting in this spectacular part of Massachusetts is the Lloyd Center for the Environment. Offering 5 walking trails over 55 acres of oak-hickory forest, freshwater wetlands, estuary and salt marsh, the center also has an observation deck named one of 15 "special places" in the Commonwealth of Massachusetts. The Lloyd Center for the Environment is located at 430 Potomska Road, Dartmouth; (508) 990-0505. From the Destruction Brook Reservation, drive southeast on Fisher Road 4.3 miles. Turn right onto Russell Mills Road, then turn left onto Rock O' Dundee Road. Turn right onto Potomska Road and continue 1.2 miles to the Lloyd Center.

40   COPICUT WOODS: Miller Brook Loop

KEY AT-A-GLANCE INFORMATION

LENGTH: 3.4 miles

CONFIGURATION: Loop

DIFFICULTY: Easy

SCENERY: Highlights include ecologically rich wetlands, vernal pools, an abandoned farmstead, and a 150-year-old scenic cart path.

EXPOSURE: Mosty shade

TRAFFIC: Light

TRAIL SURFACE: Packed earth

HIKING TIME: 2 hours

SEASON: Year-round sunrise–sunset

ACCESS: Free

MAPS: Available online at www.thetrustees.org

FACILITIES: None

SPECIAL COMMENTS: Copicut Woods is linked to the 13,600-acre Southeastern Massachusetts Bioreserve.

WHEELCHAIR TRAVERSABLE: No

DRIVING DISTANCE FROM BOSTON COMMON: 56 miles

Copicut Woods:
Miller Brook Loop

UTM Zone (WGS84) 19T

Easting: 328200

Northing: 4619523

Latitude: N 41° 42' 32"

Longitude: W 71° 03' 54"

IN BRIEF

If those who eked a living from the earth in America's early years interest you, and especially if you appreciate stonework, you will get added pleasure from this hike which explores the well-preserved woodland haunts of the Wampanoag and America's first generations of English setters.

DESCRIPTION

Seizing on a concept promoted by the United Nations' Man and Biosphere Program, the Commonwealth of Massachusetts, the City of Fall River, and the Trustees of Reservations joined forces in 2002 to create the Southeastern Massachusetts Bioreserve. Six years later, Massachusetts is soon to have boasting rights to 13,600 acres of newly protected land. The vast tract that includes forest, old farmland, vernal pools, and a watershed that supplies drinking water to more than 100,000 people in the greater Fall River area will be run under a management plan designed to protect and foster biodiversity and environmental education while encouraging recreational use.

Directions ⟶

From Boston, take I-93 to Exit 4 and join MA 24 south toward Brockton. Continue 33.4 miles. From MA 24, take Exit 7 to merge onto MA 79 south toward North Fall River/Somerset, and continue 4 miles to the I-195 east exit toward New Bedford/Cape Cod on the left. From I-195, take Exit 9 (Stanford Road) and turn left to pass under the highway. Stanford Road bears right and becomes Old Bedford Road. Turn left onto Blossom Road and follow it 1.3 miles. Bear right onto Indian Town Road and follow it 1.7 miles to the parking area on the left.

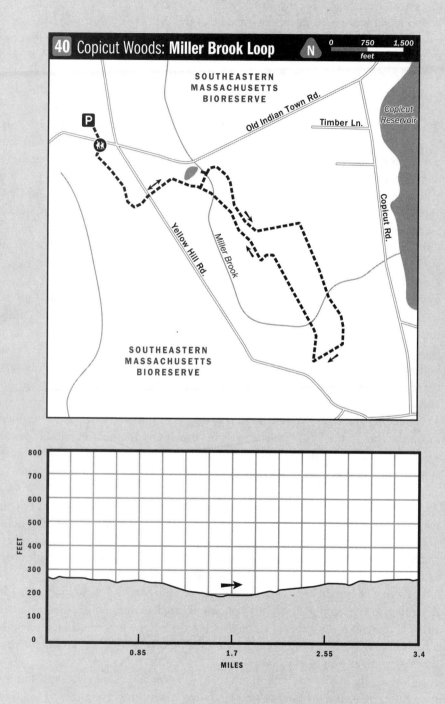

Five hundred and two acres of the land included in the bioreserve are owned and managed by the Trustees of Reservations. Named Copicut, the Wampanoag word for "deep, dark woods," the property was farmed through more than one lifetime. Today successional growth has returned the land to an approximation of its original wooded state, but among the trees, blueberries, and other shrubs lie intriguing artifacts of human industry.

From the parking lot, cross Old Indian Town Road to the trailhead opposite. Enter at the green gate marked with the number 1 beside a sign for Copicut Woods, and begin hiking along the slender path that weaves southeast through beech and pine. Downtown Fall River is 10 minutes away by car, but here in the old winter hunting grounds of King Philip's people, little but chattering chipmunks and red squirrels stirs the silence.

Ahead, after descending a slight grade, the trail reaches a paved road that appears to not have seen an automobile since all cars were black and American made. Continue across to pick up the trail where it resumes immediately opposite. This junction is marked with the number 2. From here, hike northeast alongside wetland shrouded by tangled understory. Sifting through the lovely monotony of tree parts, you will note the first of the property's impressive stonework. No longer containing knot-kneed cows inclined to wander, the line of stacked stones, however mind dulling on the one hand, is a curiosity catalyst on the other. Representing hundreds, maybe thousands of hours of labor, the wall is nothing if not a collection of a man's thoughts and choices of a century and a half ago. Shapeless rocks fighting for a resting place tell of the impatient hands that laid them, whereas geometric slabs fitted to orbs of character tell of pride and a man fully invested in his work.

Bending gently to the left the trail opens to an intersection marked number 3. Up the trail to the left is another gate beyond it Old Indian Town Road. Hike to the right to an intersection marked number 4. Here, cross the wide carriage road to reenter the woods on a newer, narrow path heading northeast.

Winding through wetland dense with brush, the path soon leads to a brook. A thick log outfitted with a handrail provides a precarious yet functional bridge over the gurgling waters. Keeping on high ground, the path dead-ends at a small kettle pond a few feet farther on. In fall, there may not be much to see other than flame-red maples, but during more lively seasons you might catch a glimpse of the flashy wood ducks encouraged to nest here.

From the pond, backtrack to the brook and pick up an unmarked path diverging to the east. Follow this recently cleared or reestablished route as it turns northeast. After meeting a stone wall to the left the path continues through a parting in another. This point marks a transition from woods of swamp oak to more ephemeral woods of white pine.

Ahead, the path runs into another route perpendicular to it. At this juncture, turn right and continue east on a moss-lined track bordered by a stone wall and a crowd of pines standing in an old pasture. Turning south, this path

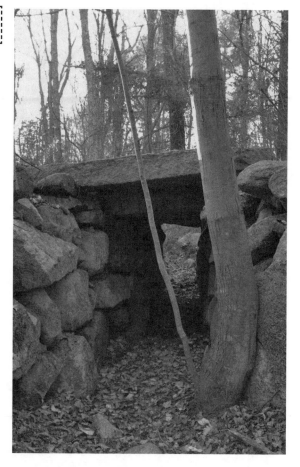

promptly leads to a brand-new post-and-beam shelter built by volunteers for the trustees.

Several paths radiate from this spot. One to the right leads to a junction marked number 5; choose the path lying between this path and the shelter and continue southeastward. A few feet along, this route passes a particularly remarkable stone wall assembled from impossibly massive stones. On the day of my hike, not far from this dazzling example of common utilitarianism taken to a high art, evidence of life and death pulled my attention back to the here and now. Looking to the ground, I noticed a ring of immaculate blue-gray feathers lying on a bed of leaves. Hours or maybe minutes earlier, having snatched a songbird from the air, a hawk had alighted here and plucked the feathers from its meal.

The path runs on its southeastern course past meadowland reclaimed by oaks, cedars, hickories, and beech until, in short time, it reaches a broad crossroads marked number 7. The expansive, grassy avenue running straight on ahead is Miller Lane, a cart path built 150 years ago. Stone walls straight as a plumb line and high enough to fence in spirited horses border the path on either side. The path's time as a working road bearing farm traffic day in and day out is long over, but the energy of the draft animals hauling loads and the men who labored with them is still present. Taken in from a stone bench set opposite the lane, the crossroads has the feel of a stage between acts.

Take the wide path to the left of Miller Lane and hike eastward. Heading on a straight trajectory outside another stone wall, the path descends on a slight incline to another junction, this one marked 12. At this split, bear right onto a scrappy trail heading southeast. Paralleling another wall, this one less intact,

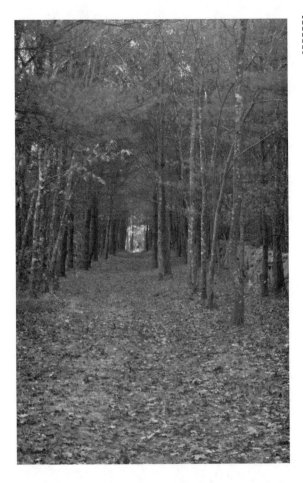

The woods have begun to retake Miller Lane.

the trail crosses meadowland giving itself up to opportunistic shrubs and saplings. Hollies and ancient fruit trees under assault by bittersweet vines stand over the bramble-ridden grassland.

Continue on this unmarked trail as it meanders southeast down a gentle slope to a small stone bridge over a stream. Leveling out, the trail runs south through woods populated by the occasional shagbark hickory and more common holly and pine. After traveling through woods, the trail soon spills from the shadows into the path of a power line. This junction is marked number 11. Leave the woods, bearing right to head southwest over grassy ground.

Climbing an easy grade, the path arrives at junction number 10. The trustees have a sign for the Copicut reservation here near a plaque adorned with exuberant vines that reads "Miller's Brook Conservation Area, in memory of Benny Costa." This point marks the southernmost end of Miller Lane.

Hike to the right, heading north to follow the many footsteps trod down this impressive road. Packed solid by the weight of loaded wagons and the tonnage of cattle and workhorses, the path has the feel of permanence only wear can produce.

Built up so that it functions as a causeway between pastures and wetland, Miller Lane has a number of interesting structures incorporated into it. The first one you'll encounter is an odd tunnel known as a "dry bridge." Narrow but tall, this tunnel was built to enable livestock to wander from one pasture to another, perhaps to have ready access to water. Bearing northwest, the path, edged by mighty stone walls, soon leads to intersection number 9 characterized by a massive corner of stone. Bear left here, continuing north.

A bit farther along, the lane encounters Miller Brook. Here, an elaborate stone grate keeps the path dry despite gushing waters visible through parallel granite slabs. Beyond the brook the lane comes to another intersection, this one unmarked. Stay with the path and hike on, now shifting toward the northwest to reach an inconspicuous path to the left marked with number 8. Leave Miller Lane here.

Follow this new slender trail south through old pasture smothered in pine. From a pastured cow's perspective the surrounding walls are even more impressive. Ignore divergent paths to reach a fork and continue to the left, heading south.

Trickling beneath tree cover this trail passes another trail on the left beside a birdhouse. Stay on track bearing right to head northwest. In a moment, the trail passes through a gap in a wall and arrives at an abandoned homestead. Lying silently in the grass, unseen at first, are several foundations. The place and the silence about it, both lovely and eerie, throbs with life.

From the wide-open junction to the north of the homestead, keeping marker 6 behind to the left, depart on the path heading west. A few hundred feet ahead on the right, this broad avenue passes the foundation of a barn. Farther still, the trail reaches junction 5, marking the path leading back to the post-and-beam shelter. Less than 0.13 miles later, the trail arrives at another familiar junction. The path to the right leads to the wood duck pond, and the one to the left leads back to the parking lot.

NEARBY ATTRACTIONS

If you would like to do some sightseeing after your hike, Tiverton Four Corners, Rhode Island, located just 11 miles away, is worth considering. Listed on the National Register of Historic Places, this rural village offers something for everyone, including antiques shopping, gourmet food, crafts, equestrian centers, beach access, and unspoiled open space excellent for hiking and biking. For more information visit **www.tivertonfourcorners.com**.

To get there, take I-95 east 1.2 miles and merge onto MA 24 south at Exit 8A. Continue 4.2 miles to Exit 6. Turn left onto Fish Road. Continue 1.4 miles and turn right onto Bulgarmarsh Road (RI 177). After 1 mile turn left onto Main Road (RI 77). Continue 3.4 miles to arrive at Tiverton Four Corners.

41 ROUND POND HIKE

i **KEY AT-A-GLANCE INFORMATION**

LENGTH: 2.33 miles
CONFIGURATION: Loop
DIFFICULTY: Easy
SCENERY: Oak and pine forest, 3 ponds, and a cranberry bog
EXPOSURE: Mostly shaded
TRAFFIC: Moderate
TRAIL SURFACE: Packed earth and some sandy areas
HIKING TIME: 1–1.5 hours
SEASON: Year-round sunrise–sunset
ACCESS: Free
MAPS: Available at Duxbury town hall (878 Tremont Street; follow Mayflower Street east to its end and turn left onto Tremont; town hall is ahead on the left). Hiking trails leading to Round Pond and North Hill Marsh are accessible immediately behind the town hall.
FACILITIES: None
SPECIAL COMMENTS: This hike is easily extended into longer hikes by linking to trails in Duxbury Town Forest and North Hill Marsh, or by using it to access Bay Circuit Trail, which leads south approximately 2 miles to Bay Farm on the edge of Duxbury's Kingston Bay.
WHEELCHAIR TRAVERSABLE: No
DRIVING DISTANCE FROM BOSTON COMMON: 34 miles

IN BRIEF

Setting out from a pond that once supplied ice to local kitchens, this loop takes you through a landscape of cranberry bogs, kettle ponds, and peaceful woodland.

DESCRIPTION

In 1627, itching for elbowroom after seven years of living within shouting distance of their fellow *Mayflower*-borne New Englanders, the Pilgrims of Plymouth Plantation spread north and south along the coast as soon as their London-based financial backers would let them. One to make the leap was Captain Myles Standish, their fearless man in arms, who was granted land situated on a cove called "The Nook" overlooking the mother plantation, which lay just a tack or two to the south.

It took some time—at first the land was used only for crops during the growing season—but inevitably the green pastures to the north lured families away from Plymouth for good. After successfully petitioning Plymouth officials for permission to build their own church, the ruddy captain, William Brewster, John Alden, and others officially founded their new village, which Standish named Duxbury after his family's estate in Chorley, Lancashire, England.

Round Pond Hike
UTM Zone (WGS84) 19T
Easting: 358195
Northing: 4655153
Latitude: N 42° 02' 08"
Longitude: W 70° 42' 47"

Directions ⟶

From Boston take I-93, merge onto MA 3 south. Take Exit 10 off MA 3 south and bear right. Follow MA 3A to the Duxbury Fire Station. Turn left onto Mayflower Street. Parking for Round Pond is about 1 mile past the Duxbury transfer station, on the left.

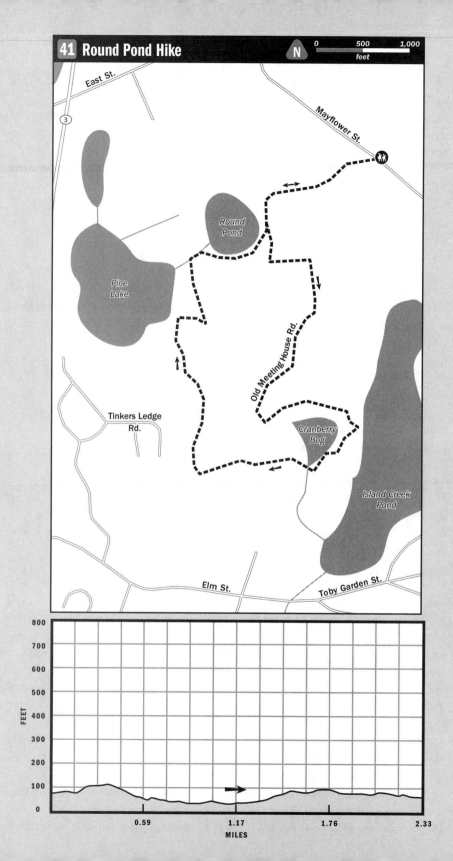

41 Round Pond Hike

N

0   500   1,000
feet

East St.

3

Mayflower St.

Round
Pond

Pine
Lake

Old Meeting House Rd.

Tinkers Ledge
Rd.

Cranberry
Bog

Island Creek
Pond

Elm St.

Toby Garden St.

800
700
600
500
400
300
200
100
0

FEET

0.59   1.17   1.76   2.33

MILES

Over the course of King Philip's War (1675–76) Duxbury was spared attack by Wampanoag warriors wielding tomahawks and torches, perhaps because the natives saw that attacking the settlement would jeopardize their chances of achieving their highest goal—the annihilation of Plymouth. In any case, Duxbury avoided conflict for well over a century.

Up until the American War for Independence, Duxbury's citizens lived quiet, productive lives as subsistence farmers, but the consequences of the country's victory over England brought rapid change. Most significant was that, following the Treaty of Paris, America secured fishing rights on the Grand Banks, which, located south of Newfoundland, was well within the reach of the enterprising citizens of New England's coastal villages.

Quick to rise to the occasion several of Duxbury's wealthy families set about building large fishing schooners. Before long, Ezra Weston, who launched his career in 1764 by turning out modest vessels, was operating a merchant fleet so profitable it earned him the nickname "King Caesar." Weston's son, Ezra II, who inherited his father's drive and sobriquet, ultimately owned both the largest fleet in America and the largest ship. Given the truly American name *Hope,* the vessel weighed 880 tons and had masts so tall they dwarfed those of sister ships and reached closer to heaven than Duxbury's church steeples.

Through the first half of the 19th century the world-renowned Weston industries employed all but the entire population of Duxbury, if not in its shipyards, sail lofts, or schooner crews, then in mills and forges, on farms, and most important of all, in lumbering operations. The hulls and masts for more than 643 ships were built of wood cut from Duxbury's old-growth forests.

Starting the hike from the parking area on Mayflower Street, set out on the Yellow Trail heading west through sparse woods of white pine and red oak. At about 0.2 miles, the trail converges with Bay Circuit Trail and bends south, passing a shade east of Round Pond.

Ahead, where Bay Circuit Trail diverts west, continue on the Yellow Trail to reach a T-intersection, where the Old Meetinghouse Road runs east and west. Incorporated into a recreational trail system in the 1890s, this road dates back to Duxbury's early days, when settlers would use it to travel from the outskirts of the village to the central meetinghouse for regular religious, government, and social gatherings. Located beside the Old Burial Ground, the meetinghouse is a 2-mile walk from this spot.

Bear left to briefly follow this route worn by the footsteps of the Pilgrims, then bear right at the next intersection to resume hiking south on the Red Trail. Dipping in elevation, the trail passes over increasingly sandy terrain. Chickadees, tufted titmice, the occasional flock of cedar waxwings, and other forest birds flit and sing among the pines and understory of low bush and dry-land blueberries, ferns, teaberry, and lady's slippers.

Opening to a pronounced dune after winding westward, the trail swings south again to pass a trail to the right. Continue to the next junction, then bear left, leaving the Red Trail for a narrower path sloping eastward into wetland,

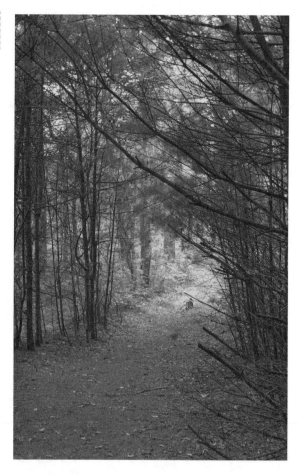

Beyond a cranberry bog the trail returns to woodland.

where species including red maple, aspen, black cherry, alder, sagebush, summersweet, highbush blueberry, sweet pepper-bush, and native azaleas grow in humus-rich soil. At the bottom of the hill, the trail spills out to one of Duxbury's many cultivated cranberry bogs.

Although called *ibimi* by the Pequot people, folk-lore has it that the Pilgrims saw in the cranberry's small pink blossoms the head and bill of a sandhill crane and hence renamed the native fruit "crane berry" How-ever it is just as likely that they recognized ibimi for kraanbere, a native of Hol-land, the country where for eleven years the Pilgrims had lived in exile before sailing to America.

Partial to the unique and highly acidic conditions found in glacier-formed peat bogs, cranberries were harvested exclusively from the wild until 1816. It was in that year that a Revolutionary War veteran named Captain Henry Hall, of Cape Cod, observed that both the plant's vigor and the quality of its fruit improved when sand is added to the peat. After some experimentation, Hall per-fected his cultivation techniques, a new industry was born when others quickly followed his lead.

Skirting the cranberry bog, the trail traces woods to reach a drive run-ning parallel to Island Creek Pond. Bear right passing a pump house, and at the southern end of the bog loop, head west to hike along a causeway that divides the bog in two.

Arriving at a crossroads where Bay Circuit Trail swings in from the north and drops south, take up this epic trail and continue west into woods. In short time, Bay Circuit Trail winds north and, after a stretch through sometimes wet lowland, gains elevation on nearing the southeast shore of Pine Lake.

Together with the cranberry bogs lying farther north and Round Pond ahead to

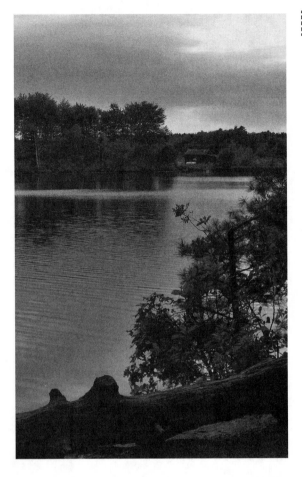

A view across Pine Lake

the east, Pine Lake attracts a full spectrum of wildlife. In the early morning and evening hours, raccoons and opossums descend from trees and upland haunts to forage at the waterside. Deer and foxes dash in and out like apparitions, and overhead, when the wind obliges and the light is right, osprey course in to swipe at schooling fish.

Follow the trail as it hugs the bank of Round Pond, pauses at a lookout, then arches northeast. Where it meets the Yellow Trail, bear right and backtrack to the parking lot.

NEARBY ATTRACTIONS

The town's beauty is reason enough to prolong your visit, but if you enjoy history two of Duxbury's historic homes provide a ready excuse to do some sightseeing. Visit Alden House Museum Historic Site (105 Alden Street, just off MA 3A). Built in 1653 on property deeded to the Alden family in the 1620s, this remarkable house has never been owned by any other family. Unlike other historic houses, Alden House has never been updated. Admission is $5 for adults 18 and over and $4 for children 3 to 17. There is a $1 discount for AAA members. The museum is open to the public between mid-May and Columbus Day, Monday through Saturday noon to 4 p.m.; the last tour begins at 3:30 p.m. Off-season hours generally are 10 a.m. to 1 p.m., but it's best to call ahead to be sure; phone (781) 934-9092.

King Caesar House (20 King Caesar Road, Duxbury) is a second historic house worth visiting. It's open July through August, Wednesday through Sunday from 1 to 4 p.m., and in September, Saturday and Sunday 1 to 4 p.m. From Mayflower Street, drive southeast to Lincoln Street. At the rotary, take the first exit onto MA 14. MA 14 becomes St. George Street. After 1 mile, turn left onto Washington Street, which becomes Powder Point Avenue. Turn right to King Caesar Road.

SLOCUM'S RIVER HIKE 42

IN BRIEF

There is no place in Massachusetts, or even the whole country, more beautiful than this reservation set on a hillside overlooking the splendidly picturesque Slocum's River. Following easements through privately owned farmland, this hike explores a quintessentially New England landscape that is as lovely now as it was centuries ago.

DESCRIPTION

Whether the river was named for Anthony Slocum in the 17th century or his descendant Joshua Slocum in the 19th century depends on whom you ask—regardless, each man is worthy of the honor.

Like the Pilgrims of Plymouth, Anthony Slocum came to America seeking opportunity and religious freedom, but by 1637, the year he arrived, the Pilgrims had secured a firm toehold and Slocum quickly found that when it came to tolerance, the Puritans were remarkably like the Church of England. All were free to embrace Puritan beliefs, and all who tipped the apple cart were free to be gone. And so the Pilgrim of Taunton indulged Slocum his

----

Directions ⟶

From Boston take I-93/US 1 south 12.5 miles. At Exit 4 merge left onto MA 24 south toward Brockton. Exit onto MA 140 south, turn right onto MA 6 west. At the fourth set of traffic lights, turn left onto Old Westport Road and follow it 0.4 miles. Bear left onto Chase Road and follow it 3.6 miles to the end. Take a right onto Russells Mills Road and follow it 1 mile through historic Russells Mills Village. Continue straight onto Horseneck Road and follow it 1.4 miles to the entrance; there is parking for about 10 cars on the left.

KEY AT-A-GLANCE INFORMATION

LENGTH: 3.87 miles

CONFIGURATION: Loop

DIFFICULTY: Easy

SCENERY: The magnificent Slocum's River, woods, wetlands, a nursery, and agricultural fields

EXPOSURE: Mostly shaded

TRAFFIC: Light

TRAIL SURFACE: Grass, packed earth with some muddy areas, and a stream or two to ford

HIKING TIME: 2 hours

SEASON: Year-round sunrise–sunset

ACCESS: Free (donation appreciated)

MAPS: Online at www.thetrustees.org/properties; maps also available on location while supplies last.

FACILITIES: None

SPECIAL COMMENTS: Dogs are welcome but must be leashed. Water-resistant boots—or better yet all-weather sandals—are recommended when the weather is warm and wet. In summer it might be a good idea to forgo the Dartmoor Wildlife Management half of the hike unless you have a high tolerance for mosquitoes, gnats, and deer flies.

WHEELCHAIR TRAVERSABLE: No

DISTANCE FROM BOSTON COMMON: 58 miles

Slocum's River Hike

UTM Zone (WGS84) 19T

Easting: 332439

Northing: 4601988

Latitude: N 41° 33' 07"

Longitude: W 71° 00' 33"

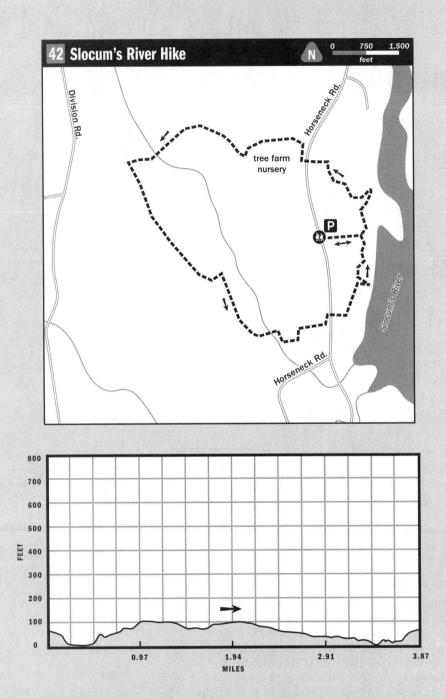

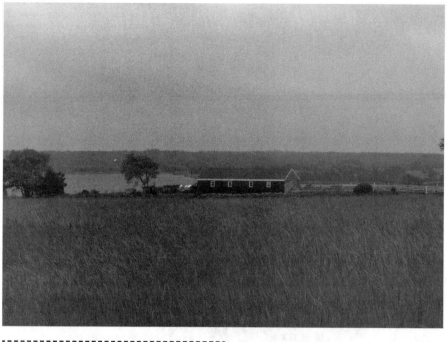

A field of grain stretches toward Slocum's River.

freedom until he joined the Society of Friends (later known as the Quakers) at which time they promptly expelled him from the settlement. Thus, in 1664, forced to find another home, Slocum went south to the coast and settled among fellow Quakers on land they purchased from Myles Standish, William Bradford, and other Plymouth officials. That same year, Metacomet—also known as King Philip, son of Wampanoag sachem Massasoit—fixed the bounds of the township and authorized the charter.

Another Slocum, also a Quaker, was forced to give up America altogether for having refused to participate in the War for Independence. Deemed a Loyalist for his pacifist ways, and therefore no longer welcome in the land of the free, he sailed for Canada in 1780 leaving America for good. Two hundred thirty-four years later, an intrepid descendent of this naturalized Canadian, Joshua Slocum, sailed into the harbor at Newport, Rhode Island, and in so doing became the first man to complete a solo circumnavigation of the globe.

The hike begins at the far end of the parking lot beside a kiosk erected by the Trustees of Reservations. As soon as you are able to free your eyes from the arresting view across fields to the river, set out along the easement that runs east between a formidable stone wall and a field planted with young fruit trees.

Where the fields and stone wall leave off, a trustees sign marks the true boundary of the reserve. Enter woods here and continue east following the trail as it leads slightly to the right then downhill beside another stone wall partially

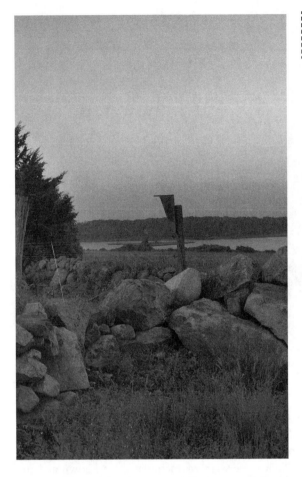

concealed by bittersweet vines and other species exuberant enough to be dismissed as weeds.

Step through first one gap in the stone wall, then another, bearing left to hike to the river over upland grown in with hearty oaks, hickories, and vigorous young sassafras. As the trail descends closer to sea level, the view clears and the south-flowing waters of Slocum's River seize center stage.

Responding to the irresistible pull of this waterway, the trail winds free of the woods and opens to a field stretched flat beside salt marsh buffered by a thin screen of trees. To get a good look at the river, follow one of the several unofficial paths that cut through to the windswept marsh—stepping carefully to avoid poison ivy.

When ready, trace the field's periphery counterclockwise to its southwest corner where the trail diverts back into woods. Take it slow to allow a chance sighting of a dazzling bluebird or oriole, acrobatic flycatcher, or wild turkey hen with hatchlings. For a good long look, take a seat on the granite bench placed among daisies and Indian paintbrush at the center of the field.

From the field hike west bearing right at a junction to continue north through woods. On emerging on the edge of privately owned farmland, bear right where the trail makes a T and follow the wide grassy avenue spotted with wild strawberries past a small meadow ensconced in trees to a trustees' sign pointing left to Dartmoor Farm. Turn here and track the reservation's northern boundary via a mowed path that leads back to Horseneck Road.

To continue the hike, navigate the iron gate on Dartmoor Farm's drive and travel north along the west side of Horseneck Road following a mowed path running between an electric fence and a wooded buffer on the farm's northern boundary. There are few trail markers; however, birdhouses with hay spilling from their circular openings line the way, and pastel-colored beehives stationed on the route indicate the easement's halfway point.

Beyond a large barn set back behind Dartmoor Farm's many rows of ornamental trees and shrubs, the trail darts north leaving solid footing for the forested wetland of the Dartmoor Farm Wildlife Management Area. Here the trail threads through tree cover staying close to the wire fence laced around a shaded grove of baby rhododendrons and azaleas. After a run to the south the trail reaches the end of the nursery and splits to the right as it nears a maintenance yard.

Now free of fencing the trail cuts a northwest course through a landscape looking something like a Rousseau painting—at least in warm months when layer on layer of green limits visibility to what is close at hand.

Covering relatively level ground the trail continues on a northwest run to eventually meet a stone wall built along a property line, whereupon it begins a gentle arc southward. Embossed with moss and fringed with ferns, the trail flirts with obscurity now and again as it disappears beneath puddles and streams. Stay the course by hiking straight on whenever faintly etched paths divert left or (most often) right.

At 0.86 miles from Horseneck Road, the trail intersects with a broad cart road running west to east. Shake off the mud and bear left onto this dry, even plane and enjoy easy walking through woods of oak and pine for the next 0.3 miles, passing an abandoned camper on the right a few hundred yards along.

Reaching a junction where the trail splits off to a clearing on the right, continue straight once again on a narrow footpath. For the next short stretch staying on track is a bit of a challenge due to fallen trees and the previous meanderings of other hikers, therefore proceed with care. Fortunately, just as the trail becomes impossibly vague, a gap in a stone wall confirms the path's direction. Once through this passage, keep the stone wall to the left and continue hiking east.

Winding onward, the trail travels through another section of stone wall and momentarily aims north passing a tremendous knotted holly tree on its left just before it reaches a cellar hole containing great flanks of granite. Hike along the right-hand edge of the cellar hole and continue a hundred or so yards to find another trail dead ahead marked with red discs.

Bear right to hike southeast on this new trail through older woods of maple and holly. Stone walls shadow to the left and right indicating pasture laboriously cleared centuries ago now once more glutted with trees.

Bending directly east, the trail loses breadth as it slopes back to wetland. Then as shadbush, blueberries, and sweet pepperbush crowd in, the trail steers straight on to startling brightness, for beyond a stream bridged by slabs of stone, it emerges to an enormous commercial hay field. Hike to the right and trace the farmland's border around this field, then head east along a mowed strip outside an electric fence to return to Horseneck Road.

Watch for traffic, then cross to a burly stone wall framing pasture. Continuing from a sign demarking another easement, hike east along a field of grazing angus to arrive at a point where four walls meet. Standing here on a hill that rises above Slocum's River like an enormous cresting wave, you can see for miles. If you are like Slocum or the many who have built replicas of Slocum's oyster sloop, *Spray,* you will feel a tug as you look downriver toward the sea. If you are an earth-bound sort, you might instead shiver, look at your watch and think about dinner.

Joshua Slocum ran away to sea as a boy of 14, then jumped from ship to ship for 58 years before finally hauling his sea chest to dry land at Martha's Vineyard—a piece of turf as like a ship as land can be. Even then, he dry-docked at his island home only through the summer months. Come autumn, when others hunkered down for winter, Slocum shuttered his house and sailed for the tropics.

To continue the hike, heed the left-pointing arrow of the trustees' sign posted beside the stone wall and cross the top of a field planted with alfalfa interspersed with oats (or another crop in rotation). Ahead, where the trail splits, bear right to hike downhill. This path leads directly to a canoe landing on the riverbank; follow the trail to its end or bear left at the fork midway.

From the left turn the trail undulates upward through a grassy meadow dotted with wildflowers to arrive at a stone seat set back from a grassy lookout. Stop to revel in the beauty, the warm sun, and misty sea air, then head north to the next fork in the path. At this junction, lengthen the hike slightly by dipping to the right. A moment later the path arrives at a stone monument dedicated to Dr. Milton A. Traverse who donated funds to maintain the reservation. Veer off to the right again to cross a meadow gone feral and right once more before swinging left to meet the path that leads to the parking lot.

NEARBY ATTRACTIONS

Two beautiful and distinctly different places are worth visiting while in the area; the 600-acre Horseneck Beach State Reservation (follow Horseneck Road south until you see a sign for the beach) and the historic village and harbor of Padanaram in South Dartmouth. For an overnight stay, consider the Paquachuck Inn located at 2056 Main Road, Westport Point (phone [508] 636-4398), just 5 minutes from Horseneck Beach. Wine lovers may also want to plan a visit to the Westport Rivers Winery, also down the road from the beach at 417 Hixbridge Road, Westport (phone [800] 993-9695).

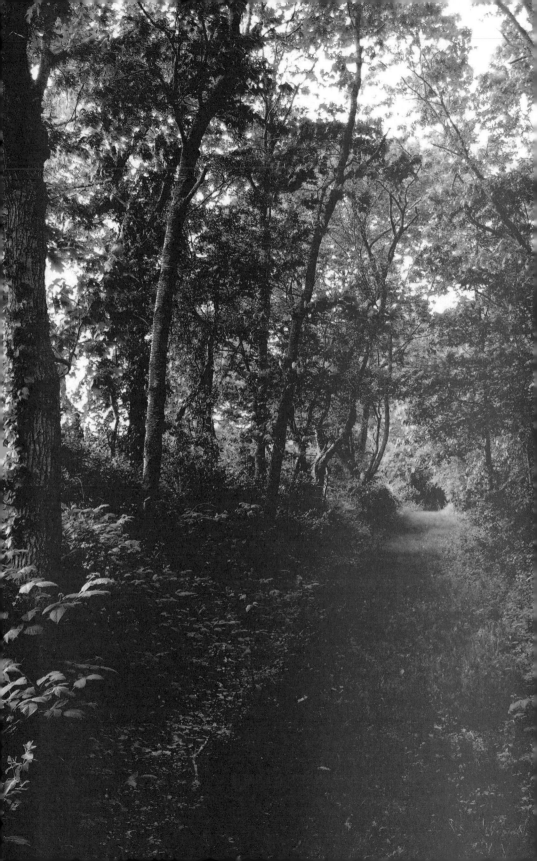

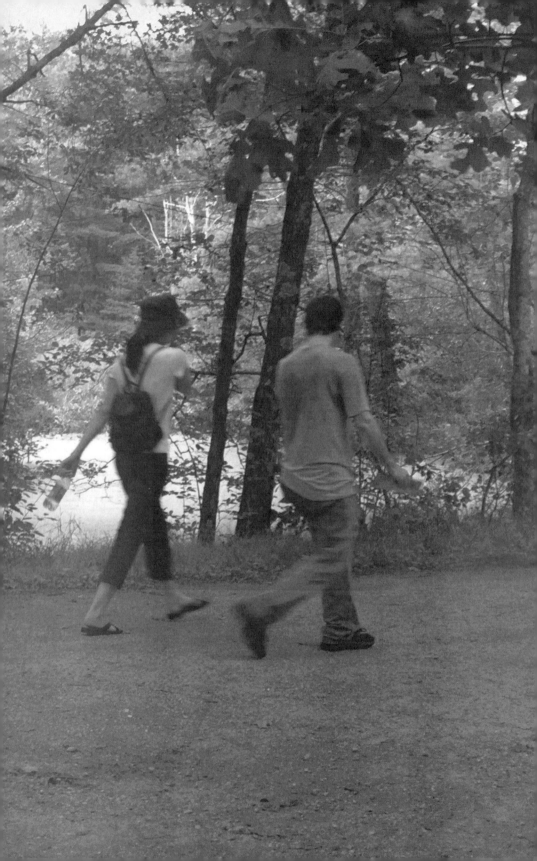

WEST OF BOSTON

43 HAMMOND POND-HOUGHTON GARDEN HIKE

KEY AT-A-GLANCE INFORMATION

LENGTH: 2.2 miles

CONFIGURATION: Loop

DIFFICULTY: Easy

HIKING TIME: 1.5–2 hours

SCENERY: Woods, a pond, and peat bog as well as a 6-acre deer park and 10-acre historic wild garden

EXPOSURE: Mostly shaded

TRAFFIC: Light

TRAIL SURFACE: Packed earth, crushed stone, and some rough wooded sections

SEASON: Year-round sunrise–sunset

ACCESS: Free

MAPS: Maps can be obtained from the Newton Conservators, www.newtonconservators.org.

FACILITIES: None

SPECIAL COMMENTS: Houghton Garden is popular among birders. Beware: This hike crosses the tracks of a streetcar.

WHEELCHAIR TRAVERSABLE: Recent rehabilitation work and upgrading has made the Houghton Garden wheelchair accessible.

DRIVING DISTANCE FROM BOSTON COMMON: 6 miles

IN BRIEF

A hidden gem, this hike passes a ten-acre pond and crosses the tracks of the country's oldest streetcar before touring a 19th-century deer park and a garden listed on the National Register of Historic Places.

DESCRIPTION

In the mid-1600s Thomas Hammond and his wife Elizabeth relocated from the coastal town of Hingham to Newton, then a part of Cambridge, where in a joint venture with Vincent Druce, they purchased several hundred acres of land. Later when they divided their holdings, Thomas Hammond claimed acreage that lies in what is now Newton's Chestnut Hill neighborhood. Immigrants from England and clearly stout of heart, Thomas and Elizabeth were pioneers in territory a hair shy of wilderness. Over time the Hammond's property passed into the hands of many others including the Webster and Houghton families. Between 1968 and 1979 the City of Newton purchased parcels totaling 113 acres to ensure that they remain open space.

Locate the trailhead at the northwest corner of the Chestnut Hill Mall parking lot next to a kiosk displaying a map of the reservation. Departing from this unlikely starting

---

Hammond Pond–Houghton Garden Hike

UTM Zone (WGS84) 19T

Easting: 307865

Northing: 4695299

Latitude: N 42° 23' 10"

Longitude: W 71° 20' 03"

Directions

From Boston by car: Take MA 9 to the Hammond Pond Parkway exit. Park at the Chestnut Hill Shopping Center. The trailhead is located in the northwest corner of the parking lot.

From Boston by public transportation: Take the D train on the MBTA Green Line to the Chestnut Hill station.

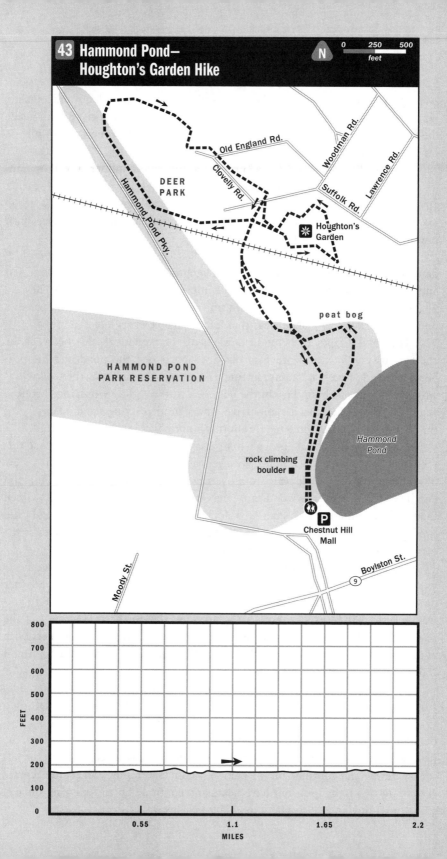

N

0   250   500
feet

Old England Rd.

Woodman Rd.

Lawrence Rd.

DEER PARK

Clovelly Rd.

Suffolk Rd.

Houghton's Garden

Hammond Pond Pkwy.

peat bog

HAMMOND POND PARK RESERVATION

Hammond Pond

rock climbing boulder ■

P
Chestnut Hill Mall

Moody St.

Boylston St.

9

FEET

800
700
600
500
400
300
200
100
0

0.55   1.1   1.65   2.2

MILES

point, set out hiking north on the wide-packed earth trail shaded by an elegant awning of hemlock boughs. Though visible from the paved ground outside, Hammond Pond quickly vanishes behind a thicket of brush once you are inside the woods. Nonetheless the trail arcs along the pond's side keeping within close range of the water.

Looking like the massive steel prow of a sinking oceanliner, a wall of granite sits incongruously to the left on a still sea of fallen leaves. A prized teacher among the area's novice rock climbers, the boulder almost always has a group lesson underway. Seasoned climbers frequent it as well, climbing during lunch hours and before or after the day's commute.

Bending northeast the trail reaches a clearing where suddenly the tannin-dark pond materializes, reflecting metallic light to the sky. Here the trail forks left and right. Bear to the right and continue into woods of oak and maple. Beyond where a minor path connects the main trail to the pond below, the trail passes a boulder so striated by glacial wear that it looks like a worry-creased brow.

The pond disappears behind a dense hedge of leatherleaf, elderberry, choke cherry, pussywillow, and other shrubs growing beside the pond and the peat bog separated from it by a dam jutting east. Staying on upland, the trail winds westward along the boundary of the bog. The trail is lightly worn and therefore vague on this section but it soon arrives at a sign identifying the land as part of the Webster Conservation Area. From this point blue blazes mark the trail.

Logs then a boardwalk provide dry passage over a wet patch. Just beyond this the trail splits. Either way will do, however the trail to the right maintains a view of the bog. Traffic sounds waft from overhead as cars whoosh by on Hammond Pond Parkway; below the woods are remarkably quiet. Track for Boston's Green Line of the commuter rail system runs along the far bank of the wetland, and from time to time a rattling train clatters by. Built around 1852, the Green Line is the oldest and most heavily traveled streetcar in America.

Ahead the trail veers west away from the peat bog and a moment later meets with its other half joining from the left. Stay with the trail as it passes another path diverting to the left and arrives at a junction. Here Hammond Pond Parkway and the MBTA tracks cross paths, forming the northern boundary of the reservation. The trail to the left fords the flow of the parkway to connect with additional Webster conservation land. For this hike continue to the right and follow blue markers over the rails of the Green Line.

The creations of two inspired and dynamic women lie on the other side: Mrs. Webster's deer park and Mrs. Houghton's garden. Set out to the left on a grassy lane to begin a tour of the two, first visiting the six-acre deer park. Bordered by the train on one side and wetland and a private garden on the other, the path leads west to a boarded-up barn behind a forbidding fence. Look to the left for a gateway and continue hiking parallel to the Green Line. The trail becomes sketchy in this tight spot, but have heart and continue on to find a set of steel stairs providing an exit to Hammond Pond Parkway.

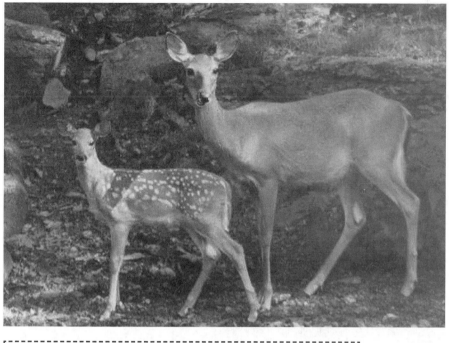

A doe and fawn at Mrs. Webster's deer park. *Photo courtesy of Carol Stapleton.*

The sprawling, unkempt meadow erupting with granite outcroppings lying ahead is the deer park. Looking around to get your bearings you will notice a sign advising visitors to refrain from scaling the fence "because deer can sometimes be dangerous," and confirming that a trail does indeed trace the park's circumference.

In the early 19th century, when Edwin Webster and his wife purchased a sizeable piece of land including these acres, Mrs. Webster, in keeping with a practice popular with European aristocracy, established the deer park. She then introduced a herd of 24 animals, mostly does with one or two bucks included to ensure fawns in spring.

A unique and valuable snapshot of the land before modernization, the rugged grazing land within the fence remains unaltered since the Webster's first took possession of it.

Follow the path around the perimeter of the park hiking first west then north beside Hammond Pond Parkway, then east to where the trail ends at an entrance to the deer park beside a private home. Managed by the Newton Conservation Commission, the deer are cared for daily by a keeper who has tended the herd for 20 years.

Leaving the deer park behind, hike east down the gravel driveway of the stately brick house beside the park to reach Old England Road. Bear right onto a horseshoe curve and continue past a gray house, then cross Lowell Lane

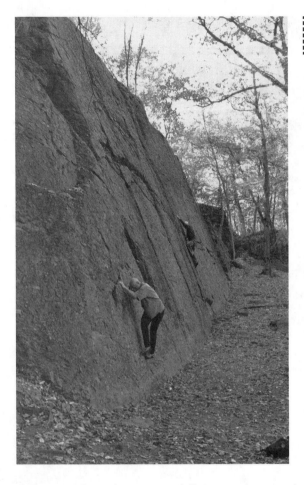

(which leads to the train tracks) to find the entrance to Houghton Garden on the south side of Clovelly Road.

Follow the path as it travels through woods to a stone bench on a hill overlooking Houghton Pond. Dressed in a ruff of rhododendrons, the bench sits atop a granite wall that forms a dramatic backdrop to an orchestrated water garden 20 feet below. From this overlook hike left at the split that travels southeast along a slender finger of water to a footbridge. Follow through with the loop on the opposite bank by bearing left at the fork in the trail.

A hundred yards or so farther on a crushed stone path enters from the street and flows west to an oxbow in the pond. Explore this extension or continue to the right to access a wooden bridge that crosses to meet an array of paths woven through an alpine rock garden on a bank beside the pond.

Martha Houghton, one of the founders of the Rock Garden Society of America, established the garden in 1919. Today members of the Chestnut Hill Garden Club in partnership with the friends of Houghton Garden and the City of Newton strive to maintain it in accordance with Houghton's high standards. Said to be one of the first of its kind, the alpine rock garden includes climbing hydrangea, lily of the valley, wood hyacinth, and exotic evergreens such as the umbrella pine.

After spending some time watching the play of light on the pond or the antics of the garden's resident warblers and orioles, follow the trail as it curves around a stone bench, climbs steps, and joins the path to the entrance.

Once back on Clovelly Road bear left onto Lowell Lane and backtrack across the Green Line to the south side of the reservation. Taking up the blue trail again, follow it southeast, staying to the right at each of its splits to return to the parking lot.

HEMLOCK GORGE LOOP 44

IN BRIEF

This hike explores the Charles River where it spills through a gorge cut by a glacier 10,000 years ago. After surveying the gorge from within a hemlock forest, the trail circles a small island in the river then crosses the magnificent Echo Bridge.

DESCRIPTION

Carved by the force of a retreating glacier 10,000 years ago, Hemlock Gorge was once Massachusetts's equivalent of Niagara Falls. Young men came in droves to ferry their lady friends out onto the sprawling waters of the Charles River in rented canoes. In the late 1800s, there were few places besides in a canoe where a couple could be together without an interfering chaperon. Nonetheless according to the *Boston Herald,* one canoe paddler was arrested and fined $20 for kissing his sweetheart on the river in 1903.

The trail that leads to Hemlock Gorge begins at the northern end of the small parking area. Follow the wide dirt road as it heads into woods between a quiet residential neighborhood to the left and the Charles River to the right. Almost immediately the road reaches a junction with another path that leads off to the left; pass this and continue

KEY AT-A-GLANCE INFORMATION

LENGTH: 1.3 miles

CONFIGURATION: Loop

DIFFICULTY: Easy

SCENERY: A view of the Charles River running through a spectacular gorge with water flowing over two dams

EXPOSURE: Shaded

TRAFFIC: Moderate

TRAIL SURFACE: Packed earth

HIKING TIME: 30 minutes

SEASON: Year-round dawn–dusk

ACCESS: Free

MAPS: Posted at various locations in the reservation and soon to be available on the Friends of Hemlock Gorge Web site, www.hemlockgorge.org

FACILITIES: Picnic tables

SPECIAL COMMENTS: Before English colonists settled the area, the gorge was the fishing ground of the Ponkapoag people of the Algonguin tribe.

WHEELCHAIR TRAVERSABLE: No

DRIVING DISTANCE FROM BOSTON COMMON: 9 miles

Directions ➤

From Boston, take MA 9 east past the MA 128 overpass, then take the first right onto the ramp over the Charles River. Take the first right onto Ellis Street and cross over the Charles River into Needham. Make an immediate right onto Hamilton Place and park at the small lot near the Hemlock Gorge Reservation bulletin board.

Hemlock Gorge Loop
UTM Zone (WGS84) 19T
Easting: 316408
Northing: 4686906
Latitude: N 42° 18' 46"
Longitude: W 71° 13' 40"

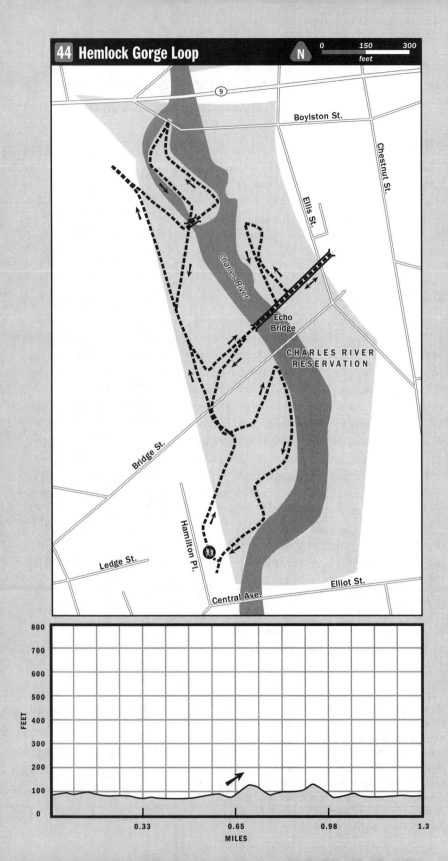

44 Hemlock Gorge Loop

N

0   150   300
feet

Boylston St.

Chestnut St.

Charles River

Ellis St.

Echo Bridge

CHARLES RIVER RESERVATION

Bridge St.

Ledge St.

Hamilton Pl.

Central Ave.

Elliot St.

800				
700				
600				
500				
400				
300				
200				
100				
0	0.33	0.65	0.98	1.3

FEET

MILES

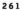

Mill buildings framed by the arch of Echo Bridge

straight, even as you meet another trail heading off to the right. A few yards farther on, under the calming canopy of the hemlocks, the whoosh of traffic on nearby MA 9 dims and blends with the sound of the river flowing below.

At the next fork, bear left and climb a steep embankment. At the top of this rise, look to your right to see Echo Bridge reaching across the water. As I passed, a lone bicyclist glided across the public promenade from the opposite bank. Have a look, or save the pleasure for later and continue following the trail as it descends back into the woods.

The hemlocks of Hemlock Gorge, most well over a century and a half old, have been under attack by an infestation of hemlock woolly adelgid (*Adelges tsugae*) for several years. Though a little haggard, the trees are now showing signs of renewed vigor, thanks to the Friends of Hemlock Gorge. After the USDA Forest Service deemed the situation beyond hope, the Friends took matters into their own hands and pressed the Massachusetts Metropolitan District Commission to finance the purchase of predatory ladybird beetles (*Pseudoscymnus tsugae*) to combat the parasite. Between May 2001 and May 2002, foresters released 15,011 ladybirds, in three batches. In the years since, experts monitoring the situation report that the ladybirds have settled in and seem to be making headway against the woolly adelgid.

Go left at the next split in the trail and make your way downhill past beech trees growing among the hemlocks. Follow the trail a short way farther to the northernmost tip of the reservation where the land falls off abruptly, and evergreen boughs block the view of the traffic opposite. The roar of water falling from the lip of a dam in the near distance will lure you to land's end.

Picking up the trail again, turn and follow it southeast against the current. Closer to the water, things quiet down, ducks paddle in sheltered coves, and almost all human noise disappears. Not far along, the trail arrives at a wooden bridge providing a route to a small island. Cross over and face south for a spectacular view of Echo Bridge and an old mill. Vintage postcards verify that this picturesque scene is nearly the same as it was in the late 1800s.

A trail loops over and around the rugged island. Following it northwest takes you to the circular dam at the end of the gorge. Follow the trail southeast to find the Devil's Den, a natural cave formed in the island's granite face, low on the western side.

Take the footbridge back to the mainland and pick up the trail to the left heading up a steep banking to return to where Echo Bridge touches land. Mount the step to this elegant piece of engineering (built in 1877 to bear the Sudbury River Aqueduct) and stroll across to the river's opposite bank.

Once on the other end, take the stairs down to the base of the bridge, cross Ellis Street, and descend one more flight of steps to get to the lookout platform below. From this stage speak or sing words to the river and listen. Keep count to see if the number of times they repeat exceeds the record 15. Afterward take the steps back up to the riverbank and look for a path to the left. Follow this short route northeast along the river to the edge of a small field, then loop back to the bridge.

Climb the stairs once more to the promenade and head back to the other side of the Charles River. Though people gave up swimming in the gorge back in the 1970s, the water flowing through is becoming healthier every year. Thanks to environmental cleanup efforts the air wafting from the turbulent river smells fresh and fortifying.

Once back on the western side, take the path to the left, which leads back down to the river's edge. Here where the river narrows and bends in an oxbow, you will find a small sandy beach edged with crab apple trees. The trail takes you close to a second dam and a reclaimed mill on the opposite bank. From here, follow the path up a hill behind a brick building and then down again to a field that stretches along the river. Traverse this acre of green to arrive back at the parking lot.

CENTENNIAL PARK LOOP 45

IN BRIEF

Just one of the many hikes possible on Wellesley's extensive trail system, Centennial Park is a place where adults can unwind while children collect pollywogs in a kettle pond and chase crickets and butterflies over rolling meadows.

DESCRIPTION

Named "Contentment" by the handful of colonials who first settled its riverside acres in 1630, expanding what was then Dedham; Wellesley has always been much coveted. Surely Algonquin chiefs Nahaton and Maugus, who sold it for three pounds of corn and five pounds sterling, failed to comprehend the full ramifications of their transaction.

Over time, due to population growth and development, settlers of Dedham's west side built a church of their own and named their new settlement Needham. By 1881 the pattern had repeated, and the town of Wellesley was born. Abandoning the name West Needham, the citizenry agreed to honor Horatio Hollis Hunnewell, the settlement's foremost benefactor, by naming their town Wellesley, after Hunnewell's beloved mansion. Hunnewell—not just a banker, railroad financier, and ardent horticulturist, but also a generous man

KEY AT-A-GLANCE INFORMATION

LENGTH: 1.58 miles

CONFIGURATION: Loop

DIFFICULTY: Easy

SCENERY: A view from Maugus Hill and woods surrounding acres of wildflower-rich meadowland maintained to provide sanctuary for breeding songbirds and other wildlife

EXPOSURE: Mixed sun and shade

TRAFFIC: Moderate

TRAIL SURFACE: Packed earth, wood chips

HIKING TIME: 1 hour

SEASON: Year-round sunrise–sunset

ACCESS: Free

MAPS: Available at kiosk by parking lot, where a map is also displayed; also at the town's Web site, www.ci.wellesley.ma.us/Pages/WellesleyMA_Trails/index

FACILITIES: None

SPECIAL COMMENTS: Landscaped by glacial action and generations of farming, the reservation includes the drumlin called Maugus Hill, an esker, a kettle pond, and kames.

WHEELCHAIR TRAVERSABLE: No

DRIVING DISTANCE FROM BOSTON COMMON: 13 miles

Directions

From Boston take MA 9 westbound to the Cedar Street ramp toward Needham/Dover (follow detour signs). Go through lights and continue on Cedar Street 0.25 miles. Bear right on Hunnewell Street and proceed 0.25 miles. Turn right onto Oakland Street and continue past Mass Bay Community College about 0.5 miles down the hill. The park is on the right marked by a wooden sign.

Centennial Park Loop

UTM Zone (WGS84) 19T

Easting: 313620

Northing: 4686339

Latitude: 42° 18' 25"

Longitude: 71° 15' 41"

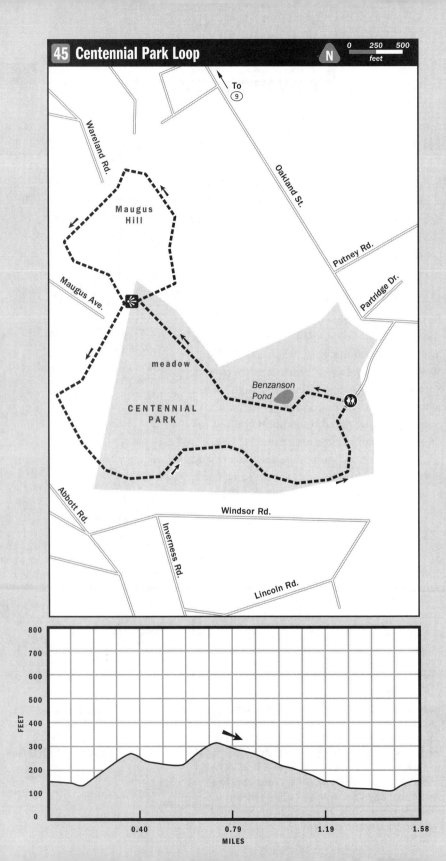

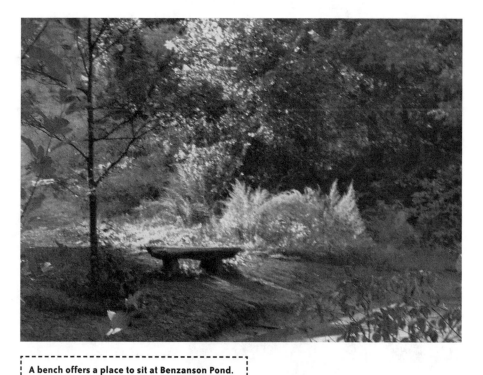

A bench offers a place to sit at Benzanson Pond.

with a romantic bent—fashioned the name from Welles, the maiden name of his of his wife, Isabella.

Fortunate to have founding fathers that had wealth, political savvy, and a deep respect for the importance of community and planning, the town got off on the right foot. Besides hiring the collaborative team of H. H. Richardson and Frederick Law Olmsted to design their train stations, in 1914 the founders made Wellesley the first town in America to adopt zoning laws.

In an inspired look to the future, on town-meeting day in the spring of 1980, the citizens of Wellesley voted to purchase the 42 acres that comprise this park. The idea was to celebrate the township's first 100 years by preserving this lovely tract of open space for now and forevermore.

The trailhead is found scarcely a foot from the parking lot, behind a notice board greeting visitors with maps, news, and a calendar of upcoming events. After a glance, head west on the sprawling trail marked with purple. Within several yards, a sign points both left and straight on to two ends of the same trail. To follow my lead, continue hiking west down an incline surfaced with woodchips to a small kettle pond. Stay on this path as it curves left, rimming the water.

On the far side of the pond, the trail, now reduced to a thin track, climbs up the face of a cascading meadow then shoots into woods. Proceeding uphill gently through a dark tunnel of trees, the path quickly emerges at the bottom of another, larger, steeper expanse of grass and wildflowers. Tall blossoms of black-eyed Susan (*Rudbeckia hirta*), Canada goldenrod (*Solidago Canadensis*), Queen Anne's lace

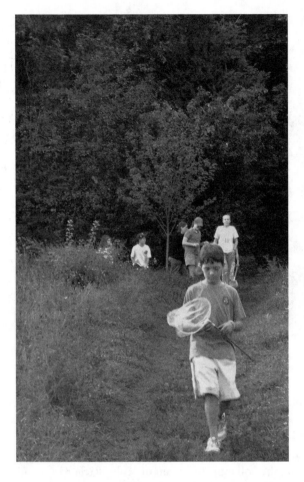

(*Daucus carota*), and lady's thumb (*Persicaria persiacria*) sway in the breeze above cow vetch (*Vicia cracca*) and purple clover. Poison ivy also shows its itch-inducing three-leaf fronds amongst the grass.

Once at the top of this rise on Maugus Hill, you will find a bench facing southeast inviting hikers to sit for a spell and take in the sweeping pastoral view miraculously free of blight. A book sealed within a watertight Tupperware box left on the bench provides an opportunity for those wanting to record their thoughts about the place or just read what others have written. This journal is for all who pass through.

From the bench, continue to the right, following purple markers. Healthy woods of sassafras, maple, pine, and oak quickly envelop the trail as it slopes around the back of the hill.

Entering a grove of beech where the trunks of the trees glint with a metallic shine, the path levels off. A quiet neighborhood sits close by to the right, its houses rendered inconspicuous by a tangle of leafy twigs and branches. A path to this neighborhood feeds into the purple-marked trail.

Bearing westward now, the path rises again from the edge of wetland back toward the top of the meadow passing a trail to the grassy peak of Maugus Hill to the right. Continue to the left, hiking southeast on the purple trail. Ahead, where the route splits, veer to the right, easing downhill again over a smooth expanse of packed earth. Squawking blue jays raise the loudest ruckus in these clean and peaceful woods that were once the home of Chief Maugus and his people.

Arriving momentarily at a broad intersection, hike through, following the purple trail to descend a steep slope Bristled swamp oak, hickories, and hemlocks grow along this stretch. Ferns and mushrooms make an appearance for the first time soon after as the trail makes a sweeping turn to the southeast.

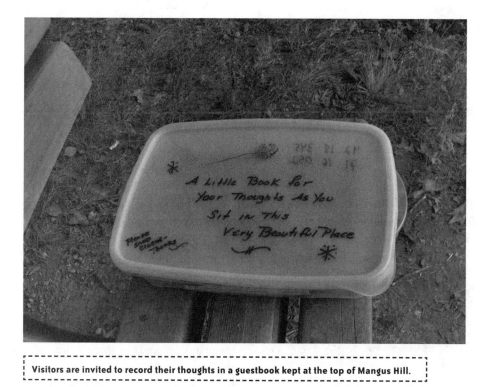

Visitors are invited to record their thoughts in a guestbook kept at the top of Mangus Hill.

Remaining on the purple trail through the next junction, continue south, tapering off the wooded hill. Gradually bending eastward, the trail curves back to meadowland. Bear right along a sliver of trail through lilting grass stalks beaded with seed, past dusty mauve-colored joe-pye weed (*Eupatorium purpureum*) to a small wooden bridge that leads through a brief bushy corridor to another small field bordered by houses.

At the end of this field, where the trail diverts left to run up a slope into woods, stay to the right. Here the trail proceeds along sandy ground on the edge of an esker to a row of birdhouses erected amongst a cultivated patch of purple coneflowers. The path drops beside a brook flowing from the left and follows beside woods festooned with wild grapes and vinca.

Reaching a split, turn left and aim north to upland flush with lady's thumb and ghostly moonflowers. Climbing ever steeply, the trail passes a magnificent oak tree left unfelled by farmers centuries ago to provide shade to herds of livestock. A few hundred yards farther along, the purple trail loops back to its beginning at the head of the parking lot.

NEARBY ATTRACTIONS

Wellesley has a tremendous number of well-maintained trails linking greenspace throughout the town. For more information and maps visit the Wellesley Trails Committee Web page at **wellesleyma.virtualtownhall.net/pages/wellesleyma_trails.**

46 ELM BANK LOOP

KEY AT-A-GLANCE INFORMATION

LENGTH: 1.86 miles

CONFIGURATION: Loop

DIFFICULTY: Easy

SCENERY: View of the Charles River as it flows beside diverse woods

EXPOSURE: Mostly shaded

TRAFFIC: Moderate

TRAIL SURFACE: Packed earth

HIKING TIME: 45 minutes–1 hour

SEASON: Year-round dawn–dusk

ACCESS: Free

MAPS: Posted at the entrance, also available at www.mass.gov/dcr/parks/metroboston/maps/elmbank.gif

FACILITIES: Restrooms available at the Metropolitan District Commission (MDC) Ranger headquarters; soccer fields; canoe/kayak launch

SPECIAL COMMENTS: The Massachusetts Horticultural Society is headquartered here. Visitors can tour the society's demonstration gardens and the Elm Bank Estate.

WHEELCHAIR TRAVERSABLE: Much of the grounds of the Elm Bank estate are wheelchair traversable; however, depending on condition, several sections of the hike described are not.

DRIVING DISTANCE TO BOSTON COMMON: 15 miles

Elm Bank Loop

UTM Zone (WGS84) 19T

Easting: 310074

Northing: 4682871

Latitude: N 42° 16' 30"

Longitude: W 71° 18' 12"

IN BRIEF

Located in an area that has maintained a charmingly rural character despite its proximity to Boston, Elm Bank's well-tended acres offer miles of hiking both along the wooded banks of the Charles River and over landscaped grounds.

DESCRIPTION

A private estate from the 17th century until the dawn of World War II, Elm Bank was given its name by one of its earliest owners, Colonel John Jones, who planted elm trees along the banks of the Charles River. The property passed through the hands of three more owners before Benjamin Pierce Cheney, a founder of a delivery company now known as American Express, purchased it for $10,000. After Cheney's death, his daughter Alice and her husband, Dr. William Hewson Baltzell, took over ownership of the estate. Together they built the neo-Georgian manor that still stands on the premises. To accent the elegant architecture, they hired the Olmsted Brothers landscape architectural company to restore and design the grounds and formal gardens. Once settled, the Cheney-Baltzells threw grand

Directions

From Boston, take the Massachusetts Turnpike (I-90 west) to Exit 14 (Weston). Follow I-95 (MA 128 south) to Exit 21B (MA 16 west). Follow MA 16 west 2.9 miles. On MA 16 west you will come to a stoplight (at a five-way intersection) in the town of Wellesley where you will bear left to continue 1.7 miles on MA 16. The Elm Bank Horticultural Center will be on your left, marked by a small green sign. The street address is 900 Washington Street (MA 16).

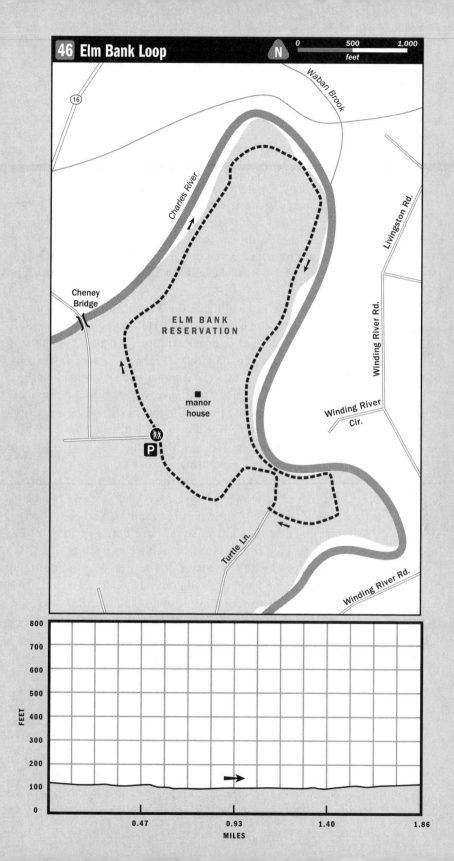

parties that spilled from the house into the gardens and to the river beyond.

Reaching her old age, Alice Cheney-Baltzell wrote in her will that upon her death Elm Bank was to be left to her nephew, but if he did not want it, the property should be offered to Wellesley College, and if the college did not want it, the land should be turned over to the Commonwealth of Massachusetts. Amazingly, each party declined, and Dartmouth College, Benjamin Pierce Cheney's alma mater, became the beneficiary when the school accepted the estate for $40,000.

Today, Elm Bank's acres, somewhat reduced in number, are owned by one of the entities that first refused them—the Commonwealth of Massachusetts. Thirty-two years after Alice's death, the state seized a second opportunity to take possession of the property and purchased it. In 1999, the Massachusetts Horticultural Society arranged to lease the buildings and gardens and made Elm Bank their new headquarters.

Starting at the parking lot located beside the Massachusetts Horticultural Society, follow the paved road northwest. As the road curves gently downhill, you will pass the Horticultural Society's demonstration gardens on the left and the red brick Hunnewell Building on your right. A short distance farther, the road makes a "T." Cross here to find the trailhead marked by a posted map.

The trail sets off immediately into magnificent woods made all the more impressive by a row of enormous white pines. Flowing northeast 21 miles from its source in Hopkinton, the Charles River lies to the left, just a few feet from the edge of the trail and down a steep slope. In May, after two weeks of record rainfall, the river ran full and faster than normal the day of my hike. According to the Charles River Watershed Association, the river's rich tea color is normal, no matter the month or recent weather. Leaves, wetland grasses, and debris from other natural sources tint the water with their tannins. Years of concerted efforts to stop dumping and other contamination have borne exciting results. Today 74 percent of the 80-mile river is clean enough for swimming.

The broad trail, cushioned with a soft layer of pine needles, continues atop the river's right bank. Before too long, the trail descends to just a few feet above water level. You encounter a narrower path splitting off to the right here. Stay with the river route to the left at this break and at each of the next intersections you come to.

Just ahead, the trail arrives at broad opening suitable for a canoe or kayak landing. On the opposite side of the trail, a few feet farther on, is a large vernal pool well fed from river overflow. Here beech and birch add lightness to the woods that earlier had been dominated by more-somber hemlocks and pines. Charged with energy from a good spring soaking followed by sunny days, the beech leaves virtually glow.

The river bends abruptly southeast at this point, creating a deep oxbow as it changes course to flow first south and then southwest. The bend is so sudden and tight that it is no wonder that, after the winter thaw and healthy rains, the engorged river redraws the map. On the day of my hike, the trail disappeared

Seasonal flooding has been known
to obscure the trail.

under a foot of water for a good 100 feet at the top of the oxbow. A passing jogger, momentarily befuddled, remarked that she had never before seen the trail fully flooded.

Happy to take our shoes off and wet our feet, my companion and I took our chances and stayed with the trail. Halfway across, I needed to roll my pants legs up closer to my knees, but the water, far warmer than expected, felt wonderful.

Looking across the river once back on dry land, you can spot private houses through the budding trees in May. By June, they will be hidden. Docks with Adirondack chairs extend onto the water from two homes.

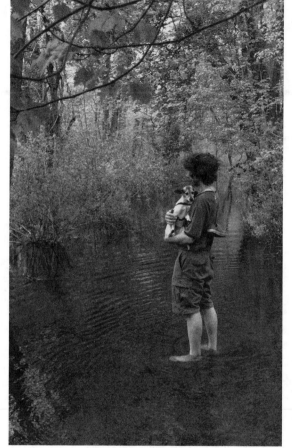

Having experienced limited cutting since the 1700s, the woods along the river are remarkably diverse. Along with species of oaks and pines, there are some tulip trees, hackberry, silver maples, and ashes, and even one towering lilac.

Once the trail has veered decidedly southwest, you will encounter a fork. Both routes lead back to the playing fields at the Elm Bank mansion. On my hike, I chose the right-hand route. This path makes a hairpin turn back to the river, heading north before turning west at another split. On this last stretch, the trail is recessed below the level of the dense woods. Mature trees cast shadows from far overhead.

Shortly the trail meets another packed-earth trail coming in from the left; stay to the right. Not much farther beyond this, the trail reaches a paved road. On the other side, you will see the playing fields. Cross here and walk to the right to arrive back at the Horticultural Society's parking lot.

47 ROCKY NARROWS LOOP

KEY AT-A-GLANCE INFORMATION

LENGTH: 3.8 miles

CONFIGURATION: Loop

DIFFICULTY: Easy to moderate

SCENERY: Views of the Charles River, forested wetlands

EXPOSURE: Mostly shaded

TRAFFIC: Light

TRAIL SURFACE: Packed earth, rocky in places

HIKING TIME: 2 hours

SEASON: Open year-round sunrise–sunset

ACCESS: Free

MAPS: Available at www .thetrustees.org

FACILITIES: None

SPECIAL COMMENTS: Rocky Narrows is a gateway to the Charles River and the Bay Circuit Trail—a 200-mile continuous greenway around Boston from Kingston Bay on the south shore to Plum Island.

WHEELCHAIR TRAVERSABLE: No

DRIVING DISTANCE FROM BOSTON COMMON: 19 miles

IN BRIEF

In this hike you will see the Charles River at its finest. Starting off from a field kept clear since farming days, the trail leads through reforested agricultural land to a canoe landing then tracks the river.

DESCRIPTION

In 1897, five years after landscape architect Charles Eliot founded the Trustees of Reservations, Frederick Law Olmsted Jr. oversaw the initial transaction that was to lead to the protection of 227 acres on the Charles River in Sherborn, property now called Rocky Narrows. Although still largely farmland producing dairy goods and cranberries for local consumers, and vast quantities of "Champagne" cider that was shipped as far afield as Texas, Nebraska, England, and Belgium, Sherborn was changing fast as the turn of the century approached. Keen on preserving the land, Augustus P. Hemenway provided the funds to purchase the first 21-acre parcel of Rocky Narrows. In the years since, others have made similar donations, with the most-recent acreage added in 1995.

Begin your hike by picking up the slender path that starts to the left of the Forest Street parking area at the head of a meadow.

Rocky Narrows Loop

UTM Zone (WGS84) 19T

Easting: 305745

Northing: 4677547

Latitude: N 42° 13' 33"

Longitude: W 71° 21' 14"

Directions

From Boston take I-90 west 16.9 miles. Take Exit 13 to MA 30 east. Turn right onto Speen Street then continue 2.8 miles and turn left onto Coolidge Street. After 1.2 miles turn right onto north Main Street. Continue 2 miles and turn left onto Goulding Street. At 0.6 miles turn left onto Forest Street; parking is on the right.

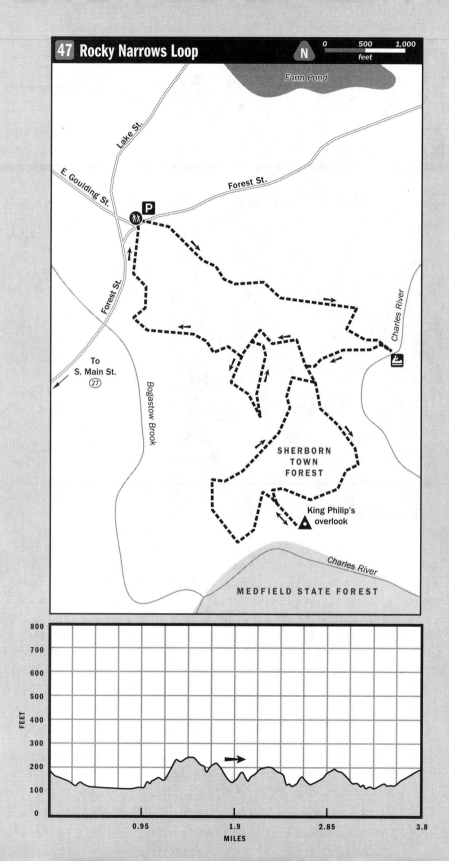

47 Rocky Narrows Loop

N

0   500   1,000
feet

Farm Pond

Lake St.

E. Goulding St.

Forest St.

P

Forest St.

To
S. Main St.
27

Bogastow Brook

Charles River

SHERBORN
TOWN
FOREST

King Philip's
overlook

Charles River

MEDFIELD STATE FOREST

800
700
600
500
400
300
200
100
0

FEET

0.95   1.9   2.85   3.8
MILES

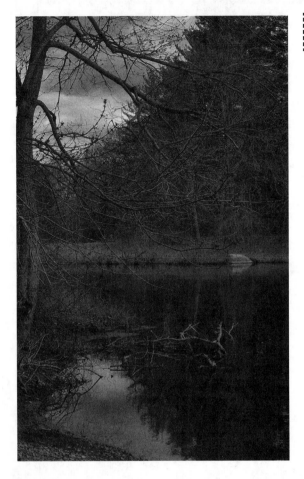

Crossing the grassy expanse to join a gravel road, bear right where the road forms a V with a rutted wagon route and continue southeast past an oak on the left and a cedar tree standing beside a stone wall opposite. From here you will notice red dots marking the way. As you hike along this open stretch songbirds will likely distract you with their song or audacity as they fearlessly fling themselves at passing hawks.

Guided by stone walls on either side, the path quickly heads into woods composed of white pine, oak, cherry, and nut trees that have grown in since Eliot and Olmsted took protective charge of the land. The walking is easy as the broad path winds down around soft bends, making a causeway as it passes through wetland. In early spring, before deerfly season, bunches of green skunk cabbage brighten the bog. Later in the season, you will see plenty of butterflies and maybe even the rare lady's slipper orchid.

When the path arrives at a split with the number 21 posted on the right, continue to the left, walking eastward. The dominant species of tree shifts to pine as the trail leads to a clearing at a "T." From here, turn right (south), noticing marker number 20. Follow as the trail tacks southwest, passing beneath tall conifers through a distinctly wetter zone. Soon you arrive at another fork. At this juncture, bear left onto the red trail.

The massive pines and hemlocks along this part spread a beautiful canopy overhead. Though old-growth trees were mostly cleared for pasture in New England, a few stands still exist in some areas, such as in this riparian zone. In a moment, you arrive at a clearing where the woods end at the sandy bank of the Charles River. The number 19 on a tree identifies this spot as the canoe landing at Rocky Narrows. It would be hard to resist a dip on a steamy day in

July, despite the possible presence of leaches (a good reason to bring salt along). A decade or two of concerted efforts to clean up the Charles River has seen impressive results. Fish are jumping again, muskrats are back in strong force, and there have been claims of otter sightings.

Leave the canoe landing, heading southwest along the river's edge. Tufted titmouse and warblers up from the tropics for the summer sing in underbrush growing between the woods and the water. Eventually the trail turns away from the river and joins a path going off to the right. Keep left and travel west up a hill. You will see the number 18 and a red dot on a tree to the left. Follow these as they direct you up a steep embankment and lead you along a hemlock-sheltered ridge high above the river. Continuing along the ridge you will pass a trail coming in from the right. A little farther on, you meet with another trail; keep to the right here, leaving the ridge to head west following the red marker.

The path widens, levels, and soon arrives at a triangular intersection marked 16. Walk straight through, staying with the red trail. Elevated above the river basin, the path is surrounded by young woods. Glimpsing the horizon, you see nothing but seemingly untouched land for miles. Follow the path downhill until you come to trail 14. Take this sharp left-hand turn back uphill to reach King Philip's Overlook.

Standing atop this granite cliff, looking across the rich valley empty of any buildings, modern or otherwise, it is easy to put oneself in the mind-set of Metacomet (given the Christian name "Philip" by his father Massasoit), the leader of the Pokanoket tribe of Wampanoag. Disturbed to see his people being killed off by disease brought by these land-hungry foreigners, King Philip (as he was nicknamed by the British) launched an all-out war against the white New Englanders in 1675.

Leaving the overlook, double back to return to the red trail, taking it downhill toward railroad tracks. The trail curves right as it nears the tracks then descends another long slope. Farther on when the trail splits at marker 12, break off to the right and climb back east before arriving at another intersection and continuing northward. In short time you will arrive at another junction, marked 26. Cross here, hiking northeast.

Partway down a rocky slope edged with pine saplings, you will come to a trail running uphill off to the right. Climb this link to where it connects with the red trail. Hike to the left, back to marker 18 then follow the red trail to where it cleaves through a stone wall. Here turn left onto a narrower trail.

When you reach a four-way intersection, turn right (northwest) and follow the path straight to marker 24 and continue on. Here, bear left to head southwest. You will pass one or two sketchy trails diverting to the left but stay on course to reach marker 25. At this intersection follow the trail left as it climbs a hill through a dense growth of young white pines. Reaching another junction, continue left and travel slightly downhill, heading northeast. Passing the green trail, continue

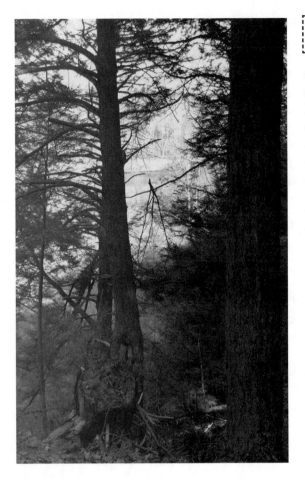

Hemlocks rooted to a steep slope at Rocky Narrows

straight ahead to reach another fork. Stay to the left here and head left again at the next split. At the next intersection, turn right onto a path running along a stone wall.

This path, marked with orange, treads between wetlands and upland to reach marker 10. From this junction head northwest on the red trail, continuing to the left at the next fork. A short way farther on, turn right to return to the Red trail. Having zigzagged your way to marker 8, the last crossroads of the hike, bear left to link back to the parking lot.

NEARBY ATTRACTIONS

After a hike at Rocky Narrows, animal lovers, peaceniks, and anyone else needing an excuse to spend an extra hour or two in beautiful Sherborn might like to stop in at The Peace Abbey Multifaith Retreat Center located at 2 North Main Street. A multifaith chapel, pacifist living-history museum, vegan-peace sanctuary, and guest house are just a sampling of what you will find at the center. But of all the center's offerings it is the Sacred Cow Animal Rights Memorial that will most likely stir your heart—perhaps even inspire you to vegetarianism. The memorial features a life-size bronze statue of "Emily the Peace Cow" who lived at the center for 8 years after escaping a slaughterhouse by leaping over a five-foot fence and evading capture by hiding out in nearby woods with a herd of deer for 40 days and 40 nights. Hours are Monday through Friday, 9 a.m. to 5 p.m., Saturday and Sunday, 10 a.m. to 6 p.m. Phone (508) 655-2143.

OGILVIE WOODS HIKE 48

IN BRIEF

Starting out in a benevolent plantation of pine, this hike becomes increasingly beautiful and intriguing as it ventures along a ridge formed by the collision of continental plates, and noses into a treacherous swamp-filled corner of an earthquake faultline.

DESCRIPTION

With 2,000 acres of protected open space, an extensive trail network, and active sustainable forestry and community agriculture programs in place, the quiet, former farming town of Weston is a national leader in land conservation and stewardship. In 1955 the town began acquiring large tracts of unbuilt land and established the Weston Forest and Trail Association to maintain trails and educate the townspeople about the forests and forest ecology. The strategy from the start was to buy "backland" and leave property owners with both homes and acreage with street frontage.

Directions

From Boston Common, start out going south on Tremont Street 0.7 miles, then turn right to stay on Tremont Street. Turn slightly right onto Marginal Road. At 0.1 mile merge onto Interstate 90 west and continue for 10.3 miles. Take Exit 15 to I-95. At 0.3 miles exit left to I-95 north. Continue 1.9 miles and take Exit 26 to US 20. Turn slight right onto US 20 east and at 0.1 mile turn slight left onto US 20 west. Follow US 20 west 1.4 miles. Turn slight right onto Boston Post Road and at 0.7 miles turn right onto Concord Road. Continue 1.6 miles on Concord Road. Stay straight to go onto Sudbury Road. The entrance to Ogilvie Woods is ahead 0.4 miles next to house number 133.

i KEY AT-A-GLANCE INFORMATION

LENGTH: 3 miles

CONFIGURATION: 2 loops

DIFFICULTY: Easy to moderate

SCENERY: Reforested farmland, swamp, and a fault zone created when continental plates collided to form the supercontinent Pangaea during the Precambrian-Mesozoic era

EXPOSURE: Mostly shaded

TRAFFIC: Light

TRAIL SURFACE: Packed earth, with rugged areas of loose gravel and exposed rock

HIKING TIME: 1.5–2 hours

SEASON: Year-round sunrise–sunset

ACCESS: Free

MAPS: Maps can be purchased at the Weston Town Hall and can also be obtained from the Weston Forest and Trail Association, www.weston foresttrail.org.

FACILITIES: None

SPECIAL COMMENTS: This forest is a veritable cornucopia of edible (and inedible) mushrooms.

WHEELCHAIR TRAVERSABLE: No

DRIVING DISTANCE FROM BOSTON COMMON: 18 miles

Ogilvie Woods Hike

UTM Zone (WGS 84) 19T

Easting: 307865

Northing: 4695299

Latitude: N 42° 23' 10"

Longitude: W 71° 20' 03"

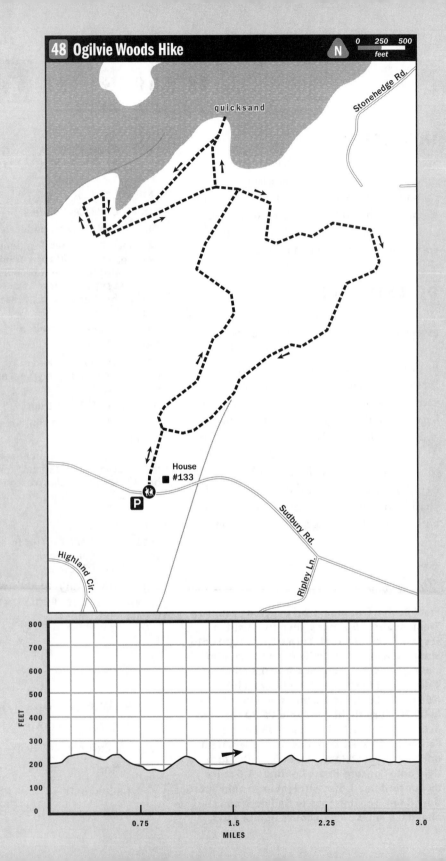

The result is neighborhoods woven together by vast tracts of unspoiled land and miles of public trails.

From the parking spot on the shoulder of Sudbury Road, locate the trailhead near a small green Weston Forest trail marker and set out hiking north into a grove of pine. Traveling in a nearly straight line past a stone wall on the left, the trail arrives at a two-way junction. Bear right here, continuing slightly uphill on a wider path edged by pines and a smattering of oaks and other hardwoods. In May, blooming wild lily-of-the-valley (*Maianthemum canadense*) and starflower (*Trientalis borealis*) light the forest floor with their tiny white petals. When the expansiveness of summer subsides into autumn, clutches of violet-capped wood blewits (*Lepista nuda*) poke through the fallen leaves and pine needles.

Undulating northeast, this grassy fire road soon leads to a two-way intersection marked 8. Continue left, aiming north under shade cast by oak, hickory, and white pine. Being well into the woods now, you'll hear none of the jarring sounds of suburbia. Nuthatches, chickadees, and other woodland birds twitter in the midcanopy, and occasionally a red-tailed hawk perches high on a dead oak limb long enough to attract a mob of crows. Otherwise, a velvety quiet settles.

As the trail descends through a void created by two ridges, note the bedrock. As extraordinary as it seems—so far away from Hawaii or Sumatra—the bedrock you see extruding from the slopes is volcanic. This "tuff" stuff is consolidated erupted molten rock and ash. This is not to say that a volcano lies under Weston; the source of the tuff is even more extraordinary. According to geologists, distinct sections of New England, including several in the Boston area, are pieces of faraway lands, including Africa and a chain of volcanic islands that once protruded from the sea above the South Pole. The volcanic rock crawling with Weston-hatched daddy longlegs and ants, then, is either of foreign origin or a local made product created when one plate of Earth's crust rode up over another. All told, Massachusetts has experienced no fewer than three such momentous collisions in the past 500 million years. Although all lies quiet today, a certain amount of instability exists along the many fault lines that radiate from these points of impact. The Bloody Bluff Fault named for a bloody scuffle between sniping Minutemen and British Regulars on April 19, 1775, in Lexington, lies nearby.

Tumbling in stop motion, a stone wall crosses down one slope, lets the trail through, then climbs to the right. Ahead where the trail splits at another junction, hike left to head northwest under hemlock cover. Rolling gradually northwest in easy undulations over gravel footing, the trail soon reaches junction 4. A hemlock stands at the crook of the "V" next to an umbrella-shaped sassafras tree. Bear right, continuing alongside intriguing ridges.

Departing the fire road at junction 3, climb over the mounded chunks of microcontinents, crystallized volcanic ash, and organic detritus, to descend to the swamp below. In crossing this spot, you'll find that flooding dictates the way. Allow dry footing to be the priority as you follow markers pointing right. The trail sidles along the swamp only temporarily; a moment later it edges back up onto the flank

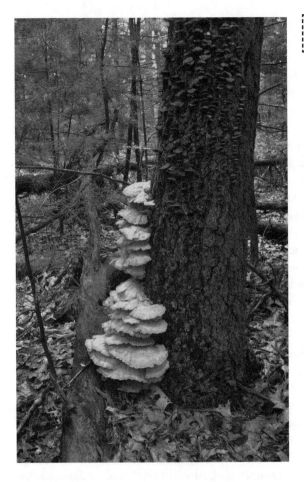

of another ridge. Ahead a sign bears the bone-chilling warning of quicksand in the lowland area beyond. The treacherous zone is an outlying tract of the Bloody Bluff Fault. For a cautious look, follow the trail down into the swamp, being sure to stop on the near side of logs serving as a makeshift bridge. The quicksand long ago trapped a horse that belonged to a farmer named Hans van Leer. Today, the animal's bones lie buried deep within the mire.

On returning to the orange warning sign, hike uphill to the right and follow the path as it switches back over the top of the ridge traced earlier. The view looking southeast from this static mass is something like that of the view from the crest of a rogue wave.

Several paths feed in from the edges, but stay with the main trail as it continues straight along the ridge beneath black oaks. As it begins to taper downhill, the trail bows left and right. Choose the right-hand route to descend along a pit used as a rifle-training range during World War II. Mushrooms pop from the gritty ground. Some, for instance, the cauliflower fungus (*Sparassis crispa*), resemble a puff of dust rising from a bullet's point of impact.

Beyond the military's borrow pit, the trail levels off as it continues on its southwest run along the border of Weston and Wayland. Across the stone wall demarcating the town line, you can see a meadow through a thin wall of trees. At the T-junction ahead, bear right for a brief foray into Wayland, on land owned by the Sudbury Valley Trustees. Take a stroll around the periphery of the meadow, keeping an eye out for raptors or fox that might be out hunting rabbits or field mice.

Returning to the woods of Weston, continue straight on across the top of the "T," heading east over acres that were once part of Hans van Leer's farm. The fire road turned hiking trail travels alongside a ravine cut by glacial outwash during the formation of Lake Sudbury. Easing into the recess, the trail arrives at junction 2. Continue to the left, hiking over floodplain to return to junction 3.

At this familiar point, keep to the left to hike southeast into the southern reaches of Lincoln. The next junction comes quickly. Here, a trail marked with the red sign of the Lincoln Trail System bears left, but bear right to remain in Ogilvie Forest. Midway up a banking, the trail forks; stay right and continue climbing. At the top of the rise, passing a stone wall likely built by Hans van Leer and sons, the trail splits yet again. Bear left, hiking eastward under pines and hemlocks. Encountering the stone wall once more, the trail continues through a gap in the stones, reaches another split, and continues straight on.

To round out a tour of the forest, the trail forges northeast toward the Lincoln border, crossing another glacial-outwash plain to access high ground. Houses are visible through trees to the left as the trail arrives at junction 9. Using drumlins and eskers as stepping-stones through wetland, continue on the route as it heads right, traveling southeastward.

Just beyond the foundation of a house on the right, the trail forks. Stay right to curve southwest. Grit washed into a mound beneath glacial ice rises to the right, facing a stone wall. Descending from this esker, the trail dips then climbs another, crossing a stream in between. Arriving at a split a moment later, stay on high ground to follow the trail as it arcs southwestward.

The rich vegetation of the swampland and the shelter provided by the ridged topography make these woods a haven for white-tailed deer. Great horned owls roosting in evergreens are less easy to spot, but pellets of coughed-up mouse fur and bits of bones at the foot of the trees are a sure sign that they are about.

At the "V" of junction 6 and the unmarked junction that follows, continue straight, hiking downhill on a gravel-strewn slope. Junction 7 comes quickly; bear left here keeping on a southwest trajectory. Having escaped the swampy ruckus of the Bloody Bluff Fault zone, the trail now returns to a far tamer landscape. Docile white pine saplings and sassafras fill sunlit spaces, and the ground lies flat. Two fully oxidized vehicles of pre–World War II vintage hide under leaves to the right of the trail. Fast returning to their most basic elements, little of these machines is recognizable besides the light sockets and rounded fenders.

Shortly beyond the automobiles' resting ground, the trail diverges left; however, bear right to continue southwest through the pinewood. On arriving at the next junction, turn left to return to Sudbury Road.

NEARBY ATTRACTIONS

Land's Sake is a private, nonprofit organization devoted to land stewardship, sustainable farming, and forestry. The organization runs a full calendar of events year-round, including maple sugaring in February and March, and a Strawberry Festival in June. Land's Sake's headquarters is located at the Melone Homestead, at 27 Crescent Street, Weston. Contact Land's Sake at (781) 893-1162, or on the Web at **www.landsake.org**.

49 CEDAR HILL TO SAWINK FARM LOOP

KEY AT-A-GLANCE INFORMATION

LENGTH: 8 miles

CONFIGURATION: Out-and-back with two loops

DIFFICULTY: Easy to moderate

SCENERY: The reserve's nearly 2,000 acres include abandoned farmland, deciduous woodland, and a drumlin next to a magnificent swamp. Birds of 38 species, including ruffed grouse, willow flycatcher, and a variety of warblers, nest on the property.

EXPOSURE: Mostly shaded

TRAFFIC: Light

TRAIL SURFACE: Packed earth, grass; boardwalks through wetland

HIKING TIME: 3 hours

SEASON: Year-round sunrise–sunset

ACCESS: Free

MAPS: Available at trailhead, at the Northborough town hall, and at the Sudbury Valley Trustees' Web site: www.sudburyvalleytrustees.org

FACILITIES: None

WHEELCHAIR TRAVERSABLE: No

DRIVING DISTANCE TO BOSTON COMMON: 35 miles

IN BRIEF

This hike travels within the borders of three towns—Northborough, Marlborough, and Westborough—crossing two abandoned farms, several drumlins, numerous streams, and a magnificent, species-rich swamp.

DESCRIPTION

From the parking lot, walk toward Lyman Street to find the Little Chauncy Trail trailhead on the left. Crossing through an abandoned farm, the flat grassy path skirts a convex meadow on the last high ground above Little Chauncy Pond. In past decades the cloven hooves of ambling cows kept this flood zone clear, now flourishing purple loosestrife and cattail grow like a bushy brow above the unblinking eye of water.

Volunteer members of Northborough and Westborough trails organizations installed a boardwalk here to provide hikers and mountain bikers passage. Not the fine grazing ground for Guernsey heifers it once was, the field has been usurped by milkweed, goldenrod, joe-pye weed, Queen Anne's lace, burdock, thistle, and hairy vetch. Today the tweed of weeds feeds a great diversity of vibrant birds and bugs from goldfinches, and bobolinks to cicadas and monarch butterflies.

Cedar Hill to Sawink Farm Loop

UTM Zone (WGS 84) 19T

Easting: 284730

Northing: 4686933

Latitude: N 42° 18' 18"

Longitude: W 71° 36' 42"

Directions ⟶

From Boston, take Interstate 90 west (portions of which are toll roads). Drive 27.5 miles, then merge onto I-495 north via Exit 11A toward Marlborough. Continue 2.7 miles before merging onto MA 9 west via Exit 23B toward Worcester. After 2.5 miles turn right onto Lyman Street. The parking lot is on the left.

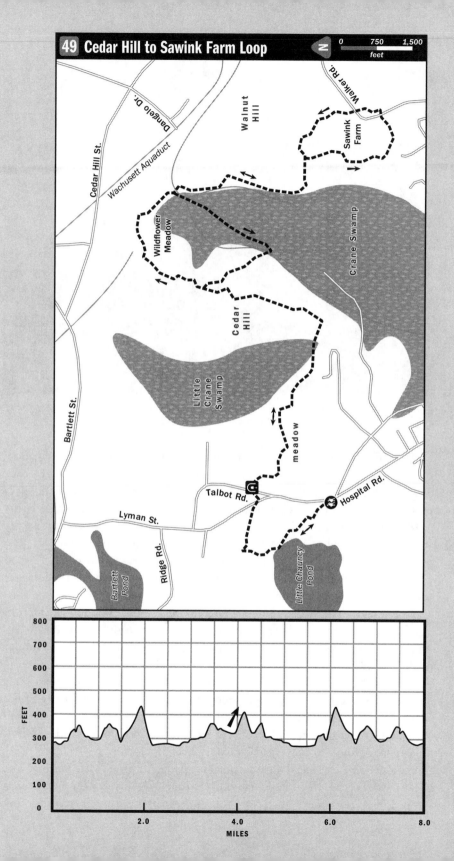

49 Cedar Hill to Sawink Farm Loop

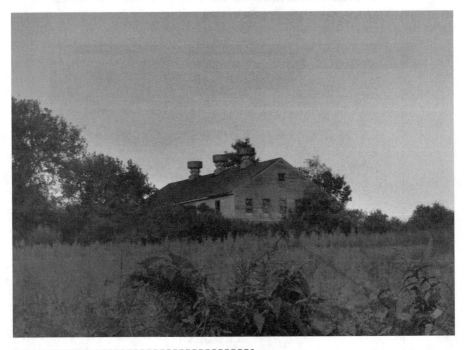

The trail passes through a dairy farm of bygone days.

Three quarters of the way along the pond, the trail climbs from the meadow into pinewoods. Follow the plentiful trail markers as they weave through enormous creaking trees, jackknife around a boulder, and head eastward. In spots the very abundance of markers makes for confusion. For clarity, keep your sights on the triangular red tags initialed "N" for Northborough, and continue eastward, staying to the left at a junction at the crown of the wood.

Easing downhill, the trail leads southeast 200 yards or so past an aspen grove to Lyman Street. To cross, stay with the trail as it bends to the left and forges its way through a tunnel.

Emerging into a thicket of maples rooted in a seasonal floodplain, the trail crosses a field over a low-slung boardwalk passing rapturous grapevines laden with purple fruit smelling like a child's sticky kiss. In the heat of a late summer day, the altitude at waist level is dense with zooming dragonflies.

Leaving the field, the trail (here called Talbot Trail) ascends into woods composed of white pine, oak, and a good number of birches, and shortly comes to a two-way junction. Bear right to continue on Talbot Trail, and when the trail splits again a short distance on, bear left. Skirting the peak of the hill, the trail cuts a narrow route through pasture consumed by Norway maples and other opportunistic species. Ahead it passes an amoral line of barbed-wire fencing. The still-taut wire pinches the fleshy girth of trees caught against it, scarring them.

As Talbot Trail continues across the slope, it passes a steep trail shooting straight to a water tower on the hilltop. Changing its trajectory, the trail then bends to meet Cole Trail ascending from the west. At this junction bear right to stay with Talbot Trail, now aimed toward a hemlock-shaded brook at the base of the drumlin called Cedar Hill. Once across the sturdy bridge built by local Eagle Scouts, follow the trail up a sandy pitch to a three-way split. Here Plantation Trail and Chestnut Trail bow off to the right, and Cedar Hill Trail branches left. Choose the latter and hike northward onto land protected by the Sudbury Valley Trustees (SVT).

Scruffy and neglected looking, this domed former pastureland is anything but. Like a Paris fashion with exposed seams or an odd cut, this hillside jumbled with weeds, unpruned fruit trees, and assorted shrubs has tremendous, if not readily apparent, value. Successional-shrub habitats such as this, created when farmland is abandoned to natural forces, are vital to a substantial number of endangered plant and animal species. In fact, the unkempt state of these 12 acres is not just intentional but carefully planned and managed. Thanks to these efforts, alert hikers might be lucky enough to see golden-winged warblers, eastern meadowlarks, brown thrashers, or American kestrels winging by. Coyotes, red fox, and not-so-shy bobcats also prowl the hillside's thickets.

From the summit of Cedar Hill, follow the mowed path north among the goldenrod, traveling downhill to reenter the woods. Pine and cedar trees frame the way, and as the trail turns northeast, birch and wizened apple trees fill in. Negotiating loosened rocks and arm-thick roots distracts, but there's plenty to see, including garter snakes on the hunt for toads and edible mushrooms such as the tasty hen of the woods (*Grifola frondosa*).

Ahead, at a junction, bear left to continue on Cedar Hill Trail. As the topography gradually levels to Crane Swamp, the trail bends around a glacial erratic the size of an elephant calf and as flat as a plains state. Beyond this, a sign points right, directing the trail under hemlock boughs on into pines shadowed by sugar maples.

After catching a glimpse of the crane nesting ground to the right, the path mounts a boardwalk to cross a stream and its overflow. Leaving this, the northern edge of Crane Swamp, the trail spills into a generous meadow sowed with 25 native wildflower species. In August the purple of the asters juxtaposed with the gold of goldenrod and the dazzling orange of monarch butterflies is gorgeously garish.

North of this rich oasis of life and color, the trail reaches a train track and the town borders of Northborough and Marlborough. Follow the trail as it bends northeast, staying south of the track. Within a few yards, the idyllically pastoral look and feel of the place is supplanted by an entirely different aesthetic and mood, for lying dead ahead, across a paved utility road, is a newly constructed water-treatment facility.

Crane Swamp Trail runs over the pavement, hugging the wooded edge of the wetland to a junction marked both with an SVT sign and the "N" of the

Northborough Trail Association. If mosquitoes are biting and time short, bear left to loop directly back to Cedar Hill; otherwise continue straight to pick up the Connector Trail that leads to Sawink Farm.

From this fork the trail runs south within spitting distance of the ziggurat-shaped water-treatment plant ingeniously disguised with native plants. Solid like a mountain with an internal spring, the monolith holds 3.6 million gallons of water.

Beyond the earthen tower, the Connector Trail continues alongside Crane Swamp through lush clover, passing a pond bulldozed to a tear shape. Farther on a sign points the way south over a small bridge. Here the land is once more untouched, or rather, untouched since its last days as a working farm.

To the left is a grove of pine set on upland and to the right a dense wood of young birch and beech. Traveling south between the two, the trail soon meets a stone wall and bends uphill to follow it. Hemlock boughs dim the light along this stretch, scenting the air with the essence of pure antiquity. Where the incline levels, the trail bears right and passes through a parting in the wall to arrive at the start of Sawink Loop.

In 1762 Edmund Brigham cut trees here and hauled stone to establish one of Westborough's first farms. Ownership changed over time, but the farm stayed in production into the tail end of the last century. After World War II, when farming was beginning to consolidate into the Midwest, Michael Sawink gave up the 35-acre tip of his farm in Northborough to the Sudbury Valley Trust-ees to ensure it would never be developed. With help from Lawrence Walkup, another local farmer, the SVT saved another 66 acres lying to the south in Westborough.

To circumnavigate these 101 acres, hike southeast on the path to the left of the sign. Traveling within the confines of a stone-wall grid, the trail jogs to the northeast between epic sugar maples. Certainly a good many steaming stacks of pancakes were dribbled with syrup boiled down from the sap of these trees. Giant pines that somehow escaped ax and saw stand in with the maples.

Ahead where the trail eases downhill, red Xs painted on stones mark the way. If you are hiking between August and October watch carefully here for the terrific blue of the flowering bottle gentian (*Gentiana clausa*).

Shortly the trail passes a meadow on the right and leads to a dirt road straight ahead. To proceed on Sawink Loop, cross the drive to the old pear orchard that now serves as a parking lot for the Sawink Farm Reservation. From the SVT kiosk exit onto the paved road and hike south 100 yards or so to the trailhead on the right.

The western side of Sawink Loop Trail, travels gently uphill over interwo-ven roots and flat stepping-stones, to reach a plateau with houses built on a cul-de-sac. From here it turns northward and descends steeply to hemlock-sheltered wetlands. Pink markers indicate the way along this section recently cleared with the help of a Westborough Boy Scout troop. After navigating the wetland rather

A monarch butterfly feeds on aster nectar at the wildflower meadow.

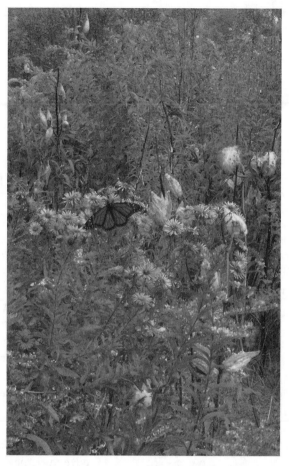

A monarch butterfly feeds on aster nectar at the wildflower meadow.

erratically through a convergence of stone walls, the trail climbs back onto dry ground. Passing sisters of the sugar maples seen earlier, the trail soon returns to the start of Sawink Loop.

From this spot, follow the Connector Trail to its end at the water-treatment plant. At the trail junction, turn left to pick up Crane Swamp Trail heading south. Forming a straight causeway across the dense swamp, the trail leads back to the eastern side of Cedar Hill. Where the hillside meets the swamp, divert onto Plantation Trail heading northwest. After crossing a small steel bridge, the narrow path makes a crooked run up the side of the hill to rejoin a section of Cedar Hill Trail, hiked earlier. Bear left at this fork and retrace your footsteps back to the parking lot on Lyman Street.

50 | IN THOREAU'S FOOTSTEPS

KEY AT-A-GLANCE INFORMATION

LENGTH: 8.67 miles

CONFIGURATION: Out-and-back with 2 loops

DIFFICULTY: Easy to moderate

SCENERY: The enormous and lovely Farrar Pond and a wooded landscape contoured by glacial ice

EXPOSURE: Mostly shaded

TRAFFIC: Moderate

TRAIL SURFACE: Widely varied, including packed earth, grassland, rocky terrain, and some pavement

HIKING TIME: 5 hours

SEASON: Year-round sunrise–sunset

ACCESS: Free

MAPS: Available through the Lincoln and Concord conservation commissions

FACILITIES: None

SPECIAL COMMENTS: If you hike with a canine friend, be sure to bring a leash. Dogs are not welcome at the Walden Pond State Reservation.

WHEELCHAIR TRAVERSABLE: No

DRIVING DISTANCE TO BOSTON COMMON: 25 miles

In Thoreau's Footsteps

UTM Zone (WGS84) 19T

Easting: 306178

Northing: 4697833

Latitude: N 42° 24' 31"

Longitude: W 71° 21' 19"

IN BRIEF

This hike links three popular hiking destinations, Mount Misery, Adams Woods, and Walden Pond.

DESCRIPTION

On Independence Day in 1845, Henry David Thoreau moved into a small cabin he had built at Walden Pond, Concord, on a woodlot belonging to Ralph Waldo Emerson. Thoreau explained, "I went to the woods because I wished to live deliberately, to front only the essential facts of life, and see if I could not learn what it had to teach, and not, when I came to die, discover that I had not lived." Each day for the two years he lived at Walden, Thoreau observed nature, wrote, and did a great deal of walking. For him, a daily walk of no less than four hours was a necessity of life. Of walking he wrote, "We should go forth on the shortest walk, perchance, in the spirit of undying adventure, never to return." Although by and large, Thoreau's compass sent him westward, it is likely that on occasion his needle spun south to Farrar Pond.

To find the trailhead, cross Oxbow Road and, bearing right, hike to a gap in evergreens

Directions

From Boston, take Interstate 90 west 11.4 miles to I-95 via Exit 15. Bear left to merge onto I-95 north. Continue 1.9 miles to Exit 26/ US 20. After 0.3 miles bear left onto Stow Street. After 0.3 miles turn left onto Main Street/MA 117. Continue 5.1 miles along MA 117 then turn left onto Concord Road. Travel 0.4 miles then turn right onto Farrar Road. Continue 0.4 miles then bear right onto Oxbow Road. There is a pulloff for parking on the left.

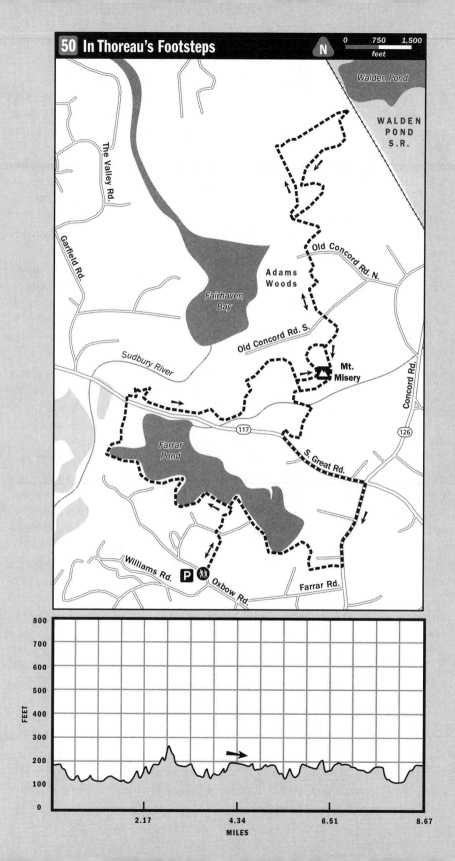

N

0   750   1,500
feet

Walden Pond

WALDEN
POND
S.R.

The Valley Rd.

Garfield Rd.

Old Concord Rd. N.

Adams
Woods

Fairhaven
Bay

Old Concord Rd. S.

Mt.
Misery

Sudbury River

Concord Rd.

117

126

S Great Rd.

Farrar
Pond

Williams Rd.

P

Oxbow Rd.

Farrar Rd.

800
700
600
500
400
300
200
100
0

FEET

2.17   4.34   6.51   8.67
MILES

framing a field. A post that may or may not be standing bears the insignia of the Lincoln Land Conservation Trust. From this corner head northeast along the edge of the field to reach a paved drive and woods beyond. Cross the pavement and resume the trail as it continues northward between two massive oaks marked with orange trail blazes.

In a rush of metaphors, one trumps all in describing what comes next. The best is Apollo's Chariot—a roller-coaster ride. Starting where the trail bears left atop an esker nearly in the clouds, the trail swerves, dips, and lurches its way to the pond below. At ride's end, a sign warning of "nuisance aquatic vegetation," feet away from a weed-ridden pool, swings shut the floodgates of adrenalin, leaving the senses wide awake but calm.

Having landed on level ground, proceed left and follow the trail as it traces the pond's perimeter. In August peaceful flotillas of Canada geese loitering in the year's last warm days paddle among lily pads, and maples looking overdressed in reds and golds.

Stay with the trail as it continues northwest on its orbit around the pond passing several trails along the way. At one bend, a fleet of canoes and kayaks lies underside up by a landing. Heading directly north, the trail leads to a peninsula then makes a hairpin turn to continue southwest. Far off at the end of the pond, traffic streams across the horizon. Except for the condominium complex built on the cusp of the hill above, Farrar Pond is remarkably undeveloped, and the few houses that are visible integrate gracefully into the landscape.

Just before reaching a private home stained the color of redwood, the trail intersects another route jutting in from the left then appears to dead-end at a gushing outlet. Here, despite the sign reading "Private," the route continues across the abbreviated bridge. A white Bay Circuit Trail marker attached to an oak indicates where the trail proceeds between a fenced-in meadow and a wispy wall of evergreens.

From a gateway with a birdhouse attached, the trail follows a driveway past a hedgerow of beach roses to a road at the foot of the hill. Aim for the Bay Circuit Trail marker next to a dirt pulloff across the road, then carefully continue around a blind curve to the right. Noting a white trail marker on a large pine, hike behind the parking area to a boat launch on the Sudbury River.

Mounting the wooded riverbank, the trail arcs back to the road where a pair of markers, one white and one yellow, indicates that the trail travels southeast alongside the road, dropping below the traffic as it skirts wetland thick with reeds. The cloven footprints of deer mark this passageway.

Emerging from the mire, the trail arrives at the solid base of Mount Misery. The Orange trail offers the option of climbing straight north. Take this route several yards to a split then ease off to the right, following a red arrow to descend back to street level. Across the parking lot in the northeast corner, the Bay Circuit Trail picks up again. Resuming this route momentarily, pass a pond then bear left on the Kettle Trail.

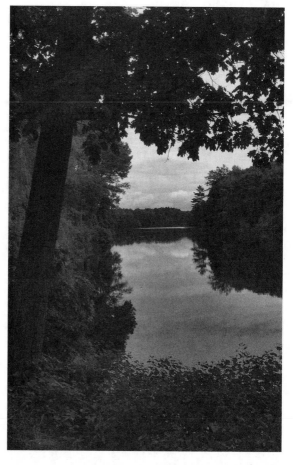

A view across the vast and beautiful Farrar Pond

After shooting straight to the top of an esker, the trail darts through an intersection, then rims a kettle pond before plunging down the other side, banking a curve, then snaking the other way to climb again.

Reaching a plateau, the trail turns southeast and, a moment later, slices across the Bay Circuit Trail. Ahead a lovely broad corridor lit by sun filtering through hemlocks and luminous beech leads to another four-way intersection. Take the Yellow trail splitting left here to spiral to the top of Mount Misery. Though a peaceful spot to enjoy a snack, the peak affords little in the way of a view.

When ready to quit the top, descend on the Yellow trail along the edge of a tremendously steep slope. At the base of Mount Misery, bear right then continue straight to a cultivated field. Trace the field's boundary to the left and enter the woods where a sign reads "Private Trail to Adams Woods." This path is private in the sense that it crosses private property, but day-hikers are welcome.

Follow orange dots as they lead past houses across a paved drive. After dipping to wetland, bear left just short of a horse paddock. This turn is easy to miss, but if you find yourself face to face with a horse standing before a brown house on a hill, you've gone too far.

Traveling north between a stream on the left and the paddock, the trail continues across a wooden bridge to meet a driveway a short distance later and Adams Woods beyond. Locate the trail to the right, marked with a hiker symbol and an orange dot.

Departing from the stream, the trail crosses through one junction to reach another distinguished by a gate on the left. When the orange trail forks just

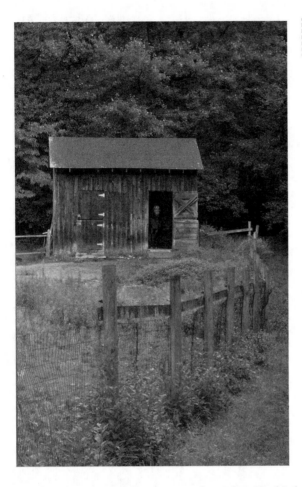

A neighbor's horse watches as hikers pass by.

ahead, stay on course to continue northwest over sandy ground above wetland. At the top of a slight grade near a kettle pond, a sign points south to Mount Misery. To press on toward Concord, round the bend to the left to another kettle pond and junction. Spurning the Andromeda Trail, hike left uphill to a fork and a sign marking the Lincoln–Concord border. Where the Fairhaven Trail breaks off to the left, veer right to continue northwest.

Having left Lincoln, be aware of a change in trail markers. The steward of these acres is the Concord Land Conservation Trust. Nonetheless, at each of the next intersections, stay to the right. On this brief stretch, the trail doubles as a steeplechase course.

Pines soften the trail's edges as it carves an arc over and between wrinkles wrought by the relentless pressure of glacial ice. Spilling to a packed mound poised above a cavity engorged with greenery, the trail pauses beside a railroad line. Emerson's Cliff at Walden Pond is just a stone's throw away across the tracks.

This junction marks the hike's halfway point. To return to Farrar Pond, continue on the orange trail to descend southward on a banking far above the outwash field. Many twists and turns lie ahead as the trail navigates all manner of ice-borne topography. Be alert for orange discs and the white medallions of the Concord Land Conservation Trust to stay on course. At a sprawling intersection where the orange trail appears to split in two, bear right.

Climbing a moraine, the trail rises above the fantastically pronounced depression left by a glacial finger and proceeds southwest on upland. After running due south through pines and oaks but nary a maple or hickory, the trail turns sharply northeast and reaches two junctions, one nearly on top of the other. Bear right at both. The second right sends the trail southwest once more.

On this downhill, fields become visible through the trees ahead, and in a moment the trail intersects another. Turn left here; this is the Orange trail you hiked earlier. Pass a sign confirming the way to retrace the route to Mount Misery.

Upon arriving at the mountain's threshold, where the Bay Circuit Trail enters from across the field, hike left to circle the base of the great hill. Rising along wetland, the trail parts a stone wall then, at an expansive intersection, heads south, following yellow markers.

A small duckweed-green kettle pond lies ahead. Crossing the causeway that contains it, the trail arrives at an intersection marked "E." Bear left here and trace the pond, traveling southeast. Where Wolf Pine Trail appears at the far bank, turn right and continue southwest, paralleling a stone wall. With yellow markers leading the way, the trail bends to the right just short of South Great Road (MA 117). Brush through ferns to reach a junction, and turn left here to meet the road.

Leaving wooded paths to temporarily join a paved bicycle route, cross to the other side and proceed 0.4 miles to Concord Road (MA 126). Make a right angle south at this intersection, and at 0.36 miles, between houses numbered 234 through 239, look for a sign marking a trail traveling east–west across Concord Road. Leave pavement and follow this well-hidden and lightly traveled path westward.

For 0.27 miles this delightful orange-marked path slips along the edges of private property to emerge at the southeastern end of bowtie-shaped Farrar Pond. On its final leg before it reaches Farrar's wooded bank, the trail darts diagonally across a driveway, passing a sculpture of granite and steel.

Once beside the water, the trail picks its way over the root-tangled shore to arrive back to where it first approached the pond hours ago. At this, the third junction, bear left and make one last push to return to Oxbow Road.

NEARBY ATTRACTIONS

To see where the "shot heard round the world" was fired—the ground on which the American Revolution began on April 19, 1775—plan a trip to Concord's Minute Man National Historical Park. Details can be found online at **www.nps.gov/mima**. Those with a taste for art will want to visit the DeCordova Museum and Sculpture Park, also in Concord. The museum is open Tuesday through Sunday from 10 a.m. to 5 p.m. and on select Monday holidays. Call (781) 259-8355 for updated information. Admission to the DeCordova Campus is $9 for adults, and $6 for seniors, students, and children 6 to 12; children 5 and under are admitted free.

51 FOSS FARM HIKE

KEY AT-A-GLANCE INFORMATION

LENGTH: 6.7 miles

CONFIGURATION: Out-and-back

DIFFICULTY: Moderate

SCENERY: Fields, woods, and riverine wetlands

EXPOSURE: Mostly shaded

TRAFFIC: Light

TRAIL SURFACE: Grass, packed earth, and boardwalks

HIKING TIME: 3 hours

SEASON: Year-round sunrise–sunset

ACCESS: Free

MAPS: Posted at the entrance

FACILITIES: None

SPECIAL COMMENTS: Waterproof shoes are recommended in wet months.

WHEELCHAIR TRAVERSABLE: No

DRIVING DISTANCE TO BOSTON COMMON: 27 miles

IN BRIEF

This hike shadows the Concord River, staying clear of its floodwaters and biting insects. Crossing through conserved farmland and a magnificent tract called The Great Meadow owned by the National Wildlife Federation, the trail passes through woods and picturesque farmsteads before rounding a large pond teeming with lily pads then doubling back to Foss Farm.

DESCRIPTION

Upon finding the trailhead at the edge of the parking lot, set out heading northeast across an open field. Rising and falling with the curve of the land, the path soon leads to two horseback-riding rings, one straight ahead and another around a corner to the left. Foss Farm is a popular destination for local equestrians who come to school their horses and to compete in horse shows held here in summer and autumn. On the fresh June day that I passed through, Amanda Brem and her Appaloosa, Lucy, flashed by at a canter.

Follow the path north past the riding ring, along the edge of a hay field planted with timothy. Reaching woods, the path turns right and heads toward gardens in the northwest corner of the field. Watch for swallows swooping low

---

Foss Farm Hike

UTM Zone (WGS84) 19T

Easting: 309544

Northing: 4709342

Latitude: N 42° 30' 47"

Longitude: W 71° 19' 07"

Directions

From Boston, take Interstate 90 west 9.4 miles to I-95 north. Continue 9.4 miles to Exit 31B/MA 4 north toward Bedford. Travel 2.8 miles; turn left onto MA 225 and continue 4.1 miles. Shortly after crossing the Concord River, look for a dirt road on the right leading to a dirt parking lot. There's a sign saying "Foss Farm" on the roadside, but it is not easy to see.

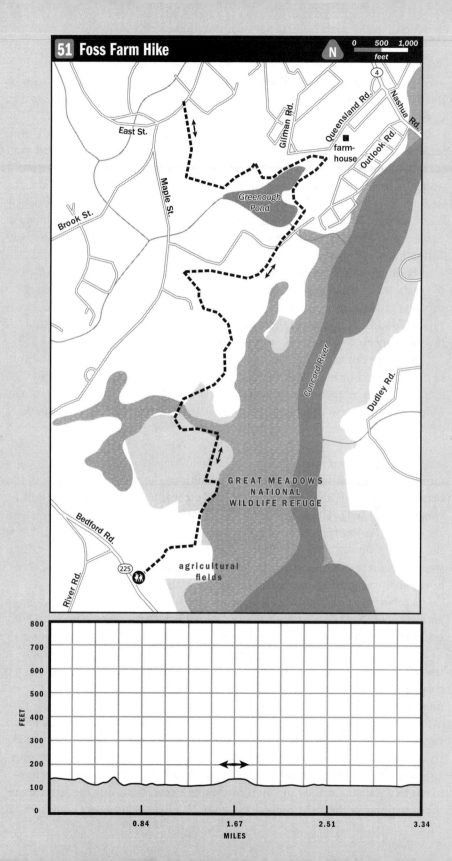

0   500   1,000
feet

N

East St.

Gilman Rd.

Queensland Rd.

Nashua Rd.

4

farm-
house

Outlook Rd.

Maple St.

Brook St.

Greenough
Pond

Concord River

Dudley Rd.

GREAT MEADOWS
NATIONAL
WILDLIFE REFUGE

Bedford Rd.

225

River Rd.

agricultural
fields

800
700
600
500
400
300
200
100
0

FEET

0.84   1.67   2.51   3.34

MILES

over the open grassland, and while swatting mosquitoes, consider that each of these aeronautic whizzes eats fours times its body weight in insects every day. Besides swallows, you are also likely to see eastern bluebirds darting by.

At the northwest corner of the field, you will find a sign marking a trail leading into the woods to the left. Turn here to leave Foss Farm and enter land owned by the National Wildlife Federation. A few feet beyond a gap in a stone wall, the path reaches an intersection. The River Trail lies to the right and the Redtail Trail to the left. Flooding forced my choice of route since tremendously heavy spring rains had the River Trail's extensive boardwalk fully submerged. Chased by a cloud of newly hached mosquitoes, I quickly rethought my plan. Teflon hides are needed for hiking the River Trail in spring and summer.

Heading north on the Redtail Trail over level ground ever so slightly out of reach of floodwater, you pass through a grove of red pines dense enough to suppress growth of any underbrush save ferns that thrive in wet, dimly lit conditions. Woodcocks also favor these parts, both for the cover they provide and for the earthworms that multiply voluminously in the forest detritus.

Weaving this way and that, the trail eventually leads to a watery mire linked to a small pond formed with the help of a dam put in place by farmers in days gone by. Here a sturdy wooden boardwalk and footbridge facilitate passage. Judging from have-a-heart-style trap submerged near the dam, the impressive depth of the floodwater is attributable in part to beaver engineering.

After crossing the bridge, bear right to continue northeast, making your way along a path that skirts the expansive Great Meadows Wildlife area. Because mowing is frequently inhibited by wet conditions, lush grasses are inclined to overwhelm the trail here. In June the humid air is filled with the ecstatic pulsing chirps of frog song. Given the wet, rich herbaceous growth, and the amphibian chorus, the setting feels more like Mississippi than New England. Farther along the tended side of the field transitions to grassland left to revert to its natural state. Though the area is open and dominated by grasses and wildflowers, aspen, birch, and pine saplings are beginning to assert themselves.

Leaving the Great Meadows, continue west along a mowed pathway through another field. Near a sign simply marked "Trail," the path splits in two. Take the trail to the left to promptly arrive at another intersection. Here, signs point back to Foss Farm and to the Pine Loop. Leave the meadows behind and continue to the left, heading west under the cover of pencil-straight pines. Traveling through this cultivated evergreen grove, the path curves northeast. Shortly you come upon a sign pointing to Maple Street, a pond, and the river to the right. Turn off here to continue northward. Still surrounded by lofty pines, you may hear a car pass on the street barely visible to the left. Rounding the knoll, glimpse the river edging into a field on the left. Just ahead, the trail dips to another fork. Continuing straight, the Pine Loop trail leads back to Foss Farm while the path to the left quits the woods and aims for Maple Street. Choosing the latter route, head east across the field toward the river. A picturesque house and barn sit

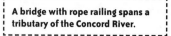

A bridge with rope railing spans a tributary of the Concord River.

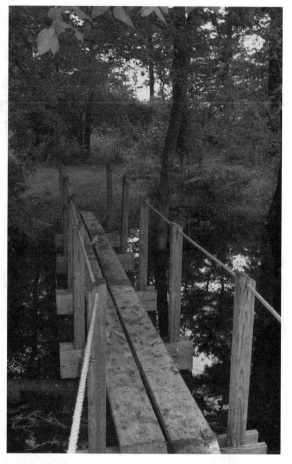

on private property to the left. Back now in the river's floodplain, brace youself for another foot soaking and attack by marauding mosquitoes.

After crossing the field, the path reenters a wooded corridor dense with oaks and pines. Several yards away, hidden by a tangled thicket, the Concord River flows southwest, meandering seaward. A sign ahead directs hikers to the right, away from private property. Behind, emerging from the bog, is the tantalizing River Trail. To the side of it, a droll sign advises dry-season use only. A sign bearing the universal stickman treading water or fending off giant mosquitoes would better convey the intended message.

Hiking a few hundred yards more on what becomes a dirt road, you will arrive at the eastern end of Greenough Pond. A dam and ruler-straight causeway bridge the water, allowing passage from the fields of Greenough Farm to the homestead just within sight. With its last crops harvested long ago, Greenough Farm is now idle conservation land, its handsome white barn and clapboard home ghostly vacant. Follow the road to the barnyard and search to the left to find a weathered post marking where the trail continues along the pond's bank.

Though overcome by weeds at the start, the trail becomes easy to follow as it encircles the pond. Looking through a veil of overhanging branches, you might see a wood duck paddle by or glimpse the blue streak of a diving kingfisher. Failing this, you are guaranteed to see redwing blackbirds, dragonflies, damselflies, and thousands of flowering pond lilies.

On the western side of the pond, the trail bends south and crosses a tributary by way of a wooden footbridge. Beyond the bridge, follow the trail now marked with red dots, as it climbs up a banking and bends away from the pond

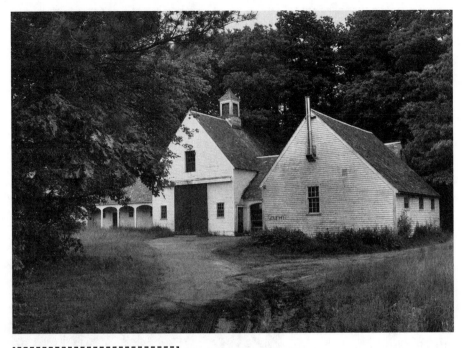

The homestead of Greenough Farm

back into woods. After crossing another stream, the trail splits at an unmarked intersection made distinct by a telephone pole at its center. Choose the trail to the right, which widens as it climbs. Beyond a break in a stone wall a sign points to the right to parking. Undulating through woods, this broad, well-traveled path leads to a bold-yellow arrow painted on a rock soon after the trail's end at Maple Street. From this terminus, turn and hike back to Foss Farm.

GREAT BROOK FARM LOOP 52

IN BRIEF

This hike provides a full tour of the nearly 1,000-acre Great Brook Farm State Park. Starting at the park's interpretive center, the hike travels over terrain varying from rugged stone-strewn slopes to boardwalk stretched across swampland. Passing the remains of a historic settlement before circling a vast glacial outwash plain, the hike ends at the center of a working farm.

DESCRIPTION

From the parking lot, set out heading north on the trail to the left of the interpretive center, passing a butterfly garden planted with bee balm and other perennials attractive to monarchs, swallowtails, and other Lepidoptera species. Ahead, junction 4 marks where two separate loop trails converge. Continue straight, crossing the gravel road to hike north on Litchfield Loop Trail. Stretching across a meadow, the trail bears right and enters woods.

Caterpillaring along over glacial mounds, the Litchfield Loop Trail leads to a sliver of meadow bordered by black-eyed Susans, Queen Anne's lace, hardwood trees, and an algae-covered kettle hole thick with cattails. Beyond this corridor, the trail broadens to another field—this one planted with corn and

KEY AT-A-GLANCE INFORMATION

LENGTH: 6.82 miles
CONFIGURATION: Loop
DIFFICULTY: Easy to moderate
SCENERY: The landscape, formed by glaciation includes vernal pools, eskers, woods, swamp, and a large pond. Established in 1939, Great Meadow State Park also features a working dairy farm.
EXPOSURE: Mostly shaded
TRAFFIC: Moderate
TRAIL SURFACE: Packed earth with loose gravel in some places
HIKING TIME: 3–3.5 hours
SEASON: Year-round sunrise–sunset
ACCESS: Parking is $2 per car.
MAPS: Maps are available at the park and also at www.mass.gov/dcr/parks/northeast/gbfm.htm.
FACILITIES: Great Brook Farm's interpretive dairy concession sells freshly made ice cream and lunch from mid-April through October from 11 a.m. until dark. Other facilities include restrooms and a friendly cross-country ski center at the Hart Barn, a rustic lodge where skiers can warm themselves with hot chocolate and a well-tended woodstove.
WHEELCHAIR TRAVERSABLE: No
DRIVING DISTANCE FROM BOSTON COMMON: 28 miles

Directions ⟶

From MA 128 north or south, take Exit 31B. Follow MA 225 west 8 miles to the Carlisle center rotary, then turn right on Lowell Street (following the sign to Chelmsford). Fern's Market is on the corner. The park entrance is 2 miles ahead on the right. The park office is on the right at 984 Lowell Street, just beyond the entrance. To park turn right onto North Road. The parking area is 0.5 miles down on the left.

Great Brook Farm Loop
UTM Zone (WGS84) 19T
Easting: 307195
Northing: 4714344
Latitude: N 42° 33' 27"
Longitude: W 71° 20' 55"

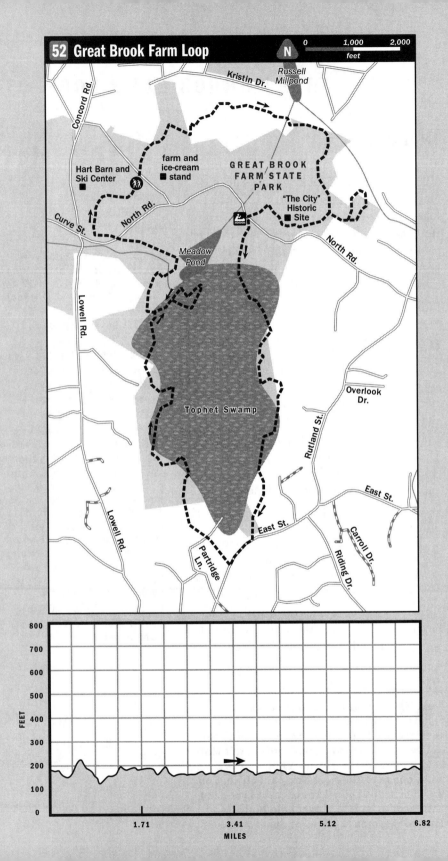

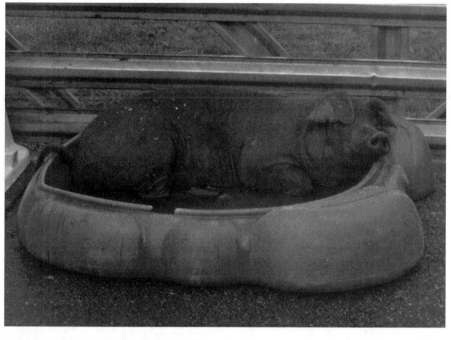

A pig naps in its bath at Great Brook Farm.

ornamented with invasive but beautiful purple loostrife. Ahead at the three-way junction (junction 6) proceed on the Indian Hill Trail marked with blue.

After some winding, Indian Hill Trail makes a hairpin turn to head northeast under pines. With eyes to the ground, you will notice sheets of granite bearing pronounced grooves etched by rubble-studded glacial ice. Reaching the top of the hill at junction 33, the trail continues straight on its northeast trajectory, gradually easing downhill.

The foot of Indian Hill marks the border between the towns of Carlisle and Chelmsford. Because the Great Meadow Farm lies entirely in Carlisle, the trail ends its north-bearing run and aims southeast, keeping flush to the town line. Several houses abutting the park are visible through the woods on this stretch. Depending on the season, the black raspberries forming a thicket on the border might slow a brisk hike to a crawl for the next few hundred yards. Keep left at the next junction, staying on the trail that doubles as a gas line, then bear right, or south, at the split that soon follows.

On encountering a brook, the trail (marked with blue) hugs the bank of the wetland, crossing first a small bridge then another wide enough to accommodate three horses walking abreast. The Indian Hill Trail runs uphill to the right at junction 10, but stay straight to continue east on the grand woodland avenue humbly named Woodchuck Trail. Flirting with wetland lying on either side, this raised trail cuts a dry, curved route south, passing a minor path or two to arrive at the butt end of a massive stone wall at junction 11.

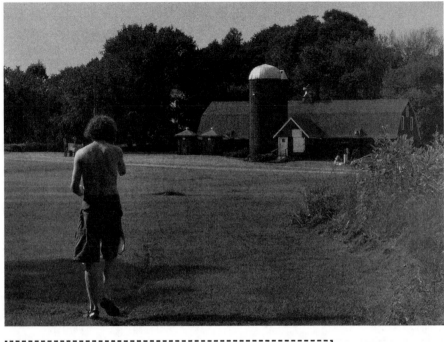

Popular and vast Great Brook Farm promises both company and solitude.

For a shorter hike, stay with the Woodchuck Trail as it veers west; or, to vary the hike with a quick jaunt on a more intimate path, detour to the left onto the Deer Run Trail. After adding a loop to the east at junction 30, the Deer Run Trail cuts west across wetland via one of the park's many boardwalks built by members of the New England Mountain Bike Association (NEMBA), then links with the Garrison Loop at junction 31. Just northwest of this crossroads, the trail leads uphill to a historic site called "The City."

Past the cellar hole of the garrison house, the trail retreats under pines and hemlocks to reunite with the Woodchuck Trail. Those interested in viewing a log cabin built by Great Brook Farm's original owner, Farnham Smith, will want to bear right at this junction; the cabin is several yards down the trail on the left. Mr. Smith inaugurated his agricultural enterprise in 1939 with the purchase of 8 acres near the Old Adams Milldam. Thanks to grit and Yankee perseverance, Smith grew his farm to more than 900 acres in less than a quarter century.

After a visit to Smith's cabin, follow the Woodchuck Trail southwest to its end at North Road. Navigate the metal gate then cross the road to reach the canoe launch at Meadow Pond—a kettle hole created by a glacial ice "calf" orphaned when the Wisconsin Glacier retreated. If it is a warm day with enough breeze to keep bugs at bay, this lovely spot may put a damper on initial ambitions. A mile or 2 of hiking is an even trade for an hour or so of sun in the company of kingfishers and iridescent dragonflies.

Pick up the Pine Point Loop Trail to the left of the canoe launch and follow this dirt cart road south along the edge of the wetland surrounding Meadow Pond. If enticed by glimpses of blooming lily pads, bear right onto the Beaver Loop, a lightly traveled trail that leads to the water's edge; otherwise continue straight to junction 15—the gateway to Tophet Swamp.

Swinging west, the Pine Loop Trail forms a causeway across a glacial outwash plain lying south of Meadow Pond. To shorten the hike by half, stay on this route; otherwise bear left to set out around Tophet Swamp. The trail begins with a length of boardwalk that NEMBA built over a section that can get particularly sticky during wet months. Beyond this, the trail makes its way through woods along the swamp's outer reaches, following the park's eastern border approximately 1.3 miles. Occasionally, neighboring homes are visible or made apparent by a barking dog or the cheerful sounds of children at play.

Emerging from woods, the trail arrives at a cul-de-sac at the end of Aberdeen Drive marked by well-groomed lawns spread before quiet homes. The change is startling but not unwelcome—like strolling out of a matinee into a glaringly sunny day. Several hundred yards up the drive, the trail reenters woods to the right. Bearing southwest, it travels through a beech grove punctuated with sassafras to reach a gate at East Street. Having left the park, Tophet Loop Trail continues to the right along the street and passes several houses before bearing right at Woodbine Road. Tracking this peaceful road to a turnaround at its end, the trail leaves pavement and forges northward.

In no time at all, the trail arrives at junction 44. Here the Heartbreak Ridge Trail bears left and the terraced Tophet Loop Trail continues to the right mirroring the swamp's irregular edge. Beeches lighten the atmosphere created by the sedate pines and swamp oak, and a rooster's cock-a-doodle-doo sears through the wood's damp shade and the twitterings of chickadees.

Beyond a boardwalk the trail winds east then west, dodging the wet to arrive at an enormous glacial erratic sitting in the center of junction 29. To stay on the Tophet Loop Trail, keep to the right. But to survey the landscape from atop a prominent esker (a ridge of sand, earth, and stone created by a stream running deep beneath a glacier), take up the Heartbreak Ridge Trail, bearing west around the boulder.

Parting swampland as it snakes northward, the trail passes a house built on a ledge, then a pond teeming with fantastic life forms, then tapers to end at junction 18 on the Pine Point Loop Trail.

Those already salivating at the thought of a triple-dip cone or sundae served at the farm's ice-cream stand will want to bear left onto the cart road (Pine Loop Trail). Traveling on a swerving beeline this road leads to the dairy by way of North Road and the Lantern Loop Trail.

However, having come this far, and knowing that as long as Great Meadow's cows give milk there will be plenty of ice cream for everyone, consider a brief tour of Great Meadow Pond's delightful southern bank.

Putting off ice cream for later, bear right at junction 18 and backtrack east to junction 16. Taking up the Tophet Loop Trail once more, bear left to hike north. After passing vernal pools and wetland glutted with weeds, the trail soon reaches its magnificent destination. Others wandering in search of the perfect picnic spot or sprinting to view a pair of wood ducks coasting in for a landing have worn light paths in all directions. The main trail, more deeply etched than the others, follows the pond's soft outline then bends south to return to the Pine Point Loop Trail at junction 17. Bear right to follow this convoluted route past the Heartbreak Ridge Trail then a cornfield encircled by the Erickson Loop.

Past junction 21, the Pine Loop Trail swings east, crossing between wetland and Meadow Pond. A neglected boathouse inhabited by bees sits to the right beside a beach popular with stick-fetching water dogs. Continuing eastward over a stone bridge, the cart road passes an idyllic picnicking spot outfitted with tables and, farther along, some timber horse jumps safely positioned off to the side.

Swing west at junction 22 to take up the clay-surfaced Maple Ridge Trail. Traveling across a wooded floodplain, this trail passes a path to the right (another shortcut to the ice-cream stand) and, after bearing left at junction 23, joins the Lantern Loop Trail at North Road.

Crossing the road on a diagonal, take up the Lantern Trail and arc northward past picturesque cornfields and the ski center at Hart Barn. Passing another horse jump east of the ski center, the trail meets junction 2. Quit the Lantern Loop Trail here and opt instead for the dirt road bearing east toward the top of the parking lot.

Note: Besides presenting miles and miles of wonderful hiking trails, Great Brook Farm offers the public a chance to see what life is like on a working dairy farm. Barn tours are offered daily on weekends. Visitors interested in learning about the park's natural, cultural, and Native American history can sign up for programs led by trained interpreters. During winter months, Great Brook Farm operates a fabulous cross-country ski rental and touring center headquartered at the farm's Hart Barn. Trails are open daily as conditions allow. The Lantern Trail offers illuminated night skiing each Tuesday and Thursday.

NEARBY ATTRACTIONS

Visitors from far afield may want to consider combining a hike at Great Brook Farm with a stay at Hawthorn Inn, located a little more than 8 miles (about 20 minutes) away in the neighboring town of Concord. To get there, take Lowell Street south to North Road, and at the next roundabout take the first exit onto Westford Street (MA 225). Turn left onto Concord Street and continue as Concord Street becomes Lowell Road and Lowell Road becomes Monument Square and Monument Square becomes Lexington Road (MA 2A). The inn is at 462 Lexington Road. For reservations, call (978) 369-5610. Concord itself is as rich

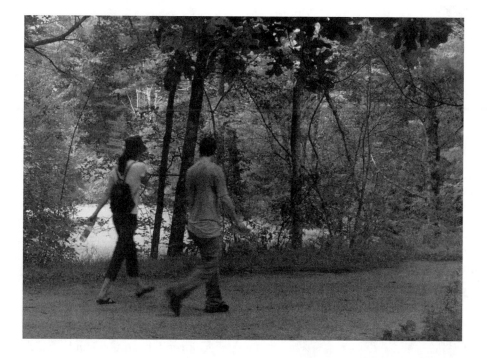

in history and appeal as any New England town, being the site of the Battles of Lexington and Concord—or the "shot heard 'round the world," as described by Ralph Waldo Emerson. As well, it is the home of Walden Pond, made famous by Henry David Thoreau and his book of the same name.

53 CALLAHAN STATE PARK HIKE

KEY AT-A-GLANCE INFORMATION

LENGTH: 7.37 miles

CONFIGURATION: Double loop

DIFFICULTY: Easy to moderate

SCENERY: Woods, reforested farm-land, a working farm, a kettle pond, and an earthen dam

EXPOSURE: Mostly shade

TRAFFIC: Moderate

TRAIL SURFACE: Packed earth with some rocky areas and mud in wet seasons

HIKING TIME: 2.5–3 hours

SEASON: Year-round sunrise–sunset

ACCESS: Free

MAPS: Maps are available from the Massachusetts Department of Conservation and Recreation Web site, www.mass.gov/dcr/parks/northeast/call.htm, and on location as supplies last.

FACILITIES: None

SPECIAL COMMENTS: The park is a favorite destination for mountain bikers, horseback riders, and cross-country skiers.

WHEELCHAIR TRAVERSABLE: No

DRIVING DISTANCE FROM BOSTON COMMON: 25 miles

Callahan State Park Hike

UTM Zone (WGS84) 19T

Easting: 296328

Northing: 4689813

Latitude: N 42° 20' 02"

Longitude: W 71° 28' 20"

IN BRIEF

This rather long hike is composed of two distinct halves. Of the two, the northern half is the more rugged and less frequented: the southern side has woods, wetlands, and tracts of meadowland—some of which are still used for agriculture.

DESCRIPTION

As interpreted by Arthur Miller in his play *The Crucible*, Thomas Danforth was a hard, self-interested man with little to no compassion, but to others, including his colleague Judge Samuel Sewell—who credited Danforth with "[doing] much to end the troubles under which the country groaned in 1692"—Danforth was not just admirable but a man of great merit.

Regardless, Thomas Danforth was one of America's first self-made men. Orphaned with the rest of his five siblings at age 15, three years after arriving from England, Danforth never went to college yet rose to become a justice of the Supreme Court, president of the Commissioners of the United Colonies, and deputy governor under Simon Bradstreet.

Directions ⟶

From Boston, take Interstate 90 west 11.9 miles then merge onto Worcester Road via Exit 12 toward Marlboro. After 1.7 miles bear left onto the Pleasant Street Connector, which becomes Firmin Avenue. Continue 0.1 mile then turn right onto MA 30. At 0.7 miles turn left onto Pinehill Road. Turn right onto Parmenter Road which shortly becomes Edmands Road. Continue 0.1 mile and turn right to stay on Edmands Road. Parking for the Sudbury Valley Trustees and Bay Circuit Trail trailhead is at Stearns Organic Farm on the right.

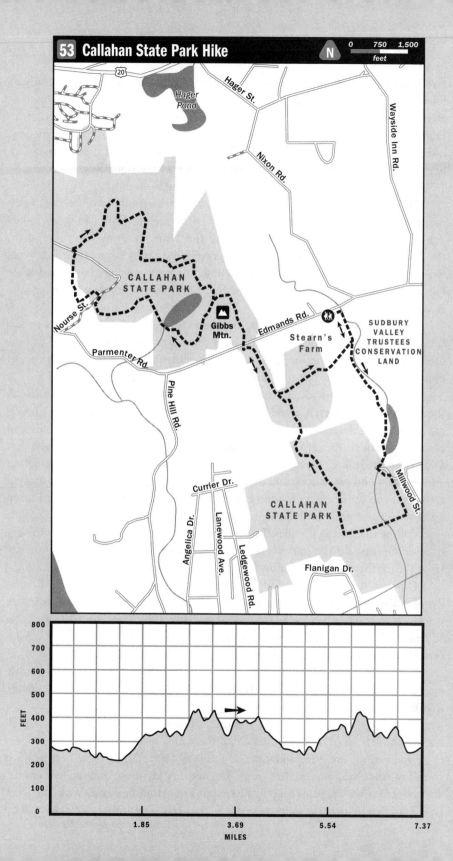

Further, by way of political savvy and hard work he expanded his father's relatively modest land holdings to more than 15,000 acres. Initially known as Danforth's Farm, Danforth eventually renamed his property Framingham after Framingham, England. Recognizing the futility of attempting to tend his vast holdings alone, Danforth recruited people to help by allowing them to establish homesteads and to cultivate the land rent free for a prescribed length of time. By 1699, on Danforth's death, Framingham supported 70 families.

From the parking area at Stearns Farm, locate the trailhead by hiking northeast past greenhouses, tool sheds, and an herb garden to find a Sudbury Valley Trustees' kiosk under trees on the edge of the farm. Entering from the north, the Bay Circuit Trail carries on its way, traveling directly south from Edmands Road along a centuries-old cart road. Follow this route past aged oaks and other hardwoods as the road parts cultivated fields and horse pasture making its way to woods.

Seepage from brooks threading through the area makes for muddy conditions as the trail leaves cleared land. The first junction comes beyond a footbridge. Here the Bay Circuit Trail swings decidedly right on a westward run, but quit this trail and bear left to continue south.

Cutting a 5-foot-wide swath through hemlocks clutching at a rocky hillside, the trail rises on an even grade above a sunken floodplain to the east. Various paths divert to the left or right from this main trail, but resist their pull and continue south to Packard Pond. At the three-way intersection ahead, bear left away from the hill. Crossing a brook via a small footbridge, the trail bears left at another split and passes a farmhouse. Unkempt orchard follows next, and beyond feral fruit trees tangled with bittersweet and brambles, the trail gains definition upon reaching a great undulating meadow tamed by regular mowing.

Follow the trail as it scales the hillside next to woods to arrive at a four-way intersection just off the park's south entrance and parking lot. Bear right away from the earthen dam and follow Moore Road downhill into a verdant basin.

Dipping to its lowest point, this no-nonsense gravel road meets Baiting Brook then cuts a straight line past Eagle Pond and open meadow to enter woods. Immediately after a boardwalk across a muddy zone, the trail splits at a V. Bear right here and hike north beneath tree cover along the edge of the adjacent meadow on the Juniper Trail.

Beyond a bridge spanning a brook that feeds into Eagle Pond, the liberally marked Deer Run Trail bears gently left. Its dual blazes (blue and red) indicate that both hikers and equestrians are welcome.

Traveling over level ground, the trail passes through woods that, though not completely devoid of hardwoods, are by and large composed of pine—a clear indication that the landscape is reforested farmland. Now and again a strand of stone wall materializes amid the maze of standing and fallen trunks.

Shortly after encountering the Fox Hunt Trail running east to west, the Deer Run Trail briefly departs state-owned land and crosses another parcel owned by

A gardener tends an herb garden at Sterns' Farm.

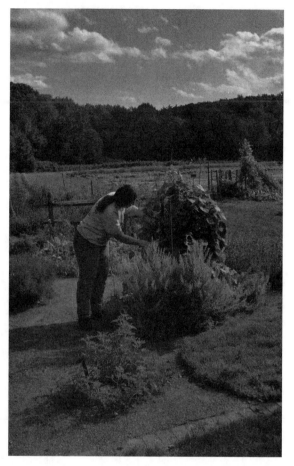

the Sudbury Valley Trustees. Here a sign informs hikers that, because of wear and tear, the trail has been temporarily rerouted.

Laid out by Eagle Scouts assisting in the restoration project, the detour through red maple wetland is clear and short. A hundred yards or so along, the new route ties in with the end of the old Deer Run Trail where a sign marks the start of the Rocky Road, a path that appears to split left and right. To shorten the hike by half, hike to the right on the true Rocky Road Trail, which travels 0.3 miles back to Stearns Farm. Otherwise, stay to the left, heading northwest on what, farther on, is identified as the Red Tail Trail.

Traveling across a drumlin's gritty slope, the trail descends, swings west on a hairpin turn, then converges with the Bay Circuit Trail entering from the east. Continuing straight, the Red Tail Trail passes private property on upland to the west as it crosses level ground to reach a gate at Edmand's Road.

From this understated entrance–exit equipped with little but a sign asserting the park's rules and regulations, stride across the two lanes of pavement to a weed-filled field lying at the foot of a farmhouse. Look for the white blazes of the Bay Circuit Trail and a small sign bearing the silhouette of a backpacker, and follow the lightly etched trail as it curves west to the foot of Gibbs Mountain.

Where marauding bittersweet backs away from the hill and its front of granite, a state park sign lends a smidgen of comfort to the austere start of Backpacker Trail. Taking the mountain straight on, the trail ascends steeply at first then eases as it winds northeast on a horizontal plane, allowing hikers to take in the setting and its natural history.

St. John's wort, mushrooms of the amanita family, and sassafras thrive on

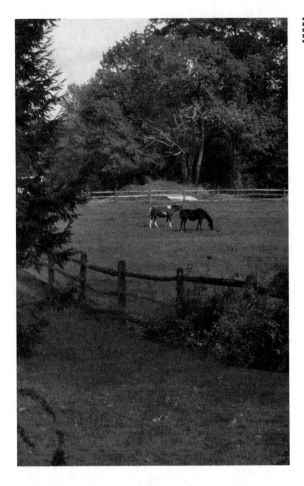

Horses graze on a neighboring farm.

the sidelines in the spotty sunlight, each translating energy and nutrients into distinct and powerful chains of DNA. St. John's wort heals, the destroying angel (*Amanita virosa*) kills—and sassafras makes a lovely tea.

Whereas the scent of cows wafts on the air in parts of the park's more pastoral south side, the air of this—the distinctly wilder north side—carries not-so-subtle hints of carnivore musk: a blend of skunk, fisher, opossum, fox, and coyote, with a dash of bobcat.

Making its way downhill, the trail passes first a path to the left and then one to the right; note these but stay on course with the Bay Circuit Trail, which, at the second junction, bears left to round the mountain's northern face. At the next intersection, which is poorly marked, the Bay Circuit Trail bears right to descend farther off the mountain. The seemingly more pronounced trail continues straight. Choose either route—they meet again farther on. To continue the hike as mapped, leave Bay Circuit Trail temporarily and bear left to travel south.

Just beyond a path cascading down a slope to the left, the trail arrives at a field. Climb along the narrow, lightly trodden route as it circumnavigates this grassland, first climbing to its high point then easing off to its western wooded border. At first glance this peaceful spot seems bereft of any living soul, which is quite to the liking of the bobolinks, bluebirds, goldfinches, and turkeys in residence.

When the path loops back north meeting the Bay Circuit Trail at a T, bear left, continuing westward. At the foot of a gravelly banking, the trail meets Beebe Pond, a picturesque glacial kettle hole neatly hidden among maples. Cross a causeway lined with hemlocks to reach a junction on the northwest side of the pond. Here, both the Bay Circuit Trail's white blazes and the park's blue markers lead uphill to the left.

Leveling off in a pine stand above the pond, the trail splits through one stone wall then tracks another out of the woods to a meadow. Hike left with confidence, despite a near-total absence of markers, and travel west along the meadow's fringe. When the sunny grassland meets woods once more, follow as the trail leads down a gentle grade and corrects its course at a hairpin turn.

Spilling into a stone-wall avenue, the trail soon meets with the stark path of a power line. Jogging left here for no more than a moment, the route then exits to the north through another stone wall at the next immediate right. Until this junction, Bear Paw Trail (blue) and the Bay Circuit Trail travel as one, but here they part ways. Forgo the path bearing abruptly left; its destination is the distant Duxbury shore. Instead follow the path heading north, marked with a blue bear claw.

Easing down a slope riddled with stones and roots, the trail soon comes to an end at an unpaved service road. Continue across on a diagonal aiming westward to pick up Acorn Trail. Don't look for a sign of any kind, for there is none—not for several hundred yards whereupon the trail is identified with a simple marker bearing a blue acorn.

Etching a thin line between a rugged rocky slope and wetland as it heads north briefly on its eastward course, the trail passes under boughs of white pine, oaks, maples, and hickories. The ample dog-ear leaves of sassafras saplings stir on the slightest breeze. Luxuriant ferns lace the air with the scent of baking oatmeal bread—or so says the nose of a hungry hiker.

Turning uphill to skirt swamp, Acorn Trail collides with Backpacker Trail. Bear right at this precarious junction and retreat downhill and across a stream. After some loopy turns, the trail straightens and travels south beside a stone wall. Tacking to the east, Backpacker Trail then passes through a lumber tract. The hardwoods were harvested long ago and replaced by fast-growing pines.

After threading through an abandoned homestead marked by fragments of stone walls and a cellar hole, the trail climbs the slope of an oblong drumlin lying crossways to the border of Framingham and Marlboro. Encountering an old north–south cart road on this hill of packed sand and gravel, Backpacker Trail accompanies it south briefly then departs east. Several undulations later it arrives at another junction at the base of Gibbs Mountain.

Having completed a loop, hike left to backtrack over Gibbs Mountain and Edmands Road to the park's south side. Follow Red-Tailed Trail to the first junction and bear left onto Wren Trail (which serves as a section of the Bay Circuit Trail). Running east across a hillside, the trail passes several ghostly birches standing like beacons among the warm gray trunks of hardwoods.

Two more junctions break the rhythm, but stay on course with the Bay Circuit Trail to head east. At the second junction, where the route is splintered by the Pipeline Trail, hike uphill several feet to find the way marked by a white

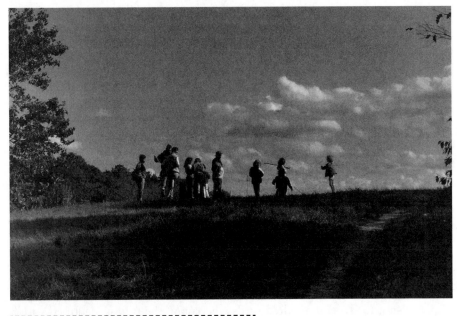

The southeast side of the park has many rolling fields.

triangle. The last stretch is sketchy but short. At the final junction, bear left and follow white blazes back to Stearns Farm.

NEARBY ATTRACTIONS

Those making a weekend of it might like to visit the nearby Danforth Museum of Art. The museum is located at 123 Union Avenue in Framingham and is open Sunday, Wednesday, and Thursday, noon to 5 p.m., and Friday and Saturday, 10 a.m. to 5 p.m. For more information, call (508) 620-0050.

MEMORIAL RESERVATION HIKE 54

IN BRIEF

Thanks to a glacier that left deep deposits of sand on the area, much of the land included in the Memorial Forest Reservation was once deemed close to worthless. Knowing better than to wrestle nature for no reward, would-be farmers turned their backs and left the forests of pitch pine and scrub oak as they remain today.

DESCRIPTION

To a Boston filmmaker out scouting locations for a spaghetti Western, finding the Memorial Forest Reservation and Desert Natural Area would be an incredible stroke of luck. Though short of cactuses, a saloon, and a sheriff's office, the location—with its scrub oak, pitch pine, and acres of sandy desert—certainly has the look of Billy the Kid's remote hideaway.

 Predictably, the reservation's unusual landscape is the handiwork of epochs of glacial action. Ages ago much of the area lay at the bottom of the now extinct Lake Sudbury. After the last glacier ceased advancing and retreated northward, leaving meltwater in its wake, filings of bedrock washed into

---

Directions

From Boston, take Interstate 90 west 11.4 miles to Exit 15; bear left toward MA 30. Turn right onto Park Road then left onto South Avenue. South Avenue becomes Highland Street. Continue 1.3 miles and turn left onto Love Lane then left onto US 20 toward Waltham/ Weston. Turn right onto Peakham Road. After 0.4 miles turn left onto Old Garrison Road. At 0.1 mile turn left onto French Road, then after 0.5 miles turn right onto Dutton Road; continue to the parking lot on the right.

ⓘ KEY AT-A-GLANCE INFORMATION

LENGTH: 5.59 miles

CONFIGURATION: Double loop

DIFFICULTY: Easy to moderate

SCENERY: Wetlands, wildlife pond, pitch-pine forest, and sandy "beaches" composed of glacial sediment that settled at the bottom of a lake created by glacial meltwater

EXPOSURE: Mostly shaded

TRAFFIC: Moderate

TRAIL SURFACE: Packed earth, sand

HIKING TIME: 3–3.5 hours

SEASON: Year-round sunrise–sunset

ACCESS: Free

MAPS: Available at www.sudbury valleytrustees.org and at www.marlborough-ma.gov

FACILITIES: None

SPECIAL COMMENTS: Those wishing to hear a whippoorwill will be glad to know that overnight camping is allowed at Hop Brook Marsh in Sudbury. The permit required can be obtained from the Sudbury town clerk or the Sudbury Conservation Commission. Contact Town Hall at 322 Concord Road, Sudbury, MA 01776; (978) 639-3351.

WHEELCHAIR TRAVERSABLE: No

DRIVING DISTANCE FROM BOSTON COMMON: 28 miles

Memorial
Reservation Hike
UTM Zone (WGS84) 19T
Easting: 297262
Northing: 4693952
Latitude: N 42° 22' 17"
Longitude: W 71° 27' 44"

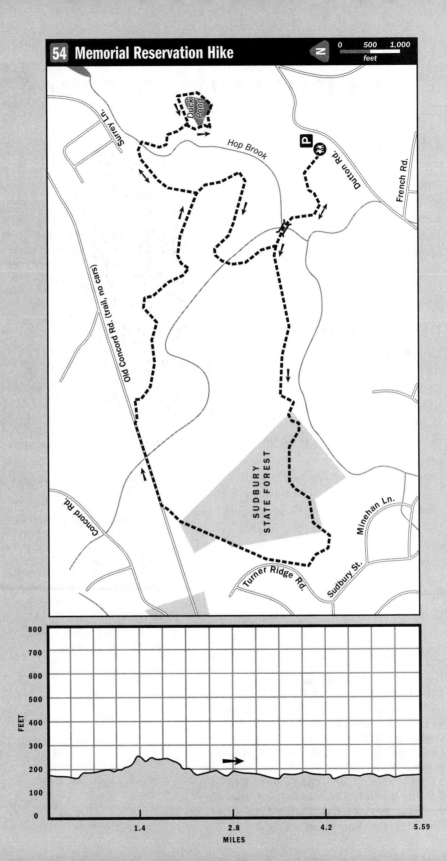

54 Memorial Reservation Hike

0   500   1,000
feet

N

Surrey Ln.

Duck Pond

Hop Brook

P

Dutton Rd.

French Rd.

Old Concord Rd. (trail, no cars)

SUDBURY STATE FOREST

Concord Rd.

Minehan Ln.

Turner Ridge Rd.

Sudbury St.

800

700

600

500

FEET

400

300

200

100

0

1.4   2.8   4.2   5.59

MILES

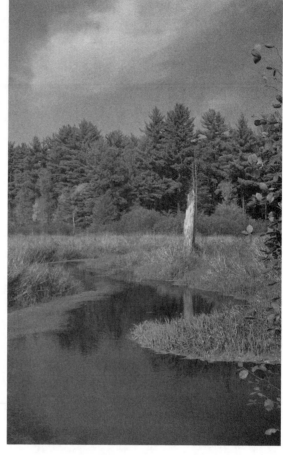

A footbridge across Hop Brook offers a spectacular view.

low-lying pockets, and was then buried as the water collected and deepened. The lake has long since vanished, but some of the glacial waters remain as swampland on the lake's poorly drained edges.

Just as Nevada and New Mexico have failed to attract farmers bent on profiting from hay or corn crops, so these sandy acres have been spurned by farmers or settlers of any kind (until suburbia crept in). Consequently, the land is comparatively free of the effects of human progress.

This being the case, it is particularly remarkable that much of Memorial Reservation was once owned by one of America's greatest industrialists—Henry Ford, who bought much of the land abutting the western Sudbury border in the 1930s. Investing time and energy in the property for nearly 20 years, Ford renovated a house and outbuildings that had belonged to the previous owner, before tossing in the towel and selling the property to the General Federation of Women's Clubs in 1950. The depth of Ford's commitment to the place was such that, when he picked up camp, his house was removed to the Greenfield Village Museum in Dearborn, Michigan.

The hike begins at the trailhead beside the kiosk situated just west of the parking lot. Taking the long way around a complex of buildings belonging to the Federation of Women's Clubs, the trail leads through a pine stand flush to wetland to reach a footbridge spanning Hop Brook. A superb gateway to the reservation, this bridge offers views north and south of a magnificent riparian landscape animated in all spheres by brook fish, flashy dragons and damselflies, flycatchers, kingfishers, and countless other fabulous creatures.

From the bridge, the trail continues westward across the mud zone emanating from Hop Brook to reach the dry footing of a moraine—a mound of debris

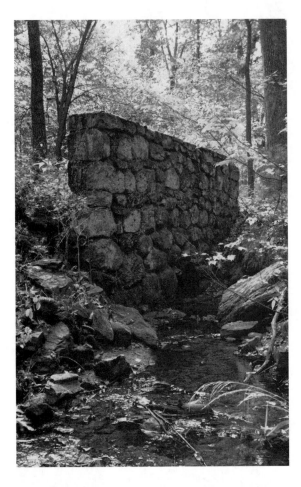

shed from the glacier as it shrank northward. At the two-way intersection marked "J" at the base of the slope, stay left to hike over the rise via the Plympton Trail (named for Thomas Plympton, the man who built the house that Ford's people had shipped to Dearborn).

Continuing west, the trail leads to junction K, where Ocean Bypass Trail offers an opportunity to hike clear across what were once the lowest depths of Lake Sudbury. But for a full tour of the reservation stay with the Plympton Trail, which before long meets an esker cut by a gas line. Here follow the trail as it jogs to the left, runs along the ridge of gravel (left from a stream running beneath glacial ice) then hikes right and eases north to junction L. Shadowing the Ocean Bypass Trail, this route runs straight to the northern border of the reservation.

If choosing to forgo this shortcut, bear left onto Sedge Hollow Link. This brief trail connects the former Ford parcel to the state-owned Marlborough State Forest. At junction M, where the link joins the Hanson Trail, bear right, away from the red maple swamp of Trout Brook.

Although still distinctly sandy underfoot, Marlborough State Forest is a good deal less austere than the central portion of the property, known to locals as "The Ocean," and its northern reaches. As the Hanson Trail continues farther west, the earth becomes more fertile. On what was once the outskirts of Lake Sudbury, glacial till (a mix of clay, sand, and gravel collected over drumlins and ledge) supports a vigorous oak forest and, best of all, an understory of low-bush blueberry and huckleberry. In turn, the abundance of acorns, pine cones, succulent berries, and peaceful acres supports a wide variety of birds, including scarlet tanagers, hermit thrushes, ovenbirds, and ruffed grouse, all favoring distinct niches. While edge habitats near brooks appeal to warblers, bluebirds and whippoorwills prefer Thomas Plympton's hard-won meadows.

A lively assortment of fur-bearing animals lives here as well. Think twice about dog footprints you may find in the sand; they are just as likely those of a brainy coyote as those of a tail-wagging Labrador. In addition to skunks, raccoons, and opossums, fisher cats are no strangers to these woods. Deer the color of spent pine needles and sand are never far away.

At junction N, a route with the intriguing name of the Witches' Cove Trail departs to the right, aiming for a vernal pool fed by spilloff from "the Ocean." The Hanson Trail broadens the tour by dipping south then climbing north along the reservation's border to junction O, where once again it converges with the Witches' Cove Trail.

Ahead, junction A marks where the Hanson Trail joins Old Concord Road—a horse and oxcart throughway of bygone days. Taking up this new route, bear right and hike northeast on a beeline to cross Cranberry Brook, not once but twice. The first crossing is by way of a massive stone bridge just off Hanson Trail, the next via a causeway just a hair beyond where the Plympton Trail emerges, at junction B. Here enterprising beavers have transformed the trickling brook to a swollen marshland alive with birds, hovering odonates (dragonflies and damselflies), and many glistening—and not so glistening— amphibians. Resident snapping turtles spend much of their lives submerged in mud, water, and weeds, but once a year females travel to the nearby sandpits to lay large clutches of eggs.

The two trails that split off from Old Concord Road up ahead offer markedly different hiking experiences. The first, the Cranberry Brook Trail, encountered at junction C, travels through a riparian ecosystem; the second, Desert Trail, bears east at junction D and transports hikers as if by magic to a dry landscape of sand and dunes.

For the sake of taking in one of Massachusetts's most unusual places, head onward to Desert Trail. Once you are across the northern end of the gas line, the ground grows increasingly sandy. The trail swings north, then south again as it opens to a great circular beach with an island of pitch pine in the center.

From this disorienting location, where rule-breaking dirt-bike riders leave deeply carved doughnuts when no one is watching, hike farther east to find a reassuring Sudbury Valley Trustees (SVT) trail marker. Continuing through woods of pitch pine and scrub oak, the Desert Trail splits in two at junction G to become the Desert Loop. To witness another startling transformation, bear left.

Arcing eastward over flat ground that glows orange when the afternoon light rests on fallen pine needles, the trail reaches junction H, which presents a link to Hop Brook Marsh. Duck between close-growing pines to find the rusted tracks of an abandoned railroad piercing the sand.

Beyond the railroad, conditions morph from parched to lush in remarkably few footsteps. Soon after bearing left at a fork, the trail finds itself on a bridge straddling spongy land—or "beaver meadow"—cleaved down the middle by Hop Brook.

A lovely pond created by a former owner of the Sudbury Rod and Gun Club lies close by. To find it bear right at the junction on the sandy slope ahead and cross to the east side of Hop Brook. Following the Ridge Trail south above the wetland, bear right at the second junction. In a moment the trail arrives at a V, where the trail splits to embrace Duck Pond.

To circle the pond counterclockwise, choose the path to the right. Fluctuating conditions make for a somewhat sketchy route; however, the path never wanders more than a few feet from the water's edge. On the pond's north side, the trail veers wide to meet other trails, but stay left to complete a full circle.

Leaving this picturesque spot, retrace your steps to the Desert Loop at junction H. Setting off again over new ground, bear left to arrive at an old sandpit. Thanks to work crews of the Sudbury Valley Trustees and others, this one-time graveyard of discarded, stolen cars and other illicit junk is now a nearly immaculate expanse of sand.

Staying on track with the help of SVT markers, continue over undulating terrain following the trail east until it approaches the marshes of Hop Brook and winds south. Quitting its brookside tangent, the trail makes a bold turn west and shoots up a gentle incline to junction I. Turn left here and ease downhill to an abbreviated boardwalk to cross the vibrant floodplain of Cranberry Brook. Climbing the swell of the upland opposite, the trail soon jogs east to meet the Plympton Trail at junction J. Back at a familiar location, turn left and follow the trail to its end beside the parking lot.

NEARBY ATTRACTIONS

No visit to the area is complete without a meal or stay-over at the historic Wayside Inn (72 Wayside Inn Road, Sudbury, MA 01776; [978] 443-1776, toll-free [800] 339-1776; fax [978] 443-8041). Operated as a "house of entertainment" from 1716 to 1861 by its first owner, David Howe, the inn was renamed by its third owner, Edward Rivers Lemon, to capitalize on the success of Henry Longfellow's book of poems titled *Tales of a Wayside Inn,* published in 1863. Longfellow visited Howe's Inn in 1862 and based many of his characters on the inn's colorful proprietor and patrons. In 1923 Cora Lemon sold the inn to Henry Ford.

WATERS FARM LOOP

IN BRIEF

Sutton is a quiet town that strives to protect its heritage as a vibrant agricultural community as it welcomes newcomers drawn to its rural appeal. On this hike you will follow paths through woods known by the Nipmuc before the arrival of colonists who felled the trees to make way for livestock and apple orchards. Sights along the way include the magnificent Manchaug Pond and historic Waters Farm, which is listed on the National Register of Historic Places and actively managed to provide visitors a glimpse of life on a 19th-century New England farm.

DESCRIPTION

In 1673, after surveying the more than 20 "Praying Indian Towns" established in the Massachusetts Colony by his initiative, the Reverend John Eliot said of Hassanamesit, then lying in what is now Sutton, "No Indian town [gives] stronger assurances of success than this [at this time]. Hassanamesit [has] become the central point of civilization and

---

Directions ⟶

From Boston, take Interstate 90 west via the exit on the left toward New York. Portions of this road require you pay a toll. Drive 33 miles then take Exit 10 toward MA 12. After 0.6 miles take the exit on the left toward I-290. Drive 0.1 mile then take the I-290 exit on the left toward Worcester. After 0.2 miles merge onto I-395 south toward Norwich, CT. Drive 5.2 miles, merge onto Sutton Avenue via Exit 4A toward Sutton, and drive 32 miles; there will be a white Baptist church on the right. Take the first right after the church onto Douglas Road. Proceed about 0.3 miles to Waters Farm on the left.

Waters Farm Loop

UTM Zone (WGS84) 19T

Easting: 269393

Northing: 4665432

Latitude: N 42° 06' 26"

Longitude: W 71° 47' 21"

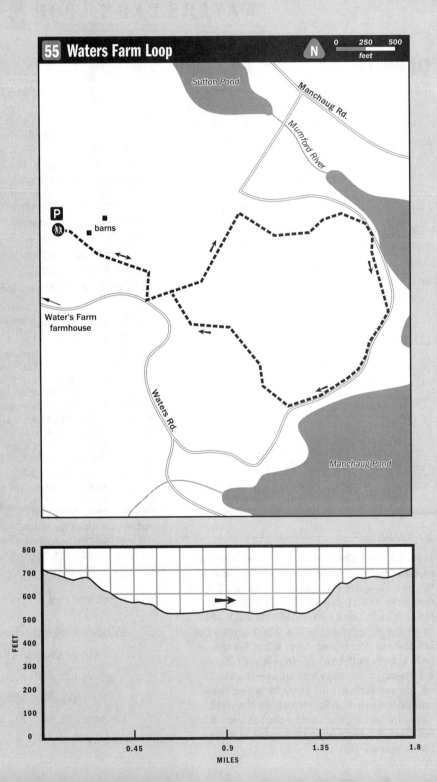

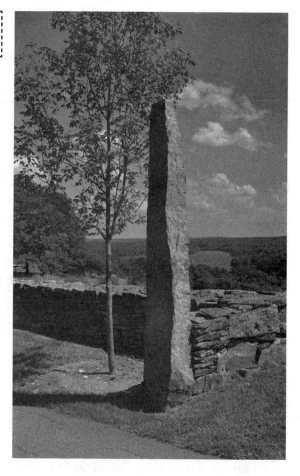

A view of Manchaug Pond looking south from the Waters Farm homestead

Christianity to the whole Nipmuc country."

Though Eliot's words sound sadly naive in hindsight, the reverend was far from ill-informed when uttering them. He was then 69 years old and a resident of Roxbury, Massachusetts, for 42 years. He had long since demonstrated his commitment to bringing God's word to the Algonquin people by mastering the Algonquin language in order to convey God's word to the people directly. Astonishingly the first book to be published in America was Eliot's full translation of the Bible into Algonquin. As his efforts prove, Eliot dearly hoped that all Indians would be converted or "saved" by Christianity. But though it is certain that Eliot was a true man of peace and sought harmony between the natives and the colonists, not all his supporters shared his altruism. Many who feared the Algonquin saw tactical sense in establishing "friendly" Indian towns in an arc around the colony since these could serve as a first line of defense in the event of attack.

Two years after Eliot's optimistic report on Hassanamesit, King Philip, the son of the Wampanoag Sachem, Massasoit, who had helped the Puritans through their first winter in Plymouth in 1620, declared war on the colonists. The year- long conflict left many settlement towns burned to the ground, King Philip dead, and most surviving Praying Indians exiled to Deer Island in Boston Harbor. Twenty-nine years later John Wampus, a Nipmuc Indian living on Boston Common, sold 8 square miles of land to a group intent on settling what was to become the Township of Sutton.

When Stephen Waters established his family's homestead on the hill beside Manchaug Pond in 1757, Sutton was on its way to becoming a thriving agricultural community. Producing apples and other goods, the Waters family

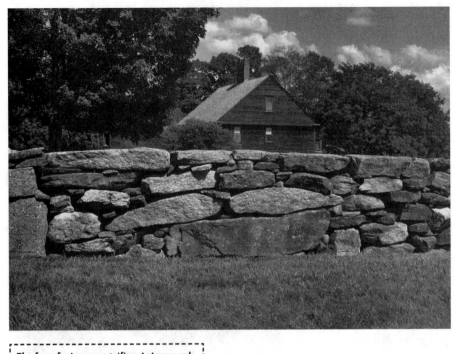

The farm features magnificent stone work.

prospered from one generation and century to the next. The Waters' remarkable enterprise finally came to an end in 1974 when Dorothea Waters Moran gave her family's 120-acre farm to the town of Sutton, 217 years after Stephen Waters first walked its ground.

Setting out from the parking area in front of the Darling Barn, hike downhill past a big red bell to a yard littered with antique farm equipment, following the gravel drive as it sweeps to the right into shade cast by overarching oaks and hickories. A house behind a meadow lies off to the right, and straight ahead is a new though rough-hewn barn. An arrow points southeast, toward the Al Beaton Trail, identified with blue markers. Here the surface of the drive changes from gravel to packed dirt. Curving southward, the path passes a curious sunken paddock fenced in by rock face on one side and stone wall on each of the others. Perhaps in farming days of old, this enclosure held a team of off-duty draft horses, or perhaps a prize bull.

Ahead you'll see a paved road on the right, but heed the arrows pointing left and follow the dirt path as it winds into woods. Shortly, the Al Beaton Trail, now identified by orange and white markers, splits off to the right, but continue straight on what is called Off the Beaton Trail, traveling gently downhill. Formerly a service road used by teams of horses and, later, tractors, this wide route now accommodates hikers, bikers, horseback riders, snowshoers, and cross-country skiers.

Farther on, the trail passes a second trail splitting off to the right. Marked informally with a pink ribbon, this trail—as of this writing—is not yet fully cleared. Regardless, stay with Off the Beaton Trail, which cuts a steeper grade as it heads northeast. After passing another trail, this one marked with white, Off the Beaton Trail arrives at a route identified with two yellow triangles posted on a birch tree. Turn right at this intersection and continue on this new trail hiking southeast.

On the August day that I passed through, the trail was somewhat rough and muddy in places, but thanks to an enthusiastic group of Boy Scouts at work clearing debris, its condition will soon be much improved. Continuing downhill, with upland to the right, the trail runs through farmland reclaimed by woods now dominated by substantial oaks. Reaching the bottom of the hill, Off the Beaton Trail merges with another route, Shore Road, which runs flush to a northwestern finger of Manchaug Pond. Continue to the right, hiking south on level ground. A large but peaceful camp is situated on the bank opposite. Power-boats and canoes are tied up to docks in this sheltered inlet that represents only a tiny portion of the 350-acre pond. As I paused to look across, a mixed flock of chickadees, least flycatchers, and a lone catbird struck up a racket as my rat terrier sniffed the whereabouts of red squirrels and chipmunks.

Making its way up a slight hill, Shore Road provides a steady view of Man-chaug's broad expanse. Big enough to have sizable islands, and whitecaps on a breezy day, Manchaug plunges 30 feet at its deepest point. Settling to level ground, the trail continues along the water, ducking behind groves of trees. Reaching a V-intersection, Shore Road travels away from the pond; the path splintering left leads to a spit of land with a wooden fishing pier built on its end. Stay on Shore Road to pass yet another trail, this one diverting to the right and marked with white. Ahead where the trail splits once more, an unmarked path traipses left toward the pond; the other, marked with a red square, lists south-west toward high ground.

In summer it's foolish to resist the lure of Manchaug's deliciously warm water, so venture down trails such as the one to the left and shed at least shoes and socks to dip your feet, or better yet, to dive right in. The rental cottage equipped with a 20- to 30-foot dock at the end of the path will likely spark thoughts of arranging an extended stay.

After enjoying the pleasures of the setting, take up the trail marked with red, following it past a horse jump on the right and a rustic camp with a picnic table on the left. Easing downhill, the trail soon meets a route, marked with pink and white diamonds, that splits off perpendicular to the pond. Turn off here to climb northwest along this winding path through scraggly brush grown in since the Waters family ceased active farming. Private individuals and Boy Scouts forged these trails and maintain them on a volunteer basis.

Continuing on its northwest course up the granite-littered hill ornamented with native laurels, the path intersects the double-white-diamond trail that climbs

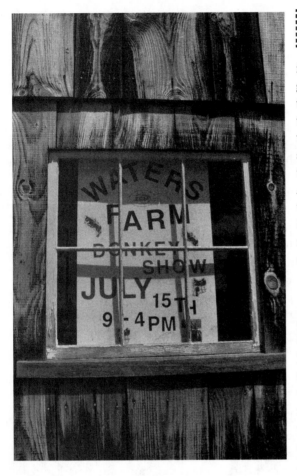

Each July Waters Farm hosts a donkey show.

farther to a broad convergence of trails. At this junction, bear left to follow the trail marked with blue and white. Hiking westward and still gaining elevation, this trail soon forms a "T" with Al Beaton Trail (marked with orange and white). Bear right onto this familiar route to return to the yard of the Darling barn.

NEARBY ATTRACTIONS

One look across Manchaug Pond will make anyone wish for more time in this wonderful place. To avoid regrets, plan to spend more than just an afternoon in the area. King's Campground, located directly on Manchaug Pond, accommodates all styles of camping including RV, camping trailer, pop-up camper, or tent. The campground has a well-stocked country store, which in addition to groceries sells housewares, beach toys, and live bait (24 Holt Road, Sutton; [508] 476-2534 or [877] 279-3206; www.kingscampground.com).

From I-395 take Exit 4A (Sutton Avenue) and go 3.2 miles. Take a right turn on Manchaug Road. Go 3 miles keeping to the right. After a dam go right on Holt Road. Go 0.25 miles to King's Campground.

BLACKSTONE RIVER AND CANAL HIKE

IN BRIEF

On this hike you will explore the Blackstone Canal following it lock by lock through tangled woods, feral meadows, and preserved farmland to the site of the recently reclaimed Stanley Woolen Mill.

DESCRIPTION

Late in the 1700s, John Brown, an industrious businessman of the family for whom Brown University is named, conceived of the idea to build a canal along the Blackstone River. Such a watercourse, he believed, would facilitate the passage of goods from the port of Providence, Rhode Island, to landlocked settlements in New England's interior. But although he handily won the backing of Rhode Island merchants, Boston businessmen fearful of competition shot the plan down.

Thirty-years later however, another wealthy Providence merchant, General Edward Carrington, made good on Brown's vision by leading a successful campaign to have the canal built. Shipping goods over land via the few, often inadequate, roads remained slow and costly. One ton of freight could be shipped to England for the cost to send it 30 miles over land. A great public works project, the building of the canal employed thousands of workers. Over the course of four frost-free seasons, men shoveled dawn to dusk six days a week to finish the job for a monthly paycheck

KEY AT-A-GLANCE INFORMATION

LENGTH: 7.4 miles

CONFIGURATION: Out-and-back

DIFFICULTY: Easy

SCENERY: The historic Blackstone Canal, with views of the River Bend Farm and the Stanley Woolen Mill

EXPOSURE: Mostly shaded

TRAFFIC: Light

TRAIL SURFACE: Packed earth and grass

HIKING TIME: 3–3.5 hours

SEASON: Year-round 8 a.m.–sunset

ACCESS: Free

MAPS: Posted at the entrance, also available at the visitor center at River Bend Farm

FACILITIES: Visitor center, restrooms, and picnic tables with grills at River Bend Farm

SPECIAL COMMENTS: Hiking is allowed in hunting season, except on Sundays. Those hiking through during hunting season are advised to wear orange reflective vests.

WHEELCHAIR TRAVERSABLE: A 0.6-mile portion of the trail from River Bend Farm to the Stanley Woolen Mill is wheelchair accessible.

DRIVING DISTANCE FROM BOSTON COMMON: 33 miles

Directions ⟶

From Boston, take Interstate 90 west to Exit 11. Turn right onto MA 122 south to Grafton. Drive 10.3 miles on MA 122 south to a light. Turn left onto Church Street. Continue 0.4 miles to the parking lot at Plummer's Landing.

Blackstone River and Canal Hike

UTM Zone (WGS84) 19T

Easting: 281902

Northing: 4667383

Latitude: N 42° 07' 40"

Longitude: W 71° 38' 20"

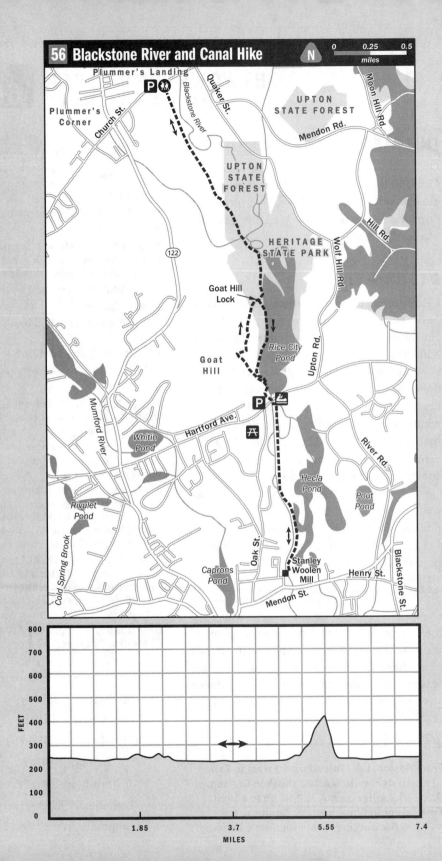

N

0   0.25   0.5
miles

Plummer's Landing

Plummer's
Corner

Church St.

Quaker St.

Blackstone River

Moon Hill Rd.

**UPTON
STATE FOREST**

Mendon Rd.

Hill Rd.

**UPTON
STATE
FOREST**

Wolf Hill Rd.

**HERITAGE
STATE PARK**

122

Goat Hill
Lock

Rice City
Pond

Upton Rd.

Goat
Hill

Hartford Ave.

Mumford River

Whitin
Pond

River Rd.

Hecla
Pond

Pout
Pond

Rivulet
Pond

Cold Spring Brook

Oak St.

Caprons
Pond

Stanley
Woolen
Mill

Henry St.

Blackstone St.

Mendon St.

FEET

800
700
600
500
400
300
200
100
0

1.85   3.7   5.55   7.4

MILES

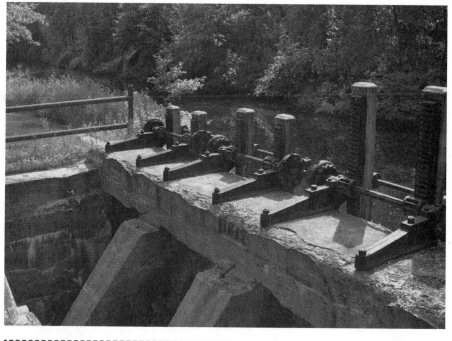

The mechanics of a lock as viewed from the trail

of $26. Much to General Carrington's satisfaction, the canal, once operational, immediately began to repay its $750,000 price tag. Barge transport up the 45-mile canal was 50 percent cheaper than shipment by horse-drawn wagons.

All was not entirely well, however. Drought, flooding, ice, and mill owners claiming infringement on their water rights made for less-than-smooth operations on the canal. In 1792 when John Brown first conceived of the canal project, there were many small gristmills along the river. But in 1793 Samuel Slater dramatically changed the tenor of life on the Blackstone when he established the first hydropowered cotton mill in the United States. Impressed by Slater's success, others soon followed suit, so that by 1800, Pawtucket, Rhode Island, alone boasted 29 cotton mills.

One of the many to take advantage of the opportunities the canal provided was a young man named Israel Plummer, who built a general store and warehouse beside a lock in 1837. Brilliantly located and managed, "Plummer's Landing" became a bustling business hub. When canal-based commerce dried up upon the establishment of the Providence–Worcester railroad line, Plummer adapted and not only survived but thrived by shifting his focus and shipping expertise from household goods to locally quarried granite. Plummer and his business are both now long gone, but the granite foundation stones of Plummer's buildings remain where they were laid well over a century and a half ago at what is now the trailhead of Towline Trail on the Blackstone Canal in Northbridge.

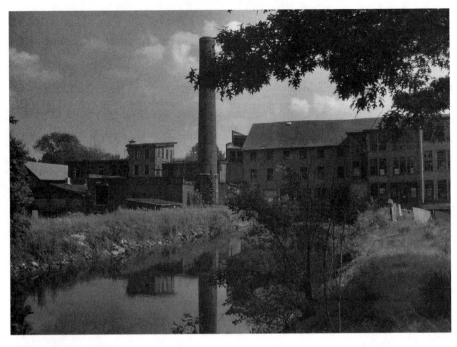

The Stanley Woolen Mill

The trail begins just beyond the parking lot to the left of the Blackstone Heritage Park sign. Follow the packed-earth path as it heads southeast along the canal. Trees have filled in between the canal and the Towline Trail, but when Plummer's Landing was open for business, draft horses in tandem hitch pulled boats loaded with as much as 40 tons of freight along this bank. Seen through tangled branches, the slow-moving, sometimes stagnant canal waters are the color of strong tea with a touch of milk added. The rushing water you hear is the freer-flowing Blackstone River that runs parallel to the canal's northern bank.

A short distance farther along a path crosses over Towline Trail, but continue straight. Though flooding or an occasional fallen tree may temporarily alter the path, there's no getting lost as it shadows the canal. As you continue on the woods to the right give way to wetland. Here and in other parts, the towpath functions as a causeway elevating you above water on either side. Breeding grounds for an array of insects and amphibians, the waterway's ecosystem also includes a wonderful variety of birds. Along with throngs of robins and catbirds, you may see a muscular kingfisher dash by. In June, dragonflies and damselflies dart about like winged jewels. Stunning iridescent aquamarine and ebony jewelwings (*Calopteryx maculat*) flit about over the canal and alight on leaves and logs.

After running tight with the river for a stretch, the trail swings to the right to pass through a small meadow. A remnant of farming days, this shrinking patch of grassland is now giving way to wildflowers and shrubs. Sweet pea, vetch, tansy, and milkweed bloom in this sunny spot. Before rejoining the river, the trail crosses a tributary by way of a short, elevated boardwalk. Farther on the trail turns east to cross a small dam. From here the causeway between the river and the canal becomes more pronounced as it straightens again on a southeastward course.

Well maintained by work crews, the trail varies from packed soil to gravel brought in to add reinforcement after washouts. The day my partner and I hiked through, we noticed an entire wooden footbridge hanging precariously from trees on the opposite riverbank after it was washed there by especially heavy spring rains. A few yards later we found the void left in the trail and had to backtrack to a detour of half-submerged logs.

Once past this section where the Blackstone runs particularly fast and strong, Towline Trail splits from the river following the canal instead. Hickory, beech, and pine cast shade. Ferns, bamboo, and other wetland plant species conceal toads and baby snapping turtles.

Soon the trail bends to the left to meet the river's edge. Here you will notice big pieces of carved-out granite blocks. These are remnants of stone quarried to construct the canal's lock system. A few yards on, where the trail dead-ends upon reaching Rice Pond, you encounter lock 25 at Goat Hill. When boats still traveled on the canal an attendant would collect a toll and then, by opening and closing massive oak gates, adjust the water level to allow the boat to proceed to its north- or south-bound destination. To lift a boat past Goat Hill, the water level at lock 25 would be raised nearly 10 feet.

On the other side of the lock, the trail ascends to an intersection. Take the trail to the left and continue hiking along the bank of the river gaining elevation as you go. Soon you arrive at an imposing granite boulder to the right of the path. Stopping to look, you will notice stonecutters' tools stuck in a long crack at eye level. Apparently the rock refused to break according to the worker's plan and the wedges remain where they were driven.

Continuing on its southeastern trajectory, the trail undulates along in a cleft between the Blackstone wetlands and Goat Hill under a canopy of beech, oak, hickory, and pine. Looking down the banking to the left, you will see what was once a 100-acre storage pond for the Taft Central Mill, which later became the Stanley Woolen Mill. Dammed after the Blackstone Canal Company shut down, the waters covered the towline until a hurricane came through in 1955.

Ahead, Towline Trail meets another route coming down the hill to the right. On the left, a stone wall forms a clean 90-degree angle enclosing a meadow of bygone days now grown in. Just beyond here the trail leaves the woods and crosses a field to arrive at Hartford Avenue. Across to the right is a visitor center. As you make your way over this quiet road you can hear the water rushing through the remains of the mill owner's dam-control gate.

At the canoe landing on the eastern side of Hartford Avenue, pick up

Towline Trail again, and follow it as the river is diverted slightly northward. From here the towpath causeway is particularly pronounced as it approaches the bridge at River Bend Farm. Across the pond to the right sits an enormous red barn that once housed one of the largest dairy herds in the region. The farm started with its first herd of Holsteins before the Revolutionary War and carried on with descendants of those cows until 1974.

Continuing south from River Bend Farm to the trail's end at the Stanley Woolen Mill, there is an unmistakable change in the canal. After the Blackstone Canal Company shut down, the owner of the Stanley mill, Moses Taft, obtained water rights so that he might increase water flow to his machines. To accommodate the greater volume of water, the trench was deepened and its banks reinforced with rock.

After taking in the picturesque mill and reading the informational plaque posted at the trail's end, return to the towline path and retrace the trail back to Goat Hill. To vary your return trip, split from the towline path at Goat Hill and follow the trail northwest as it climbs to the left, away from the canal. Follow blue markers, continuing northwest to the top of the hill. Soon the trail turns due north and descends steeply, flush with a stone wall. Soon after reaching the stone wall's great end-stone, the trail arrives at a junction. Continue to the right and walk a short distance to find Goat Hill Lock. From here, follow the Towline Trail 1.7 miles back to Plummer's Landing.

PURGATORY CHASM HIKE

IN BRIEF

This hike takes the backdoor entrance to the spectacular Purgatory Chasm, explores the geologic curiosity from within, surveys the fissure from cliffs above, and explores the surrounding woods. Those interested in lengthier hikes can access the Sutton State Forest from linking trails.

DESCRIPTION

From the map and information board at the head of the parking lot, set out to the left, hiking southeast. Beyond a large sheltered picnic area and swing, you will find a short stretch of paved road leading to Charlie's Loop trailhead, named for Charles Gravlin, who oversaw care of the park for many years. Starting off wide and gravel-topped, this route passes under hemlocks as it rises and falls, twists and turns, then settles to level ground. Along the way a handful of paths split off to the right. The work of bushwhackers, these more than likely lead to the chasm. Try your luck with one if curiosity drives you, or stay on track to follow the faint yellow markers of Charlie's Loop.

Before long the trail makes a determined turn to the right and is met by another path. Continue northwest on Charlie's Loop along pancake-flat terrain passing numerous

KEY AT-A-GLANCE INFORMATION

LENGTH: 2.14 miles

CONFIGURATION: Loop

DIFFICULTY: Easy to extremely treacherous

SCENERY: Wooded trails, with views of a rugged chasm with cliffs as high as 70 feet

EXPOSURE: Mostly shaded

TRAFFIC: Light

TRAIL SURFACE: Packed earth, except inside the chasm, where the trail meanders over and between great slabs of stone

HIKING TIME: 1.5 hours

SEASON: Year-round sunrise–sunset

ACCESS: Free

MAPS: Posted near the parking lot and available at visitor center

FACILITIES: Restrooms at the park offices, picnic tables with grills

SPECIAL COMMENTS: Hikers are advised to wear rubber-soled shoes or hiking boots because the rocky path through the chasm is slippery.

WHEELCHAIR TRAVERSABLE: No

DRIVING DISTANCE FROM BOSTON COMMON: 48 miles

Directions

Take Interstate 90 west 39.8 miles to Exit 10A toward US 20 to Worcester. After 0.9 miles turn right and merge onto MA 146 south. After 7.1 miles take the Purgatory Road ramp toward Northbridge/Whitinsville. Just ahead take the Purgatory Road ramp toward Purgatory Chasm and bear right onto Purgatory Road. Parking is 0.8 miles ahead.

Purgatory Chasm Hike

UTM Zone (WGS84) 19T

Easting: 275586

Northing: 4667672

Latitude: N 42° 07' 45"

Longitude: W 71° 42' 54"

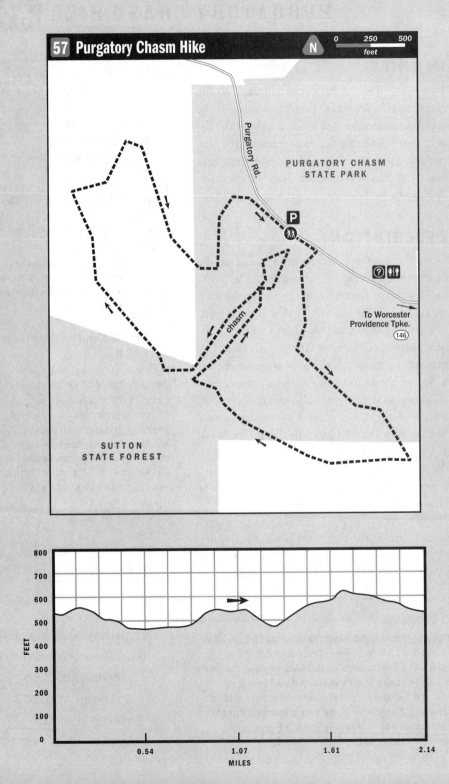

offshoots. Don't let the yellow markers at each of these paths mislead you: Charlie's Loop runs straight until it reaches a wide, open junction. Here a trail marked with blue continues straight while two other trails diverge right. Take the more extreme right and proceed on the gravel path that narrows quickly as it bends around a clutch of two-story-high boulders.

Accessing the chasm through this backdoor entrance feels like making a journey back in time. The benign woods through which the trail passes to reach this spot seem miles and ages away as monolithic chunks of rock bedecked with all manner of ancient ferns and mosses envelop you.

Some say that the chasm was formed by glacial action 14,000 years ago when geological movement let loose meltwater locked within bedrock. A folkloric legend attributes the enormous fissure to an incident involving the Native American devil, Hobomoko, and an unruly woman. But another intriguing notion is that the powerful earthquake that ripped across the land on November, 18, 1755, forged the chasm. Mr. Whitin, who previously owned the land, claimed that he discovered the fissure while out hunting in the days after the earthquake's tremors had subsided. Water trickling underfoot and over the giant stones littering the fissure's floor adds an element of excitement and danger since mosses and lichens slick with moisture make each step riskier than the one before.

A few yards ahead, the trail delivers you to the Devil's Coffin, a deep, dark void surrounded by slabs of dour quartz-freckled, feldspar-veined granite. Poke your head inside or pass quietly by, following the blue dashes of paint that indicate the recommended path to take over and between the chaos of stone.

Heading north, the crack in the earth deepens, its walls rising higher and higher until they reach 70 feet. Ancient pines thrusting skyward beside the rockface grow impossibly straight until they encounter stone buttresses jutting into their path, whereupon the trees engulf the granite or bend to it, protecting their heartwood with bulging bark calluses.

Halfway through the chasm, you come to the Devil's Pulpit, a rock formation favored by the many rock climbers who come to Purgatory Chasm in all seasons. Beyond the pulpit, a sign on the left alerts you to the heart-quickening cliff known since the very day of Custer's Last Stand as Lover's Leap. On this day in July 1876, Wesleyan University professor George Prentice and his wife came to this scenic spot to picnic. Before departing, Prentice's wife, tightly corseted despite the informal setting, strolled to the cliff's edge for a last look. Perhaps she caught a heel, or simply slipped—no one knows. But despite the official report, which asserted that she had been overcome by fumes, fainted, and fell to her death—historians believe it is more likely that her tight bodice was to blame. Regardless, two weeks later, Mrs. Prentice died of her injuries and shortly thereafter her greatly distraught husband, George Prentice, ended his life.

Just before arriving at the northern end of the chasm, the trail passes His Majesty's Cave. "His Majesty" may be an ogre, bear, or bat—it's up to anyone gutsy enough and equipped with a headlamp to say.

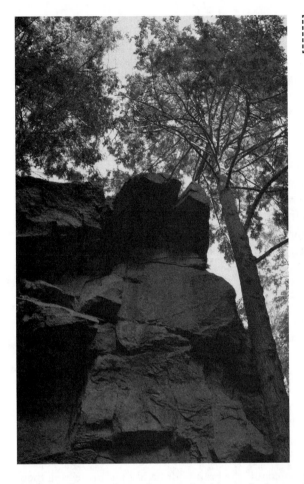

In 1865, word of a "huge beast" at the chasm compelled Henry David Thoreau to investigate. He traveled by horse cart many miles over rough roads to search the woods but found no hint of the fierce animal others had spoken of. Far from disappointed, Thoreau is said to have been charmed and delighted to find a nesting wood thrush.

Emerging from the chasm, you find yourself back at the park entrance. To continue your hike, turn left and look for a sign for Charlie's Loop. The trail travels west through sparse woods growing on the edge of the cliff far above the chasm. The path veers far enough away from the tear in the earth that nothing within view alerts you to it. To get a look down into the chasm you must leave the trail and tread carefully over uneven sheets of granite. Surprisingly, there is nothing between the woods and the chasm's void—no wall, handrail, or rope, just an understated warning sign or two. Hikers are allowed to get as close to the edge as their nerves allow.

Follow Charlie's Loop as it heads south to deliver you back to the far end of the quarter-mile-long chasm. At this broad intersection (you will recognize from passing through earlier), turn right to pick up the Forest Road Trail, which is marked with blue. Continuing uphill, stay on this trail when it bears right upon meeting another trail, which heads left to Purgatory Brook.

Traveling northward now, the trail persists up a steep slope for a third of a mile or so. Upon reaching a steel gate continue to the second of two intersections. Leave the Forest Road Trail, taking the trail off to the right. A short distance farther, at another junction, go right again to continue on a narrow trail that weaves through woods over grizzled roots and loosened stones. Follow this

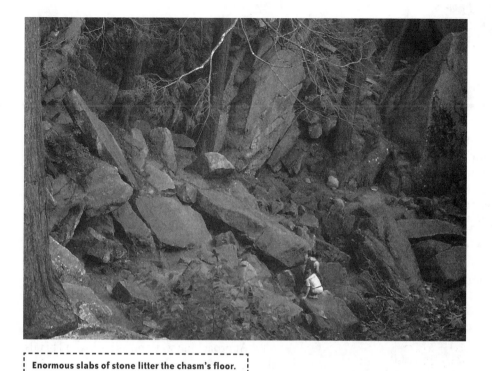

Enormous slabs of stone litter the chasm's floor.

thin ribbon, which parts the trees on its upward trajectory, to reach a two-way split. Here both trails are marked with blue, but take the path to the right also marked "PC" for "Old Purgatory Chasm Trail," and continue hiking eastward. The trail soon curves south and emerges at an open pine grove nearly devoid of underbrush. As the trail winds northward, the woods thicken again and the trail scales a ridge as it approaches a paved road to the left. Just after a park building on the left, you arrive at a parking lot slightly north of the chasm entrance. Walk along the wide shoulder of Purgatory Road to return to your starting point.

58 MOUNT PISGAH HIKE

KEY AT-A-GLANCE INFORMATION

LENGTH: 4.75 miles

CONFIGURATION: Double loop

DIFFICULTY: Moderate

SCENERY: Hardwood forest on abandoned farmland, two gorges, and two scenic vistas; Boston's skyline visible on clear days

EXPOSURE: Mostly shade

TRAFFIC: Light

TRAIL SURFACE: Packed earth with some rocky areas

HIKING TIME: 3 hours

SEASON: Year-round sunrise–sunset

ACCESS: Free

MAPS: Available online at www.town.northborough.ma.us/ntrails/index.htm

FACILITIES: None

SPECIAL COMMENTS: Fishers, a fierce relative of the weasel, are frequently seen on the trails. These chocolate-brown, nimble animals are quick on their feet and can weigh up to 30 pounds.

WHEELCHAIR TRAVERSABLE: No

DRIVING DISTANCE FROM BOSTON COMMON: 39 miles

Mount Pisgah Hike

UTM Zone (WGS84) 19T

Easting: 280028

Northing: 4693158

Latitude: N 42° 21' 35"

Longitude: W 71° 40' 16"

IN BRIEF

Located in one of the state's more rural areas, this hike travels through a landscape that though once tamed by axes and ploughs, has the feel of unfettered wilderness.

DESCRIPTION

Begin by setting out from the parking lot on the Mentzer Trail. Aiming straight toward the summit, this broad trail ascends nearly imperceptibly through woods regrown on land laid bare for pastureland. A stone wall, proof of the hill's former life, runs parallel 20 feet or so to the right.

Approaching wetland as it dips and bends to the northeast, the route crosses Howard Brook. High-bush blueberry, swamp azalea, sweet pepper bush, arrowwood, pungent skunk cabbage, and rare swamp oak grow here, supporting game such as fierce fisher cats, coyotes, bobcats, and black bear.

At a split just ahead, bear right on the Sparrow Trail which is marked with red blazes,

---

Directions ⟶

From Boston take Interstate 90 west to Exit 11A and merge onto I-495 north toward Marlborough. After 8.1 miles take Exit 25B to merge onto I-290 west toward Worcester. Drive 2.5 miles to Exit 25A toward Hudson Street. Turn right onto Solomon Pond Road, drive 0.3 miles, then head right onto Bearfoot Road. Go 0.9 miles, turn left onto Whitney Street, make a sharp right onto Washburn Street, and turn left to stay on Washburn. Continue straight to reach Mohawk Drive, turn left onto Howard Street, make a sharp right onto Green Street, and continue to the top of Ball Hill. Turn right onto Smith Road. A sign on the right designates a parking area for the trails.

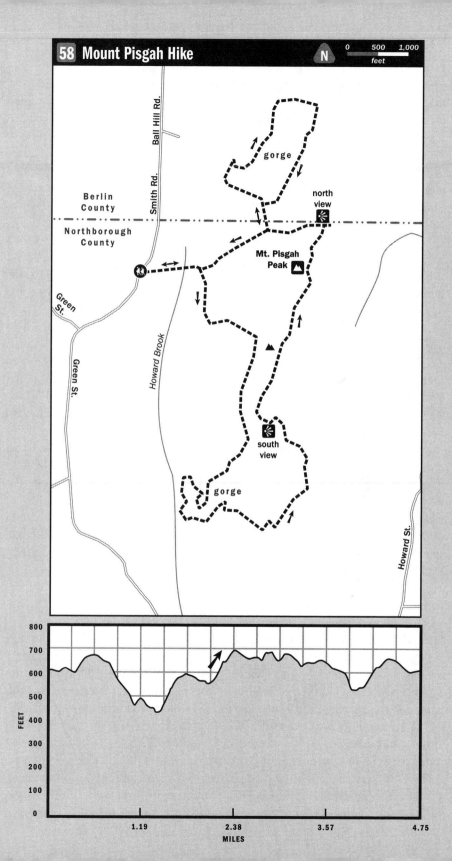

then continue south along the base of the hill. Narrower, with easy dips and rises, this section of trail serves as a warm-up as it winds through a wood distinguished by pine, oak, birch, beech, and most notably, thriving sugar maples.

Shortly after winding eastward, the Sparrow Trail meets the Berlin Road Trail. Turn right here to head south again, this time following blue blazes. Here, in late summer, you might catch the lemony smell of witch hazel (*Hamamelis virginiana*) wafting on the air. With a smell as tantalizing as lemon meringue pie, it's no wonder cottontail rabbits, white-tailed deer, ring-necked pheasants, beavers, and even burly black bears hanker after its fruit.

Coasting downhill on an easy grade, the Berlin Road Trail soon enters a wildlife-management area. Here the trail arches eastward, passing a kiosk and the start of the Howard Ridge Trail, identified by yellow markers. Leave the Berlin Road Trail at this junction and continue southeast along the rocky spine of an esker, the left side of which falls precipitously into a deep ravine.

A short distance ahead, the trail meets the Howard Brook Trail, which diverges to the right. Follow the blue markers of this new trail to descend the esker's western slope. A few feet farther, at another split, continue to the left and hike downhill on what is quickly revealed to be a particularly whimsical route. Winding among multitrunk ash, birch, and hemlock up and over glacial debris, the trail eventually leads to Howard Brook and then reunites with the Howard Ridge Trail. Here the Green Street Trail, marked with red, departs to the right.

From this intersection hike east, following the yellow arrows of the Howard Ridge Trail a few yards to find the South Gorge Trail, marked with red. Turn right here to leave the ridge and head for the dramatic gorge beside the esker. Near the start of the trail sits a wooden footbridge looking like a barge on a sandbar. Once past the bridge, the trail bends sharply northeast and climbs out of the gorge along its far banking. Almost sheer rock through and through, this slope has a forbidding feel. Nothing but hemlock, which somehow get their nutrients from the stone ledges, grows here.

Looping to the right at a twisted oak high above the gorge, the trail divides at an intersection. Add the South Ridge Loop to your hike by continuing southwest, or stay enroute with the South Gorge Trail, heading south.

After the split, the South Gorge Trail settles on level ground and enters benign woods of beech and pine. Moody hemlocks are scarce here, where rocks are buried deep under humus. Winding left and to the east, the trail reaches another junction. The Vernal Pool Trail forks off in two directions from this spot, and the South Gorge Trail veers to the right to feed into the Fisher Trail.

Getting under way, the Fisher Trail jogs to the left to make a near-straight run north. Except for minor bumps and dips, the trail stays level and dry, crossing through sunlit groves of young birch, beech, and sometimes hemlock. Someone with a keen eye might even single out American chestnuts sprouting here. Plagued by blight caused by a fungus of Asian origin, *Cryphonectria parasitica*, the American horse chestnut has essentially been wiped out as a commercial

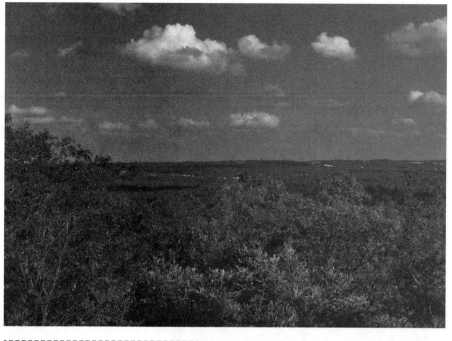

The view from the peak of Mount Pisgah

species since 1926, when its entire range was deemed infected. However, the blight affects only the aboveground parts of the tree. Living root systems of ancient trees long since "dead" regenerate to produce sprouts that grow into promising saplings. Sadly though, *Cryphonectria parasitica* rages on, invading the young trees through weak patches of bark.

Leaving a decrepit stone wall behind, the trail curves northwest and arrives at a stack of stones with a trail marker. Look for the red triangles of the Fisher Trail and make a quick turn to head up a steep slope. Winding over packed earth, the trail soon reaches a grassy plateau.

From this peak, pick up the Tyler Trail, heading northwest away from The Sparrow Trail (also marked with red). A half mile along, when these two trails intersect, continue on along the Tyler Trail. The hiking is easy along the top of this timeworn hill, but when the blueberry bushes are full of ripe fruit late in the summer, there's no need to hurry.

Ahead the land slopes gently, like the dip in a horse's back between the rump and the withers. Tracing the contour, the Tyler Trail edges higher and soon reaches Mount Pisgah's highest point. No doubt more impressive back in farming days, when the peak at 715 feet was cleared of trees, the point nonetheless maintains the distinction of being the highest elevation in Northborough.

Continuing north beyond the summit, the Tyler Trail rubs shoulders with remnant stone walls as it tapers downhill to meet the top end of the Mentzer

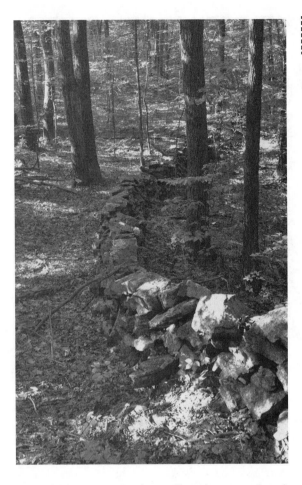

A graceful stone wall winds through reforested pastureland.

Trail. Before following the yellow markers of this trail west, take a few more steps to the east for a view from Mount Pisgah's northernmost point. From the northern lookout return to the Mentzer Trail and follow its rocky course to a nearby intersection with the Berlin Road Trail.

The parking lot lies less than 0.5 miles ahead on the Mentzer Trail, so if the sun is low, hike on through. But if the sun is high and the weather fine, veer right onto the rutted cart road running northwest to the Northborough–Berlin border.

A short distance ahead, the road reaches a stone wall lying along the town line. A gap in the wall makes way for the road as it continues northwest, passing a trail to the right and a sign posted by the Berlin Conservation Commission.

Once you are in Berlin, the Berlin Road Trail narrows and looks more like a footpath than a cart road. Although its course remains clear, trail markers are few and far between. Making its way through pinewoods, the path soon swings abruptly to the right, zigzagging around two mammoth pines. A few yards farther along, the path passes a house on the left that, though well concealed by trees, startles nonetheless.

Beyond the house, the trail reaches a junction. One route, marked with yellow, continues along a stone wall; the other cuts to the right to head east. Choose the latter, following it downhill to where it meets the North Gorge Trail, splitting to the right at a tree decorated with three markers—two yellow and one white.

Rough, wild, and haunting, the view within the gorge is the most beautiful of the hike. Pale yellow blazes, difficult to see in fading light, mark the route as it

Hikers and horses share the trail.

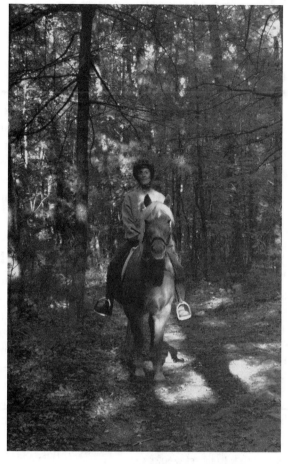

weaves south along a rocky ridge above a brook and broad floodplain. Toward the southernmost end of the gorge, the trail descends to the brook and a chaotic convergence of stone walls. From this deep cleft in the land, the trail bends westward as it climbs free of the shadowy recesses. Reaching level ground, the trail arrives back at the Northborough–Berlin border.

From here, bear left to return to where the Mentzer Trail bisects the Berlin Road Trail. At the junction, follow yellow markers southwest down an easy grade through woods that transition from pine to red oak. White pine is known to grab a foothold soon after farmland is abandoned. By the early 1900s, mature "old field" pine stands, like the one to the right of the trail, were harvested for "boxboard," the precursor to corrugated cardboard. Once the pines were thinned, fast-growing red oak took over, as it did in the woods to the left. As time passes and the woods mature, other shade-tolerant species will supplant the red oak, and the forest will look strikingly different. On the last stretch of trail, wild grape climbs in great tangles on any and all available branches. In the end of summer the air is sweet with the smell of their succulent fruit.

59 MOUNT WATATIC– NUTTING HILL LOOP

KEY AT-A-GLANCE INFORMATION

LENGTH: 3.5 miles

CONFIGURATION: Loop

DIFFICULTY: Easy to moderate

SCENERY: Woods of hemlock, birch, and beech, with a magnificent view from the bald peak of Mount Watatic

EXPOSURE: Mostly shaded

TRAFFIC: Light to heavy, depending on the season and day of the week

TRAIL SURFACE: Packed earth and a great deal of granite in the form of gravel, glacial erratics, or exposed sheets

HIKING TIME: 2 hours

SEASON: Year-round sunrise–sunset

ACCESS: Free

MAPS: Available through Friends of Wapack at www.wapack.org

FACILITIES: None

SPECIAL COMMENTS: The peak of Mount Watatic is a fabulous place to watch hawks migrate from September through the first weeks of November. On average, 7,700 fly over Mount Watatic in a given season. Because of the odd break-in, hikers are advised to not leave valuables in their cars.

WHEELCHAIR TRAVERSABLE: No

DRIVING DISTANCE FROM BOSTON COMMON: 54 miles

IN BRIEF

Providing a hiking experience like that offered by New Hampshire's White Mountains, this hike makes a strenuous ascent to the peak of Mount Watatic. Continuing northward to scale the lesser peak of Nutting Hill, the route swings west on reaching the Massachusetts–New Hampshire border then eases back to the start.

DESCRIPTION

A list-topper among destinations favored by Boston's hiking crowd, Mount Watatic offers not only an exhilarating get-away-from-it-all day hike, but also the chance of doing as Henry David Thoreau urged. Get your affairs in order and, once so freed, set out indefinitely—for it is a portal to two epic routes, the Midstate and the Wapack trails.

From its starting point on the edge of Rhode Island, Midstate Trail travels north 95 miles, clear across Massachusetts, to its end at Nutting Hill on the New Hampshire border. At 21 miles long, Wapack Trail is comparatively modest in length but equally inspired and worthy. Like most good ideas, the Wapack Trail originated in the mind of one but took shape and became real with the help of a small group of like-minded people

---

Mount Watatic– Nutting Hill Loop

UTM Zone (WGS84) 19T

Easting: 262087

Northing: 4731246

Latitude: N 42° 41' 49"

Longitude: W 71° 54' 16"

Directions ⟶

From Boston, take MA 2 west 34.1 miles to MA 31, then take MA 31 north 2.4 miles to MA 12. Drive 5.6 miles on MA 12 to Ashburnham, turn right onto MA 101, and continue to the intersection with MA 119. Turn left onto MA 119 west. The difficult-to-spot parking lot is 1.5 miles ahead on the right.

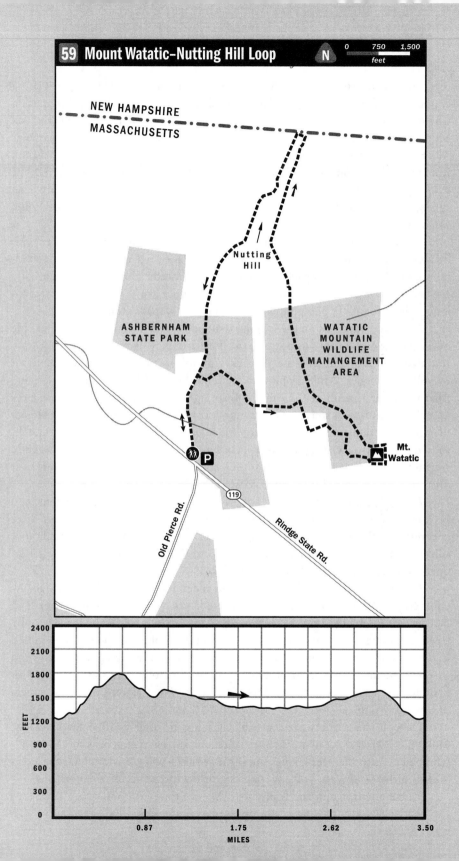

59 Mount Watatic–Nutting Hill Loop

N

0   750   1,500
feet

NEW HAMPSHIRE
MASSACHUSETTS

Nutting
Hill

ASHBERNHAM
STATE PARK

WATATIC
MOUNTAIN
WILDLIFE
MANANGEMENT
AREA

Mt.
Watatic

119

Old Pierce Rd.

Rindge State Rd.

2400
2100
1800
1500
1200
900
600
300
0

FEET

0.87   1.75   2.62   3.50
MILES

ready to roll up their sleeves. And so, in the summer of 1922, while writing his book *The Annals of Grand Monadnock* in Jaffrey, New Hampshire, Allen Chamberlain dreamt of a trail that would connect New Hampshire's North Pack Monadnock to Massachusetts's Mount Watatic. A friend, the local factory owner Albert Annett, disseminated the notion to two key agents—local farmer Frank Robbins and his companion Marion Buck, a champion lumberjack. Incredibly, by early December of the same year, the Wapack Trail was fully cleared. In spring, it was ready for the hikers and cross-country skiers, who, in short time, came in droves.

It was Marion Buck, the lumberjack, sheepherder, and mold breaker who by blending the "Wa" from Watatic with the "Pack" from North Pack Monadnock coined the name Wapack. Immediately embraced by all, Wapack eventually replaced the original name for the mountain range traversed by the trail. No longer the "Boundary Mountains," it become the Wapack Range.

This hike starts out on the logging road behind the metal gate at the far side of the parking lot. From this point to the border of New Hampshire, the recently rerouted Midstate Trail and the Wapack Trail follow the same course, identified by yellow triangles. After dipping to wetland dammed by beavers, the logging road reaches a turnoff at 0.23 miles. Bear right here and continue uphill over an obstacle course of tree roots to a map kiosk that, because the map is almost illegible, functions more as a benchmark than an information source (though, subsequent to this writing, the map may have been replaced). After this gentle warm-up and adjustments to clothing or backpack straps, follow the trail as it drops to cross a stream then climbs eastward under hemlocks.

As it progresses up the side of Mount Watatic, the trail broadens and becomes rocky, with lengths seemingly paved with loose cobblestones. After becoming markedly steeper and exposed, the trail bends to a gentler pitch and, slinking back under hemlock cover, emerges at an outcropping the size of an opera box, with a view of Mount Monadnock.

Beyond the lookout, the trail rises to meet a stone wall along a ridge. As counterintuitive as it may seem today, these lands were indeed once farmed. In fact, when Thoreau visited the area in 1852, the rolling landscape was virtually treeless. Though only madmen would try to take a plow to the granite-riddled higher elevations, more than a few reasonable men and women grazed cattle and sheep in the mountains. Marion Buck was one. She told more than one story of helping run sheep herds from Massachusetts to New Hampshire in summers during her youth.

Once at this stone wall, the trail levels off to offer another terrific view, looking out over what was likely pasture but is now a sparse wood of wind-whipped oaks. A few feet farther on, if the weather obliges, Mount Wachusett is visible in the southwest. Soft, overlapping peaks spread across the horizon.

Turning east again, the trail cuts over the stone wall and heads back into the hemlock wood, passing a swampy grove thick with vivid green ferns. On

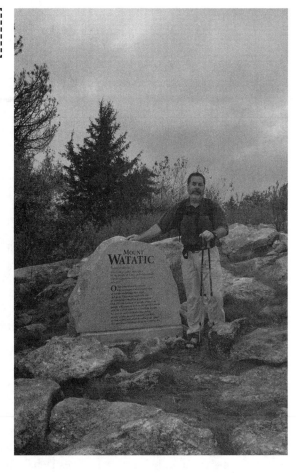

the upland to the left, maple saplings mix with young effervescent pines, and ahead, a boggy glade provides a surprise respite. Continuing southeast, the trail makes a stumbling ascent over granite chunks to the remains of a shelter crumbled amid hemlocks.

Climb from this plateau up one more thigh-testing slope to reach the top. The almost entirely bald 1,832-foot peak provides a stunning panoramic view of all points, including Boston. Since a fire tower was removed in 1997, and the rope tows of the ski areas that once operated on the western side of the mountain were dismantled, the monadnock has been free of man-made obstructions. And as of 1:30 p.m., July 10, 2002—thanks to a Herculean effort by the State of Massachusetts Department of Environmental Management and Division of Fisheries and Wildlife, the Ashby Land Trust, and the Ashburnham Conservation Trust—the mountain is forever protected from development.

From the meadowlike peak, take the partially constructed gravel road north several yards to a narrow path running off to the left. Starting downhill, this trail joins a stone wall as it fixes on a northwest trajectory. Forming a "U" like the humps of a camel, the trail links the peak of Watatic to the knob of Nutting Hill. If hiking in the well-chosen month of July, plan to picnic here on the hill's sun-stroked flanks of granite; abundant blueberries will be your dessert.

Here and there, minor, or "social," paths feed in from the edges but continue over the contours of Nutting Hill, following yellow triangles. Ahead at the intersection, heed the arrows pointing to the right, toward New Hampshire. Cut wide to accommodate cross-country skiers. This grassy, comparatively rock-free section eases downhill a short way then nearly levels as it projects northeast.

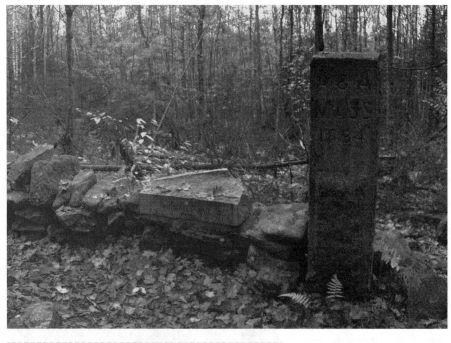

Stone markers on the Massachusetts–New Hampshire border

Stone walls on either side pencil in this well-traveled road. Farther on to the left, it passes the foundation of what might have been a shepherd's shelter. Farther still, the trail passes a T-junction, where a path marked with white enters to the right through a gap in a stone wall. Continue past each of these distractions—the next being "Dave Loves Deb," carved into the mouse-gray side of one of many beech trees standing along the edges—to a junction at the New Hampshire border.

This is the jumping-off site, where those who have their affairs in order, as well as water, some trail mix, and a headlamp with fresh batteries, may decide to toss fate to the wind and head for New Ipswich, Pack Monadnock, and beyond. Sprightly arrows pointing straight ahead to a road-wide path make such wanderlust hard to resist.

However, if your plan was to stay with the plan, bear left to hike northwest. A trail marked "Midstate Express" barrels in from the left and right, conveying hikers to the start or the finish of their cross-state trek. A hundred yards or so ahead, flush to a stone wall, the trail leads to two granite blocks, one engraved "ANA Mass 1894," and the other "The Midstate Trail 1985."

To finish the circuit back to the parking lot, bear away from the stone wall and hike southwest under hemlocks that shut out daylight like lashes blinking over an eye. Swatches of varying shades of blue blaze this spindly trail as it meanders like a nosy goat along the gentle slope of the Nutting Hill. At the next junction double

This marker can be found beneath leaves near the Midstate Trail.

blue arrows point right, to MA 119, and the parking lot 0.79 miles away. Pick up this rugged logging trail— the very one on which the hike began—and follow it south to the start.

NEARBY ATTRACTIONS

The pioneers of the Wapack Trail, Marion Buck and Frank Robbins, operated a popular ski lodge in New Ipswich, New Hampshire, from 1924 to 1958. Following their lead, Al Jenks, a Wapack Trail devotee, started his own ski center in 1972. Called "Windblown," the center is 10 miles up the road (NH 123A) from the Wapack trailhead off MA 119 in

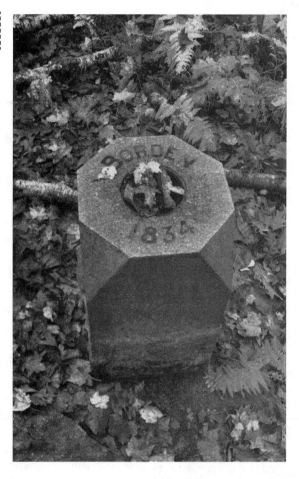

Ashburnham. Windblown has 25 miles of trails and offers rental equipment, a lodge, hearty food, and even rustic lodging. The telephone number is (603) 878-2869, and the owners request you call only between 7 a.m. and 9 p.m.

60 MOUNT WACHUSETT LOOP

KEY AT-A-GLANCE INFORMATION

LENGTH: 5.74 miles

CONFIGURATION: Loop

DIFFICULTY: Mostly moderate with some easy and some difficult sections

SCENERY: This hike loops around Mount Wachusett, at 2,006 feet, Massachusetts's highest peak. The top offers a spectacular view of the Berkshires to the west, Mount Monadnock to the north, and Boston's skyline to the east.

EXPOSURE: Mostly shaded

TRAFFIC: Moderate

TRAIL SURFACE: Packed earth

HIKING TIME: 3.5 hours

SEASON: Year-round without restrictions

ACCESS: Free

MAPS: Available at www.mass.gov/dcr/parks/central/wach.htm

FACILITIES: Picnic tables

WHEELCHAIR TRAVERSABLE: The trails in this hike are not wheelchair traversable; however, the peak is made accessible by a paved service road.

DISTANCE FROM BOSTON COMMON: 59 miles

IN BRIEF

This hike loops around Mount Wachusett, eventually climbing its northeastern face to reach a spectacular view from the peak.

DESCRIPTION

Refusing defeat in his war against the English settlers in 1675, Wampanoag leader King Philip and his army of allied tribes—composed of men, women, and children—retreated from the coast and headed to Mount Wachusett. Though he had won the support of the Narragansett and Pocumtuc tribes, Philip was faced with the tragic reality of having no food to feed his fighters.

So it was that on Thursday, February 10, a group of Nipmunk and Narragansett Indians set on the small town of Lancaster, Massachusetts, looking for supplies. Ironically the town's minister, Joseph Rowlandson, was away in Boston, where he was pleading for his government's protection. Thirty-seven people, along with Reverend Rowlandson's wife, Mary, and their three children, crowded into the Rowlandson's heavily fortified house hoping to fend off assault. The settlers huddled close, bracing themselves as the Indians attacked with gunfire. But when flames engulfed the house, the settlers burst from cover into a hail of bullets.

Mount Wachusett Loop
UTM Zone (WGS84) 19T
Northing: 4709764
Easting: 262728
Latitude: N 42° 30' 19"
Longitude: W 71° 53' 04"

Directions

From Boston, take MA 2 to Exit 25 (MA 140 south). Follow MA 140 south 2 miles. Turn right onto Mile Hill Road. Follow Mile Hill Road 0.5 miles to the split in the road. Bear left at fork onto Mountain Road. Follow Mountain Road 1.25 miles to the top of the hill. The reservation entrance is on the right. The Mount Wachusett visitor center entrance is immediately on the left once you enter the reservation.

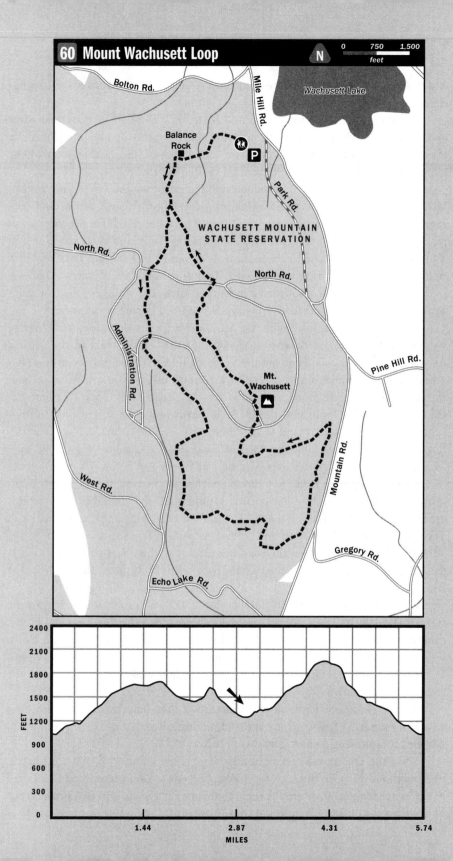

Many were killed instantly; others including Mary and the Rowlandson's children, were taken captive.

For three months, King Philip and his people traveled in search of cover and sustenance taking their hostages with them. Not staying any one place long they traveled north to New Hampshire and Vermont and farther west to the Connecticut River, all the while pursued by English troops.

In spring King Philip led his people and their captives back to Mount Wachusett. Through scouts Reverend Rowlandson learned of his wife's status and courageously arranged negotiations with Philip to have her freed. Finally the parties reached an agreement that on May 2, 1676, King Philip and the English met at a location thereafter called Redemption Rock, and for a ransom of 20 English pounds, Mary Rowlandson was released. Two of her children, whom she had not seen since the raid, were also freed a short time later. The youngest, the Rowlandson's six-year-old daughter, died of wounds sustained during her capture.

From the parking lot beside the Mount Wachusett ski lodge, walk northwest to find the start of Balance Rock Trail located to the right of the ski lift. As you step into the woods on a quiet morning in April, with no one around but a handful of workmen and a couple of mountain bikers, you are likely to hear the sound of loon calls from the lake across the parking lot. A few feet onto the trail, thanks to the loons and the shade of hardwoods, the stilted resort atmosphere vanishes. Two diamond-shaped markers—one blue, one yellow—identify the trail as two routes, blue for Balance Rock Trail and yellow for the 92-mile Midstate Trail which passes over Mount Wachusett.

Rising steeply at first, the broad, packed-earth trail winds as it climbs under hemlock bows. Mountain laurels punctuate the underbrush in wetter areas. About 0.25 miles on, the trail is interrupted by a sandy, unpaved road. Turn right at this intersection and follow the road a few yards to a sign on the left for Balance Rock. Leave the road here and take this short path for a look at this geological spectacle. A glacier's handiwork, this sculpture outdoes any artist from da Vinci to di Suvero.

Loop back to the road on Balance Rock Trail and look south to find the start of Old Indian Trail. Worn from the passage of many moccasins and boots, this trail ascends steeply over roots and rocks 1.3 miles to the summit. For a less direct route, switch off to Semuhenna Trail when the two trails meet at a V. Here Old Indian Trail continues straight while Semuhenna Trail runs to the right, heading southwest.

At this elevation the wind whistles through the bare treetops. In autumn, scores of migrating hawks wing overhead, taking advantage of these strong wind currents as admiring birders gawk from below.

Soon the trail passes between a gap in an old stone wall that runs seemingly without purpose through the trees. The cows it once confined in cleared pastures are long gone, as are the region's farms. But the springs that greened the herd's forage still flow, even in the driest of Aprils.

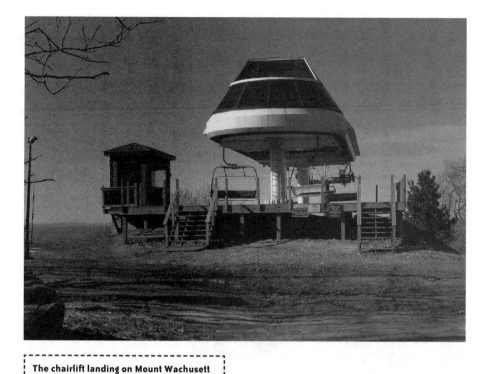

The chairlift landing on Mount Wachusett

After making its way south through the shelter of hemlocks, the trail reaches the mountain's auto route. Follow the painted footsteps across to stay with Semuhenna Trail. From here, the level trail passes through a stand of young beeches. A series of small bridges offer dry footing as the path climbs just short of the peak. Coming into the open, Semuhenna Trail passes a group of picnic tables and signs for other trails. Having approached the mountain's highest point, Semuhenna Trail crosses a paved road then ducks off to the southeast.

Ringing the mountain at a constant elevation just shy of the peak, Semuhenna Trail turns eastward. Dark flanks of granite make a wall to the left, moss-covered fallen trees and displaced boulders lie to the right on the downhill slope.

When the trail arrives at an intersection, leave Semuhenna Trail and turn right onto Harrington Trail, heading west. A short way along this route, you will come to another junction. Turn left to proceed on Lower Link Trail. Hiking south now, on flat ground, you next arrive at Jack Frost Trail. Picking up this new path, follow it left to travel eastward. Narrower than the previous routes, Jack Frost Trail winds uphill past laurels growing beside rivulets diverting from a brook. A series of wooden bridges guarantee dry crossing through this mud zone.

From a wet plateau, Jack Frost Trail takes you on a climb up a pocked and grizzled slope. Emerging from this trail, you find yourself at another crossroads. Turn right here to hike downhill on High Meadows Trail. As its name suggests, this route takes you southwest across land previously used for grazing cattle that

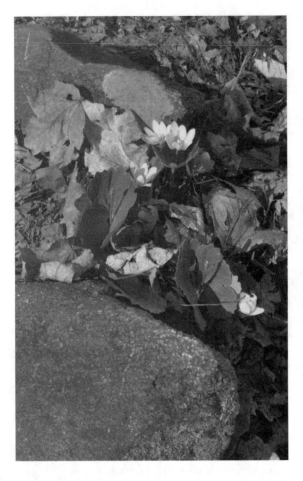

must have been lean, well-muscled beasts, judging from the thin layer of sod stretched over the granite substrate.

Winding over the curve of the hill, the trail leads to two plateaus edged by stone walls. Leaning as if in a stop-action fall, ancient oaks spread shade over each other. Cows with knees aching from grazing on an incline spent many hours chewing their cud under their branches.

Farther on, you arrive at a junction where High Meadow Trail meets Bicentennial Trail. Change course here, turning left to take Bicentennial Trail northeast. Continue downhill, picking your way along the rough path past the occasional wizened oak and younger black cherry trees. If you are hiking through in April or May, you may be lucky enough to see bloodroot (*Sanguinaria canadensis*) blooming. This elegant, small white flower with 8–16 petals and bright yellow stamens is rare and prized for its medicinal properties. Indians used the rich red "blood" of its roots as a potent antibiotic, antimicrobial agent. Today the plant is used commercially in toothpaste and in the treatment of cancer. The FDA however, has classified bloodroot as an unsafe herb.

As the slope of the mountain eases to flat, you will hear cars motoring by on a road a short distance to the right. After traveling along level ground for a spell, Bicentennial Trail reaches an intersection with Mountain House Trail. Continue on to the next junction to find Loop Trail. Take this turn to double back, heading southwest. Instead of walking, you will now find yourself straining uphill to scale boulder after lichen-mottled boulder, peering warily into the many caves you pass.

This rigorous stretch works your every sinew before finally letting up upon your arrival at a junction with Mountain House Trail. Turn right here to leave the rocks behind and take a direct shot at the peak, heading northwest. Stay with this path as it converges with the Jack Frost, Midstate, and Link trails.

Emerging from thinning woods, the trail crosses a paved road then makes one last run northward to reach the mountain's top. Wide-open and bare, Mount Wachusett's peak provides a fantastic view of seemingly all of Massachusetts and the southern edge of New Hampshire. It is for this reason perhaps, that King Philip sought refuge for his people here.

After scaling the lookout tower and having a sandwich or several handfuls of trail mix, cross to the northwestern side of the peak to find a marker directing you to Old Indian Trail. Following this gentle path through the woods, you soon come to a ski lift, which in all seasons—but especially spring—resembles George Jetson's spaceship.

From here, trace Old Indian Trail's crooked trajectory downhill to where it crosses the auto route. Hike left, looking for painted footsteps, and resume the trail on the other side of the pavement. Continuing on, the trail leads through woods and three times crosses ski slopes before meeting Semuhenna Trail and Balance Rock Road. Walk a few yards downhill on the sandy road to find Balance Rock Trail on the left. Having returned to the first trail of the hike, follow it back to the parking lot.

Note: Mount Wachusett offers superb hawk watching from September through November, with 12,000 hawks sighted per season over the last 24 years. Autumn is a wonderful time to hike Mount Wachusett, but if you are planning to venture into the woods between mid-October and mid-December, play it safe and wear bright colors, preferably orange, and avoid wearing white or brown. For a precise hunting schedule for Massachusetts, visit **www.mass.gov/dfwele/ dfw/dfwpdf/dfw_hunting_dates.pdf.**

NEARBY ATTRACTIONS

Those spending a weekend in the area might consider visiting the nearby Wachusett Meadow Wildlife Sanctuary located at 113 Goodnow Road, Princeton. Managed by the Massachusetts Audubon Society, the sanctuary offers 12 miles of trails and an abundance of wildlife in addition to a wheelchair-accessible nature center. Admission is $4 for nonmember adults and $3 for nonmember children ages 3 to 12 and senior citizens. For more information, call (978) 464-2712.

APPENDIXES
AND INDEX

APPENDIX A:
RECOMMENDED READING

Boston: A Topographical History, by Walter Muir Whitehill, The Belknap Press of Harvard University, 1959.

Boston's Gold Coast: The North Shore 1890–1929, by Joseph E. Garland, Little Brown & Co., 1981.

The Complete Guide to Boston's Freedom Trail, 3rd ed., by Charles Bahne, Newtowne Publishing, 2005.

Inventing the Charles River, by Karl Haglund, MIT Press, 2002.

Judge Sewall's Apology: The Salem Witch Trials & the Forming of an American Conscience, by Richard Francis for Fourth Estate, HarperCollins, 2005.

Narrative of the Captivity and Restoration of Mrs. Mary Rowlandson, by Rowlandson. Available for downloading at Project Gutenberg, **www.gutenberg.org/etext/851.**

Of Plymouth Plantation, by William Bradford, Dover Publications, 2006.

Plum Island: The Way It Was, 2nd ed., by Nancy V. Weare, Newburyport Press, Inc., 1996.

The Saga of Cape Ann, by Melvin T. Copeland and Elliott C. Rogers, Bond Wheelwright Co., 1960.

The Town on Sandy Bay: A History of Rockport, Massachusetts, by Marshall W. S. Swan. Published for the Canaan, NH, Town History Committee by Phoenix Pub., 1980.

Winthrop's Journal: History of New England 1630–1649, Elibron Classics Adamant Media Corporation, 2005.

APPENDIX B:
OUTDOOR SHOPS

Hilton's Tent City
272 Friend Street
Boston, MA 02114
(617) 227-9242; toll-free, (800) 362-8368
E-mail: htc@hiltonstentcity.com
Store hours: Mon.–Fri., 9 a.m.–9 p.m.;
Sat., 9 a.m.–6 p.m.; Sun., noon–6 p.m.
www.hiltonstentcity.com

Joe Jones Wilderness House
1048 Commonwealth Avenue
Boston, MA 02215
Phone: (617) 277-5858
Store hours: Mon.–Fri., 10 a.m.–9 p.m.;
Sat., 10 a.m.–7 p.m.; Sun., noon–6 p.m.
www.joejonessports.com

Maynard Outdoor Store
24 Nason Street
Maynard, MA 01754
(978) 897-2133
Store hours: Mon.–Wed., Sat., 9 a.m.–
6 p.m.; Thurs.–Fri., 9 a.m.–9 p.m.;
Sun., noon–5 p.m.

Moor & Mountain
3 Railroad Street
Andover, MA 01810
Store hours: Mon., Tues., Wed., Sat.,
9 a.m.–5 p.m.;
Thurs., Fri., 9 a.m.–8 p.m.; closed Sundays
(978) 475-3665
www.moor-mountain.com

Natick Outdoor Store
38 North Avenue
Natick, MA 01760
(508) 653-9400
www.natickoutdoor.com

Store hours: Mon.–Wed., Sat., 9 a.m.–
6 p.m.; Thurs.–Fri., 9 a.m.–9 p.m.;
Sun., noon–5 p.m.

New England Backpacker
6 East Mountain Street
Worchester, MA 01606
(508) 853-9407
www.newenglandbackpacker.com
Store hours: Mon.–Tues., 10 a.m.–6 p.m.;
Wed.–Fri., 10 a.m.–8 p.m.; Sat., 10 a.m.–
5 p.m.; Sun., noon–5 p.m.

Eastern Mountain Sports
www.ems.com
(multiple locations)
Boston
855 Boylston Street
Boston, MA 02116
(617) 236-1518
Store hours: Mon.–Sat., 10 a.m.–8 p.m.;
Sun., noon–6 p.m.

Boston
1041 and 1045 Commonwealth Avenue
Boston, MA 02215
(617) 254-4250
Store hours: Mon.–Sat., 10 a.m.–9 p.m.;
Sun., noon–6 p.m.
www.ems.com

Cambridge
Harvard Square
1 Brattle Square, Second Floor
Cambridge, MA 02138
(617) 864-2061
Store hours: Mon.–Thurs.,10 a.m.–8 p.m.;
Fri.–Sat., 10 a.m.–9 p.m.;
Sun., 11 a.m.–6 p.m.

Hingham
Anchor Plaza
211 Lincoln Street
Hingham, MA 02043
(781) 741-8808
Store hours: Mon.–Fri., 9:30 a.m.–9 p.m.;
Sat., 9:30 a.m.–6 p.m.; Sun., 11 a.m.–6 p.m.

Newton
300 Needham Street
Unit #1
Newton, MA 02464
Phone: (617) 559-1575
Store hours: Mon.–Fri., 10 a.m.–9 p.m.,
Sat., 9 a.m.–9 p.m.; Sun., 11 a.m.–6 p.m.

Peabody
Northshore Mall, Routes 128 and 114
Peabody, MA 01960
(978) 977-0601
Store hours: Mon.–Sat., 10 a.m.–10 p.m.;
Sun., 11 a.m.–6 p.m.

REI, www.rei.com
(multiple locations)
Boston
401 Park Drive
Boston, MA 02215
(617) 236-0746
Store hours: Mon.–Sat., 10 a.m.–9 p.m.;
Sun., 11 a.m.–6 p.m.

Framingham
375 Cochituate Road
Framingham, MA 01701
(508) 270-6325
Store hours: Mon.–Sat., 10 a.m.–9 p.m.;
Sun., 11 a.m.–6 p.m.

Hingham
98 Derby Street
Suite 470
Hingham, MA 02043
Phone: (781) 740-9430
Store hours: Mon.–Sat., 10 a.m.–9 p.m.;
Sun., 11 a.m.-6 p.m.

Reading
279 Salem Street (exit 40 off Route 128)
Reading, MA 01867
Phone: (781) 944-5103
Store hours: Mon.–Fri., 10 a.m.–9 p.m.;
Sat., 10 a.m.–8 p.m.; Sun., 11 a.m.–6 p.m.

APPENDIX C:
CONSERVATION ORGANIZATIONS

Appalachian Mountain Club
AMC Main Office
5 Joy Street
Boston, MA 02108
(617) 523-0655; fax: (617) 523-0722
www.outdoors.org

Audubon Society
Massachusetts Audubon Society
208 South Great Road
Lincoln, MA 01773
781-259-9500 or (800) AUDUBON
www.massaudubon.org

Essex County Greenbelt Association
82 Eastern Avenue
Essex, MA 01929
(978) 768-7241; fax: (978) 768-3286
E-mail: ecga@ecga.org
www.ecga.org

AVIS
(Andover Village Improvement Society)
P.O. Box 5097
Andover, MA 01810
www.avisandover.org

Bay Circuit Trail
For general information
about the Bay Circuit Alliance contact
Alan French, Chairman Bay Circuit Alliance
3 Railroad Street
Andover, MA 01810
(978) 470-1982

Charles River Conservancy
c/o EF Education
EF Center Boston
One Education Street
Cambridge MA 02141
(617) 619-2850; fax: (617) 619-2856
E-mail: crc@thecharles.org;
www.thecharles.org

Dartmouth Natural Resources Trust
Dexter Mead, President
P. O. Box P-17
404 Elm Street
Dartmouth, MA 02748
(508) 991-2289; fax: (508) 991-4044
E-mail: info@dnrt.org;
www.dnrt.org

Friends of Hemlock Gorge
1094 Chestnut Street
Newton Upper Falls, MA 02464
www.hemlockgorge.org

Friends of Lynn Woods
P.O. Box 8216
Lynn, MA 01904
(781) 593-7773
www.flw.org

Manchester-Essex Conservation Trust
Helen Bethell, Executive Director
P.O. Box 1486
11 Jersey Lane
Manchester, MA 01944
(978) 526-7692; fax: (978) 526-1104
E-mail: helen.bethell@verizon.net
www.mect.org

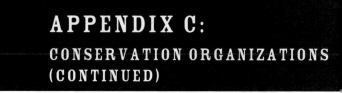

APPENDIX C:

CONSERVATION ORGANIZATIONS (CONTINUED)

Friends of Middlesex Fells
4 Woodland Road
Stoneham, MA 02180
(adjacent to the Spot Pond Visitor Center)
(781) 662-2340
E-mail: friends@fells.org
www.fells.org

Midstate Trail
E-mail: rockypond@charter.net
www.midstatetrail.org

Sudbury Valley Trustees
18 Wolbach Road
Sudbury, MA 01776
(978) 443-5588
E-mail: web@svtweb.org
www.svtweb.org

Trustees of Reservations
572 Essex Street
Beverly, MA 01915-1530
(978) 921-1944; fax: (978) 921-1948
E-mail: information@ttor.org
www.thetrustees.org

Trust for Public Land
New England Regional Office
33 Union Street, 4th Floor
Boston, MA 02108
(617) 367-6200; fax: (617) 367-1616
www.tpl.org

Friends of the Wapack
P.O. Box 115
West Peterborough, NH 03468
E-mail: info@wapack.org
www.wapack.org

Waters Farm Preservation, Inc.
For general information contact Pam
Gurney Farnham
E-mail: warefarnham@aol.com
For information about the annual donkey
and mule show contact Deb Kovac
(508) 765-9573 (after 2 p.m.)
E-mail: debkovac@charter.net
www.watersfarm.com

APPENDIX D:
HIKING CLUBS

Appalachian Mountain Club Main Office
5 Joy Street
Boston, MA 02108
(617) 523-0636; fax: (617) 523-0722

Blue Hills Walking Club
Download information at:
**www.mass.gov/dcr/events/blue hills
walking club.pdf**

Boston Hiking Club
www.bostonhiking.org

Breakheart-Fells Hiking Club
Download information at:
www.mass.gov/dcr/events/breakfells.pdf

Massachusetts Sierra Club
100 Boylston Street
Boston, MA 02116
(617) 423-5775; fax: (617) 890-0338
www.sierraclubmass.org/index.html

INDEX

Page references followed by *m* indicate a map.

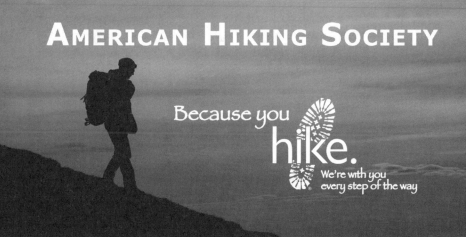
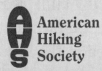

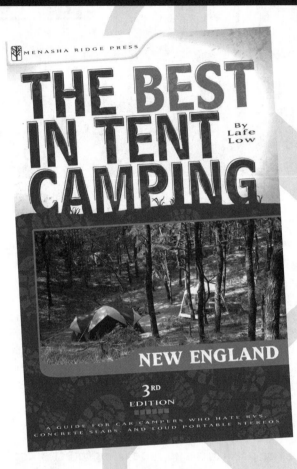

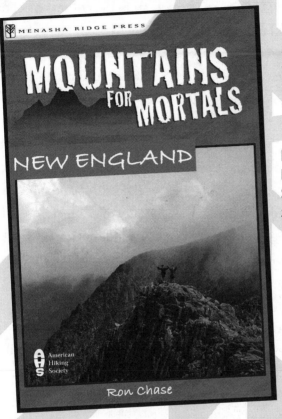

MOUNTAINS FOR MORTALS
New England

by Ron Chase
ISBN 978-0-89732-621-6
$19.95
224 pages

This guide is the quintessential New England hiking book with meticulous directions, comprehensive trail descriptions, detailed maps, precise orienteering data, and exhilarating photos.

Every New England state is represented and many trailheads are just a short distance from major metropolitan areas. Others, such as Camel's Hump in Vermont and Mount Lafayette in New Hampshire, are located in remote, pristine wilderness settings. Each climbing description includes trail conditions, weather advice, lodging and camping options, ideal hiking times, and other pertinent information.

DEAR CUSTOMERS AND FRIENDS,

SUPPORTING YOUR INTEREST IN OUTDOOR ADVENTURE, travel, and an active lifestyle is central to our operations, from the authors we choose to the locations we detail to the way we design our books. Menasha Ridge Press was incorporated in 1982 by a group of veteran outdoorsmen and professional outfitters. For 25 years now, we've specialized in creating books that benefit the outdoors enthusiast.

Almost immediately, Menasha Ridge Press earned a reputation for revolutionizing outdoors- and travel-guidebook publishing. For such activities as canoeing, kayaking, hiking, backpacking, and mountain biking, we established new standards of quality that transformed the whole genre, resulting in outdoor-recreation guides of great sophistication and solid content. Menasha Ridge continues to be outdoor publishing's greatest innovator.

The folks at Menasha Ridge Press are as at home on a white-water river or mountain trail as they are editing a manuscript. The books we build for you are the best they can be, because we're responding to your needs. Plus, we use and depend on them ourselves.

We look forward to seeing you on the river or the trail. If you'd like to contact us directly, join in at www.trekalong.com or visit us at www.menasharidge.com. We thank you for your interest in our books and the natural world around us all.

SAFE TRAVELS,

Bob Sehlinger

BOB SEHLINGER
PUBLISHER